ILLUSTRATED ADVANCED ANTERIOR SEGMENT SURGERY

A STEP-BY-STEP GUIDE FOR CHALLENGING CASES

ILLUSTRATED ADVANCED ANTERIOR SEGMENT SURGERY

A STEP-BY-STEP GUIDE FOR CHALLENGING CASES

Iqbal K. Ahmed, MD
Professor, Department of Ophthalmology and Vision Sciences
University of Utah, Salt Lake City, Utah
Assistant Professor, Department of Ophthalmology and Vision Science
University of Toronto, Toronto, Ontario, Canada
Director of Research, Kensington Eye Institute, Toronto, Ontario, Canada
Head of Ophthalmology, Trillium Health Partners, Ontario, Canada
Medical Director, Prism Eye Institute, Ontario, Canada

Xavier Campos-Möller, MD
Glaucoma and Advanced Anterior Segment Surgery
Assistant Professor, Ophthalmology
Memorial University, St Johns, Newfoundland, Canada
Head of Glaucoma and Advanced Anterior Segment, Department of Ophthalmology
Western Health Memorial Regional Hospital, Corner Brook, Newfoundland, Canada

Manjool Shah, MD
Clinical Assistant Professor, Kellogg Eye Center
Division of Glaucoma, Cataract, and Anterior Segment Disease
University of Michigan, Ann Arbor, Michigan

Arsham Sheybani, MD
Washington University
St. Louis, Missouri

SLACK
INCORPORATED

SLACK
INCORPORATED

SLACK Incorporated
6900 Grove Road
Thorofare, NJ 08086 USA
856-848-1000 Fax: 856-848-6091
www.slackbooks.com

Senior Vice President: Stephanie Arasim Portnoy
Vice President, Editorial: Jennifer Kilpatrick
Vice President, Marketing: Mary Sasso
Acquisitions Editor: Tony Schiavo
Managing Editor: Allegra Tiver/Jennifer Cahill
Vice President/Creative Director: Thomas Cavallaro
Cover Artist: Katherine Christie
Project Editor: Dani Malady

Illustrations in the book were created by Sebastian Campos-Möller.

Library of Congress Cataloging-in-Publication Data

Names: Ahmed, Iqbal Ike K., author. | Campos-Möller, Xavier, author. | Shah, Manjool, author. | Sheybani, Arsham, author.
Title: Illustrated advanced anterior segment surgery : a step-by-step guide for challenging cases / Iqbal K. Ahmed, Xavier Campos-Möller, Manjool Shah, Arsham Sheybani.
Description: Thorofare, NJ : SLACK Incorporated, [2021] | Includes bibliographical references and index.
Identifiers: LCCN 2020026681 (print) | LCCN 2020026682 (ebook) | ISBN 9781630911843 (hardback) | ISBN 9781630911850 (epub) | ISBN 9781630911867 (web)
Subjects: MESH: Anterior Eye Segment--surgery | Ophthalmologic Surgical Procedures--methods | Atlas
Classification: LCC RE334 (print) | LCC RE334 (ebook) | NLM WW 17 | DDC 617.7--dc23
LC record available at https://lccn.loc.gov/2020026681
LC ebook record available at https://lccn.loc.gov/2020026682

Printed in the United States of America.

Last digit is print number: 10 9 8 7 6 5 4 3 2

Dedication

This book is dedicated to my late mentor, Alan S. Crandall, MD, who has inspired generations of anterior segment surgeons to push the limits and to do so with humility and love.

—Iqbal K. Ahmed, MD

- To my wife, Patricia, for the creative insight, relentless support, and comedic intermissions throughout this project.
- To my daughter, Kasha—may this one day serve as inspiration for whatever you decide to become.
- To my parents, Clara and Xavier, for teaching us that anything is possible and for always placing their children's needs before their own.
- To Ike Ahmed, teacher/friend—meeting and working with you has been the privilege of a lifetime.
- To my patients for trusting me with their most precious gift of vision.
- To my brother, Sebastian, for the tremendous work put into our illustrations.

—Xavier Campos-Möller, MD

To my wife, whose humility and empathy are an inspiration. To my patients, who teach me courage. To my colleagues, mentors, and trainees who stand with me as we encourage surgical excellence and educational growth.

—Manjool Shah, MD

I dedicate this to my mentors who taught me patience while teaching; to my father for showing me the value in training physicians and my mother for allowing me to push boundaries; to my wife, who keeps me motivated to be better; and to my children, who force me to be a good role model.

—Arsham Sheybani, MD

Contents

About the Authors

Iqbal K. Ahmed, MD is Professor, Department of Ophthalmology and Vision Sciences at the University of Utah in Salt Lake City, and Assistant Professor at the Department of Ophthalmology and Vision Science at the University of Toronto, Ontario, Canada, where he is Director of Research at the Kensington Eye Institute, Head of Ophthalmology at Trillium Health Partners, and Medical Director at Prism Eye Institute. Dr. Ahmed has become world renowned for his skills and ground-breaking work in the diagnosis and surgical treatment of highly complex eye diseases including glaucoma and surgical complications. He is recognized as being one of the most experienced complex eye surgeons in the world and has trained numerous surgeons in innovative surgical techniques.

Furthermore, he has been at the leading edge of novel treatments for glaucoma, cataract, and lens implant surgery. Patients are referred to him locally, nationally, and from around the world. He has been invited to perform surgery in 4 continents across the globe.

Dr. Ahmed has a keen interest in the development of advanced microsurgical devices and techniques in glaucoma surgery and complicated cataract extraction, and is actively involved in research and medical education at a national and international level. He has received research grants to study glaucoma medications, glaucoma laser and surgical devices/techniques, angle closure glaucoma, anterior segment and retinal/optic nerve imaging in glaucoma, cataract surgical techniques and devices, and intraocular lens designs.

Dr. Ahmed has designed innovative glaucoma diamond scalpels for surgery, microsurgical instrumentation, and devices, implants, and techniques for the management of the dislocated cataract, iris reconstruction, and glaucoma implant devices. He has done pioneering work in innovative glaucoma surgery, developing and coining the term "Micro-Invasive Glaucoma Surgery (MIGS)" as a new genre of surgical approaches and devices. He also performed the first laser cataract surgery in Canada. As a result of his innovative expertise, Dr. Ahmed has been asked to consult for a variety of companies and manufacturers, especially pertaining to the development of new devices and technologies.

Xavier Campos-Möller, MD is head of the Glaucoma and Advanced Anterior Segment Surgery division of the Department of Ophthalmology at Western Memorial Regional Hospital in Corner Brook, Newfoundland, Canada.

Dr. Campos-Möller completed his ophthalmology residency at the Asociación para Evitar la Ceguera in Mexico and a fellowship in Anterior Segment Surgery at the Instituto Nacional de Rehabilitación, in Mexico City. He later completed a Glaucoma and Advanced Anterior Segment Surgery fellowship with Ike Ahmed at the University of Toronto in Ontario, Canada. He currently runs a busy surgical practice in Corner Brook, Newfoundland, focusing mostly on cataract, complex anterior segment, microinvasive, and traditional glaucoma surgery. He is committed to the eradication of blindness and frequently travels overseas for humanitarian surgery missions.

Manjool Shah, MD serves as a clinical assistant professor of Ophthalmology and Visual Sciences at the Kellogg Eye Center, University of Michigan in Ann Arbor. Additionally, he is the Medical Director of the Division of Glaucoma, Cataract, and Anterior Segment Disease as well as the Director of the glaucoma fellowship program. Dr. Shah completed his residency training at the Casey Eye Institute in Portland, Oregon, and fellowship training in Glaucoma and Advanced Anterior Segment Surgery at the University of Toronto, Ontario, Canada. He is active in teaching residents and fellows at his own institution, participates in surgical education missions around the world, and is an active participant of various national and international societies dedicated to sharing knowledge. His specialized interests include performing and teaching novel and traditional glaucoma surgeries, as well as the management of complex anterior segment challenges.

Arsham Sheybani, MD is an avid teacher but balances his life working with residents and fellows by chasing adventure and spending time with his wife and children.

Foreword

Effective management of cataract surgery complications, whether in "routine" cases or complex scenarios, is a fundamental goal of every ophthalmic surgeon. Over the past 3 decades, several gifted ophthalmologists have selflessly shared their surgical experience and educational skills to assist the global community of ophthalmologists seeking better outcomes for their patients. Following pioneering video lectures by Robert Osher, MD, a group of talented new speakers emerged in this field, and few have been more renowned than Ike Ahmed, MD, whose extraordinary surgical skills and insights, engaging lecturing style, and immersive videos have captivated and educated countless eye surgeons around the world. Dr. Ahmed is an especially gifted teacher, able to walk his audience through his logical approach to a variety of challenging anterior segment cases. The flow of pearls of wisdom is akin to trying to get a drink of water from a fire hydrant!

Dr. Ahmed and his team have written this book that serves as an outline and playbook for surgeons approaching a challenging case or faced with an unexpected complication. Surgical photos, graphic overlays, and illustrations, as well as procedure steps provide the reader with a nuanced understanding of each case. This foundational approach enables the surgeon to intelligently adapt to inevitable variations of surgical challenges as opposed to being limited to a rigid cookbook approach. The book is conveniently laid out in separate chapters for the various complications, facilitating its use both for individual video review as well as preparation for tackling that particular challenge preoperatively.

In addition to providing a comprehensive analysis of complex cases, Dr. Ahmed and colleagues have devoted an invaluable section to the ergonomics of eye surgery. Such considerations are important in routine cases, but especially so for the longer durations of complex cases. Surgeon comfort and surgical technique are enhanced by meticulous analysis of foot/leg/arm/hand/neck and microscope positioning and movement. Just as a pilot would be unprepared without a fundamental understanding of aerodynamics, a surgeon cannot perform at peak level without these empowering pearls of ergonomic insight.

Dr. Ahmed is to be commended for this invaluable new book that enables surgeons to face so many anterior segment surgical challenges with understanding and confidence.

—Barry Seibel, MD
Seibel Vision Surgery
Los Angeles, California

CHAPTER 1

INTRODUCTION—HOW TO USE THIS BOOK AND PLOTTING OUT A FLIGHT PLAN

HOW TO USE THIS BOOK

We set out to create a book that was visually exciting and easy to use as a quick "how to" guide when planning procedures. For this, we cut down on text and provided more images, mostly from surgical videos. Accompanying text provides additional insight into what cannot be seen directly in the images or specific points that we believe need to be highlighted. We suggest that you go over every image during and after reading the entire chapter; the technique and image sequence will be clearer the second time around. That is the way this book was designed because we want to provide a quick visual reference that can (and should) be reviewed over and over again, especially the day before or the morning of a complex procedure. This will ideally create a visual memory that will give the reader a "déjà vu" familiarity with the complex situations that may present.

We do encourage that you read the entire book, but we also understand that sometimes you only need to learn or review a specific technique. This book's chapters are titled "How to [insert technique]" to help you quickly find the solution to your patient's problem. If you prefer to read individual techniques, we encourage that you first read the introductory chapters to maximize utilization of this work's resources.

1 **INTRODUCTION**

KEY POINTS 2

3

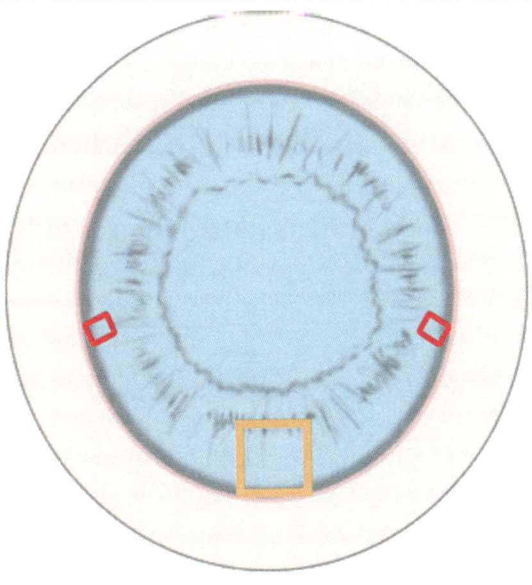

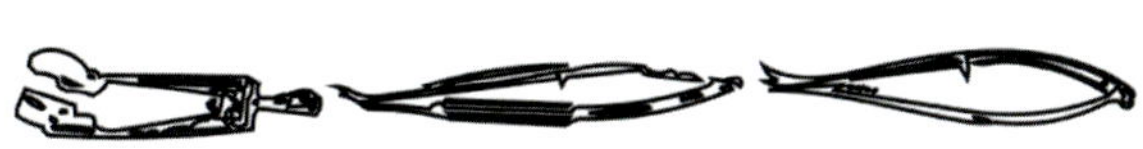

4

The first page of each chapter is loaded with important information and should not be overlooked. It is divided into 4 sections:

1. Introduction: This section provides a very brief overview of what the chapter is about and a general scenario in which the technique may be utilized.
2. Key points: These are the technique's main points that must always be at the top of mind. This section can be a "quick reminder" when reviewed before each case to freshen up key concepts.

Ahmed IK, Campos-Möller X, Shah M, Sheybani A. *Illustrated Advanced Anterior Segment Surgery: A Step-by-Step Guide for Challenging Cases* (pp 1-4).

3. Incisions: We have designed an "incision template" format to aid visualization of where and how incisions are to be placed. It is a quick-glance reference that can be reviewed before each case. Each incision type has been assigned a specific color throughout the book, thus providing continuity and helping to create a visual memory of incision types and locations. Please note that these are just templates and incision design should not be cast in stone. Individual adjustments must be made to account for individual characteristics of both patient and surgeon, such as ocular and orbital anatomy, instrument variation, and hand positioning. The incisions chapter provides additional information on each type of incision and the reference icon that represents it throughout the book.
4. Toolbox: This section is aimed to help you with preparing yourself and your staff by having the necessary instruments and devices on hand. A complete ophthalmology set (standard cataract tray) is assumed to be present, so this section will only focus on the extra tools that are specific for the technique in question.

The rest of the pages in each chapter will dive straight into the technique. All of the important steps are represented by an image, complimented by text, and sometimes expanded on with the aid of illustrations. Due to space limitations within each page, some explanations may not be directly adjacent to the images that they correspond to, for which we suggest that each chapter be read twice. It should not be time consuming because all of our chapters are concise and to the point. We chose a "graphic novel" aesthetic to present a different, novel approach to learning. We intentionally decided to divert from the traditional format used in standard scientific publications to make this book more visually appealing and a fun experience. However, we are not suggesting that this book be read instead of scientific publications—they complement one another.

"Magic Hands"—wide-angle photos taken from the surgeon's point of view—are interspersed throughout the book. These are here to help the reader understand the hand positioning that was used for the particular case presented. These hand grips and positioning images are simply a reference, as hand positions should be individualized for each case.

Ultimately, this book is simply a guideline and an overview of the key concepts and techniques that have helped us succeed in specific complex cases. However, every case is unique, and therefore, we leave it up to the surgeon's discretion to adjust and modify accordingly.

PLOTTING OUT A FLIGHT PLAN

Anterior segment surgery can be highly complex. Despite the relatively small size of the human eye, one may encounter a myriad of diseases and surgical approaches, all with their own technical challenges. As physicians, we must first aim to do no harm—avoiding complications starts with proper preoperative planning.

The first step of any successful surgery is elucidating an accurate history and exam. Surgical planning begins when the patient and physician first meet.

An accurate history reveals insights into not only the technical steps but also elements around the surgery that may be equally as important. For example:

- Medications (prior allergies to oral carbonic anhydrase inhibitors may mean that a more aggressive removal of viscoelastic at the end of the case is necessary)
- Previous surgery and surgical complications (an anterior capsular tear may mean that optic capture may not be possible)
- Patient experience with prior surgeries (consider the choice of anesthesia based on the planned procedure as well as the patient's comfort with previous care)

Based on a careful history, it is paramount to rank the patient's complaints in order of priority and severity. This can guide the surgical decision making to follow. For example, the plan for treating the positive dysphotopsia with a diffractive lens might be straightforward, but this plan may be altered if the patient is actually more bothered by the negative temporal dysphotopsia.

Eye exam—beyond a thorough eye exam (we will not list all components), here are pearls we have found useful in guiding our decisions:

- Orbital anatomy identifies challenges in anterior chamber access; prominent orbital rim, orbital fat atrophy, and small palpebral fissures may make incision placement and instrument access difficult.
- Ocular surface evaluation can reveal other causes of dysphotopsia and glare.
- Identifying endothelial changes and guttata are useful not only in preoperative planning, but also may be the reason for positive dysphotopsias instead of the lens or intraocular lens (IOL).
- Gonioscopy:
    - Look for asymmetry in the angle beyond just the grade of opening. Careful attention to pigmentation may suggest iris chafing in a pseudophakic patient with asymmetric glaucoma.
    - Using dilated gonioscopy has been an invaluable tool to view beneath the iris, especially in complex anterior segment cases.
- Retroillumination is also a very useful tool to diagnose iris chaffng and otherwise invisible iris defects, as well as the status of the lens capsule or lens position.
- Iris examination is used to not only assess size and pupillary function but also to identify atrophy or thinning that may result in significant transillumination defects with stretching or cheese-wiring with suturing.
- Careful documentation of the type of IOL, rotational position of the haptics, position relative to the capsule, status of the anterior and posterior capsule, and size of anterior and posterior capsulotomies can be helpful in choosing the appropriate IOL exchange and/or fixation techniques.

Diagnostic studies—these do not replace the exam, but add data:

- Corneal analysis:
    - Corneal topography is useful in determining more than just astigmatism; it can be used for identifying dry eye, determining optimal incision placement, or identifying higher-order aberrations.
    - Endothelial cell counts: For low cell counts (absolute or compared to the other eye), we may opt for posterior fixation of lenses; however, we would plan on techniques that minimize the amount of irrigation in the eye. An anterior chamber maintainer may be detrimental for these patients, for which pars plana irrigation may be necessary.
- Anterior segment optical coherence tomography (OCT) is useful for an objective angle assessment when clinical identification of structures is difficult.
- Ultrasound biomicroscopy is useful in delineating anatomical structures and implants behind the iris where OCT cannot penetrate. It is also useful for visualizing the ciliary body size and position.
- Posterior segment imaging:
    - Fundus photography: Aside from documenting posterior pole pathology, reviewing fundus photos can help identify pathology initially missed on clinical exam.
    - Macular OCT: Even subtle changes on exam should prompt an analysis of macular structure. Untreated mild macular edema may worsen after surgery.

Managing expectations is paramount. No matter how easy or how difficult the case, our patient's expectations must be aligned with reality, and they should be made aware of the uniqueness of their situation and the challenges that may lie ahead. Complex anterior segment surgery requires a team-based approach, and recruiting the patient to be on your team will make the entire process easier. While we always aim to improve the patient's functional status, one cannot always expect a complete resolution of all symptoms. For example, operating on a patient for glare due to a large iris defect may improve symptoms with a pupilloplasty, but depending on the state of the iris tissue, those symptoms may not fully resolve.

PLANNING AN APPROACH

Every step of the surgery must be planned ahead of time. Online video resources can help plan a surgical approach. Mental visualization of every step prior to surgery can help guide incision placement and help sequence the steps. Some additional questions to consider and address prior to surgery are as follows:

- How will the patient be positioned?
- What is the anesthesia plan?
- Where will the surgeon sit?
- Where will incisions be located, and what type of incisions are to be used?
- Will the lens be addressed first or the glaucoma, or the iris?
- Types of ophthalmic viscosurgical devices needed? Mechanical pupil dilators? Capsule support? Capsule or IOL suturing devices?
- Is vitrectomy anticipated?
- Will triamcinolone or trypan blue be required?

PLAN B(ACKUP)

For advanced anterior segment surgery cases, as for routine procedures, having a backup plan is an absolute necessity. What should be done if the primary and secondary surgical plan are not successful? Do additional lenses or devices need to be preordered? Discuss with the patient if there is a high likelihood of additional surgery, and any additional visits or costs that may arise from this secondary plan.

SURGICAL SETUP

In the operating room, incision placement requires careful attention. Orbital anatomy should have been addressed during the preoperative visit. When needed, additional paracentesis incisions may be necessary. In complex cases, consider hovering an instrument over the eye with the intended hand grip prior to making the paracentesis incision in order to determine ideal incision placement.

Remember the prioritized list of patient complaints as well as the surgical plan, and address concerns in a logical order. As with even basic intraocular surgery, every step can have a dramatic effect on subsequent steps, so take the appropriate time to be methodical with every aspect of the case.

Postoperative management of the intraocular pressure is critical after successful surgery. If there is any doubt that there is a significant amount of viscoelastic remaining in the eye, oral carbonic anhydrase inhibitors should be considered depending on the patient's tolerance. Intracameral injections of medications or sub-Tenon's placement of medication should be considered if the patient may not be able to administer medications reliably.

CHAPTER 2

ERGONOMICS, HAND POSITIONING, AND INSTRUMENT GRIPS

INTRODUCTION

As eye surgeons, we have learned to function in a high-magnification world. We are able to focus on micrometric structures and perform maneuvers in extremely confined spaces. This makes it easy to forget about what is happening outside the field of view of the surgical microscope.

As well as reducing the risk of back and neck injury, good ergonomics will guarantee surgical success by increasing precision and reducing tremor. This chapter is about zooming out and focusing on yourself, the surgeon, for an instant before zooming back into your next complex case.

Ahmed IK, Campos-Möller X, Shah M, Sheybani A. *Illustrated Advanced Anterior Segment Surgery: A Step-by-Step Guide for Challenging Cases* (pp 5-19).

We spend most of our days sitting. There is increasing evidence to support the health risk of prolonged sitting, especially in an incorrect posture. The first recommendation is of course to get a good stool, but even with the best stool, an incorrect posture can lead to back and neck injuries. Furthermore, sitting incorrectly could be the reason why some procedures or maneuvers seem harder to perform.

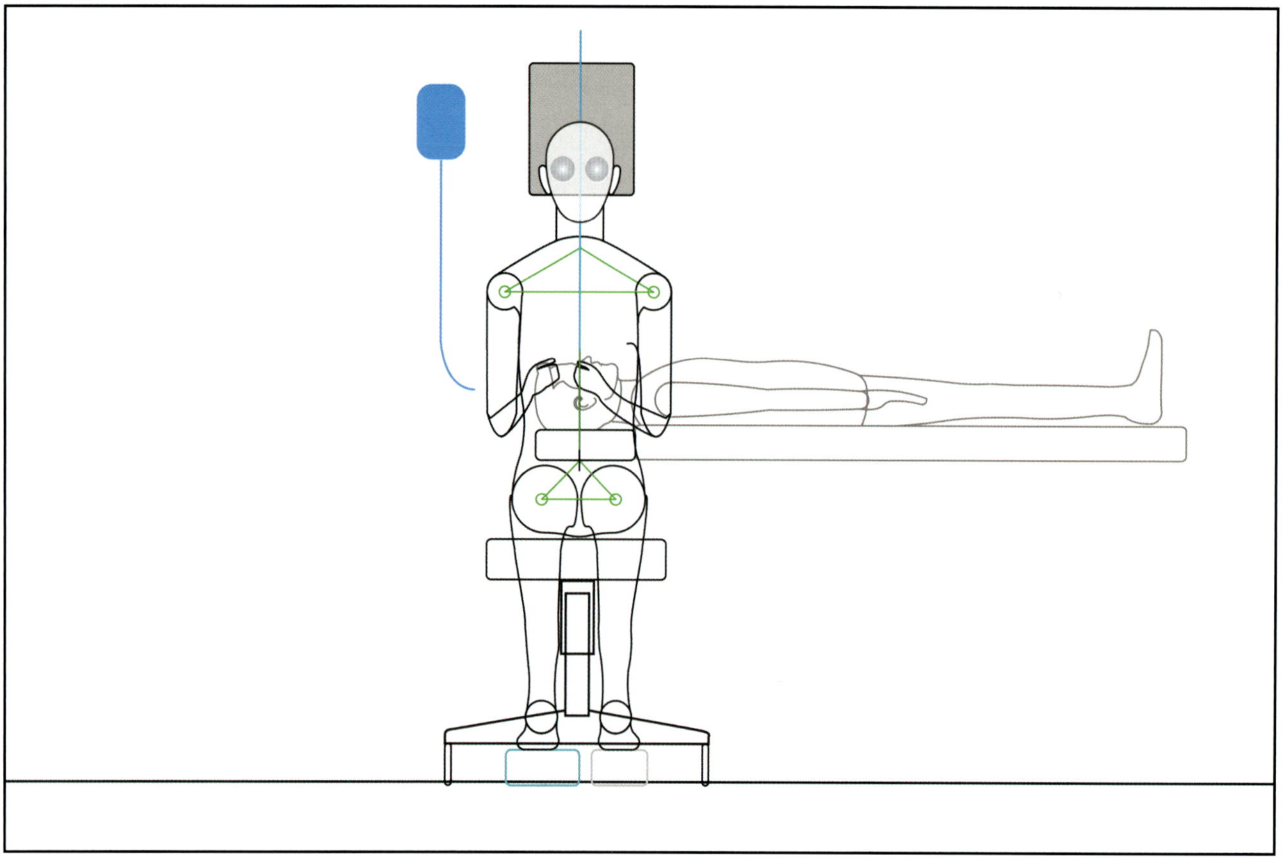

A good way to think about body alignment: Viewing the sitting surgeon from behind, draw 2 parallel horizontal lines (one for the shoulders and one for the hips) and 1 vertical line, going down through the spine. The angle between the vertical and horizontal lines should approximate to 90 degrees. Any disruption in this angle means that either shoulders or hips are tilted sideways, or the spine is not vertically aligned.

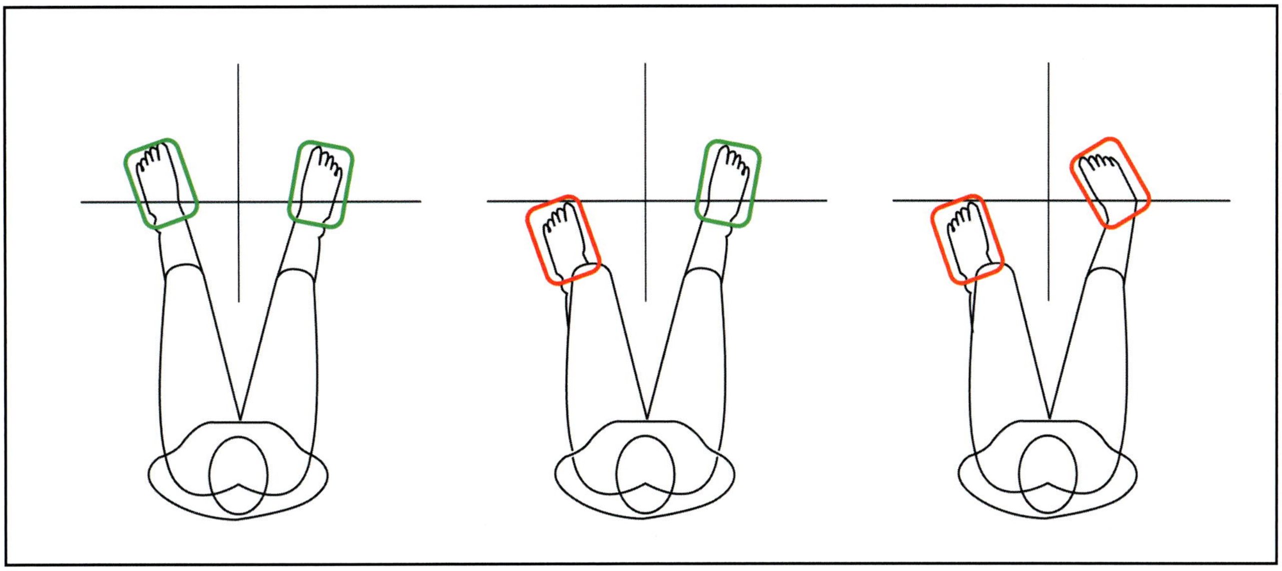

Pedal positioning is very important for good ergonomics. Having both pedals pointing straight ahead and right next to each other is not ergonomic because it brings the thighs together and makes it easier for the pelvis to tilt from side to side (think of a wide-based triangle vs a triangle balancing on its apex). Having an internally rotated pedal (toes pointing inward) is also detrimental to hip health. An ideal position is to have a slight "duck stance." It is also important to have both pedals aligned in such a way that both knees have similar degrees of flexion. Stretching one knee out more than the other could lead to pelvic rotation and lumbar spine lesions.

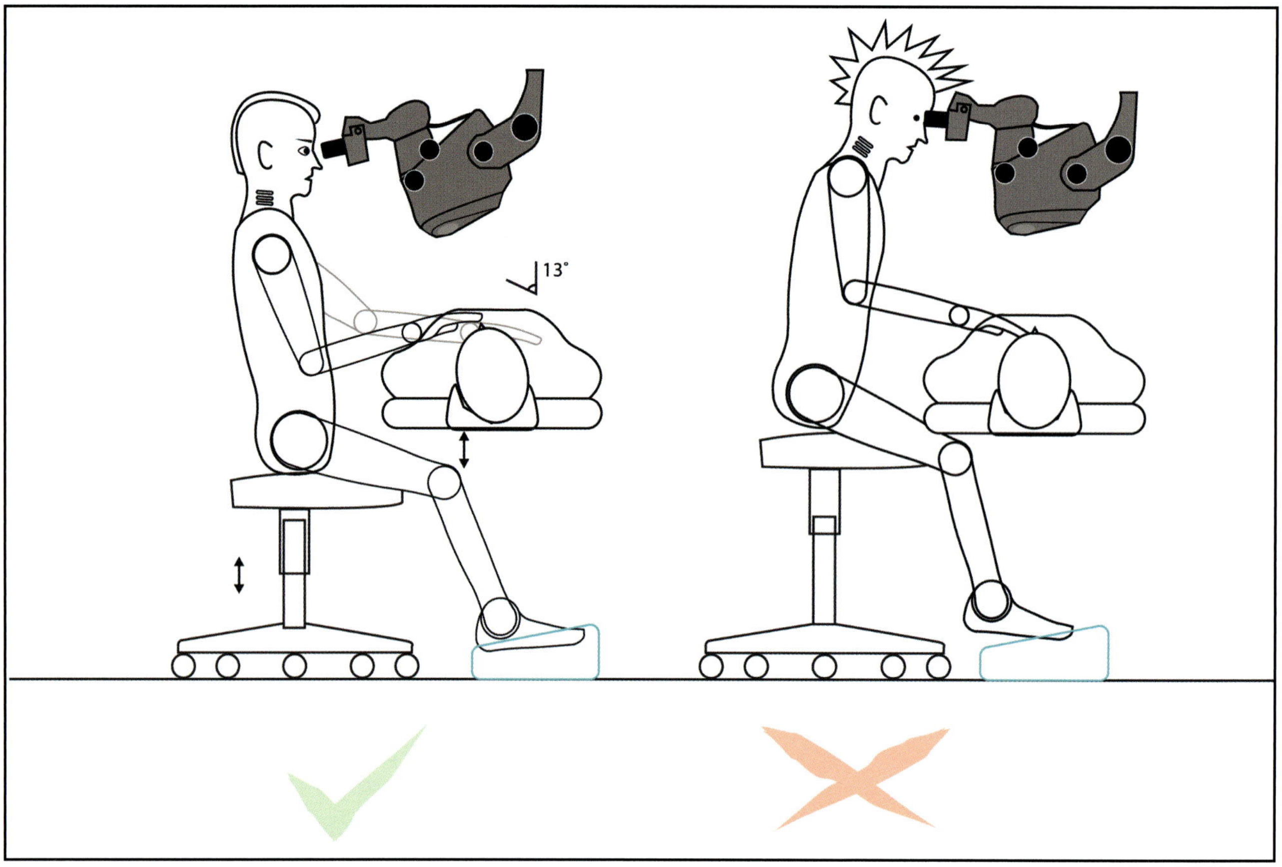

The image on the left represents all aspects of adequate positioning.

The image on the right represents all aspects of incorrect positioning.

The posture on the right can be drastically improved by 2 simple modifications: lowering the seat height and tilting the microscope 13 degrees toward the surgeon.

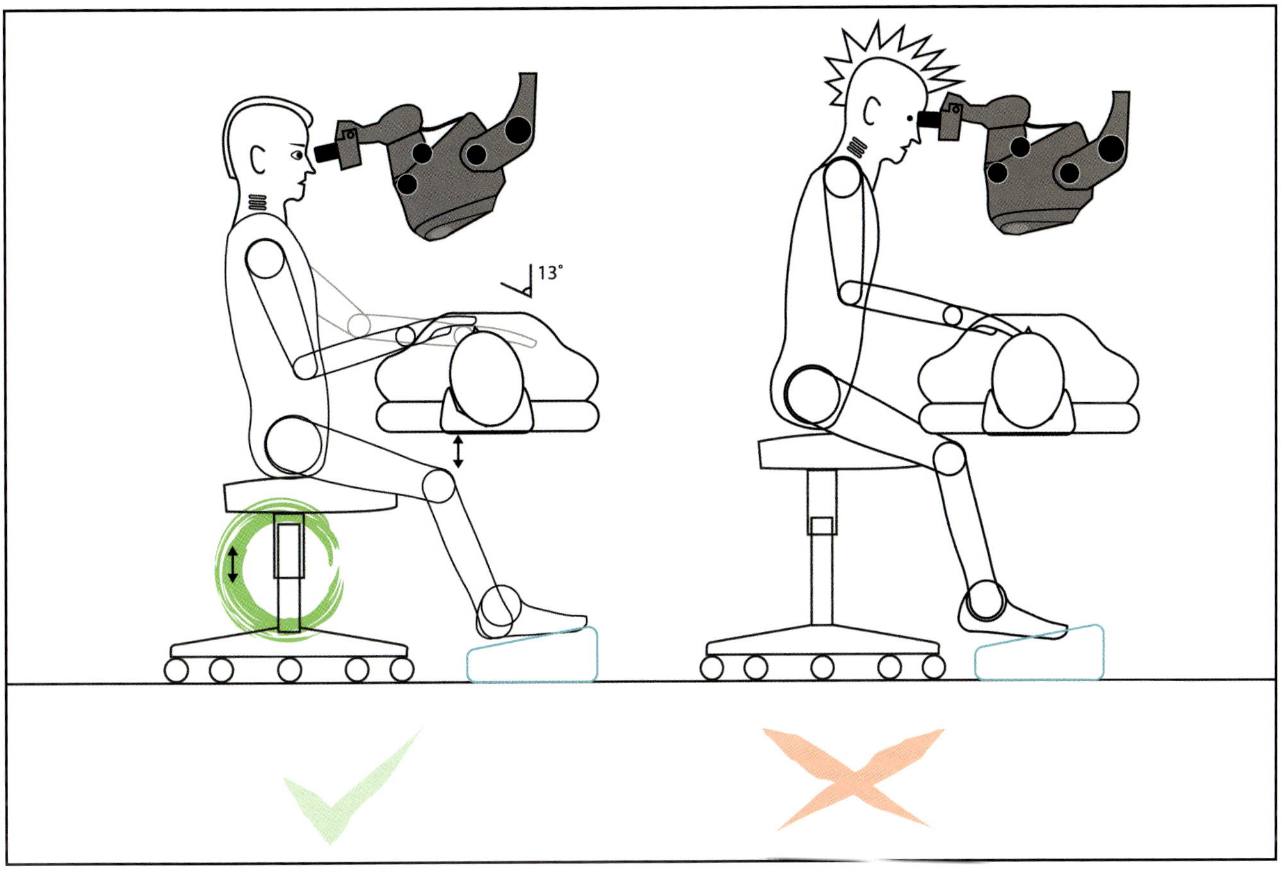

1. Lower your seat height. Your seat height should allow for your heels to touch the ground with about a 30-degree angle of flexion at your knees. This ensures that you have a stable base and are not falling over on a high stool.
2. Adjust the height of the patient's bed so that your elbows are slightly below the patient eye level (PEL) when your arms are hanging naturally to the side of the body. If the elbows are below the PEL, you will be able to keep your hands comfortably at eye level without pushing down on the eye. When adjusting the bed height, remember the simple formula to adjust for bottle height for phacoemulsification: 15 cm of height = 11 mm Hg change in intraocular pressure.

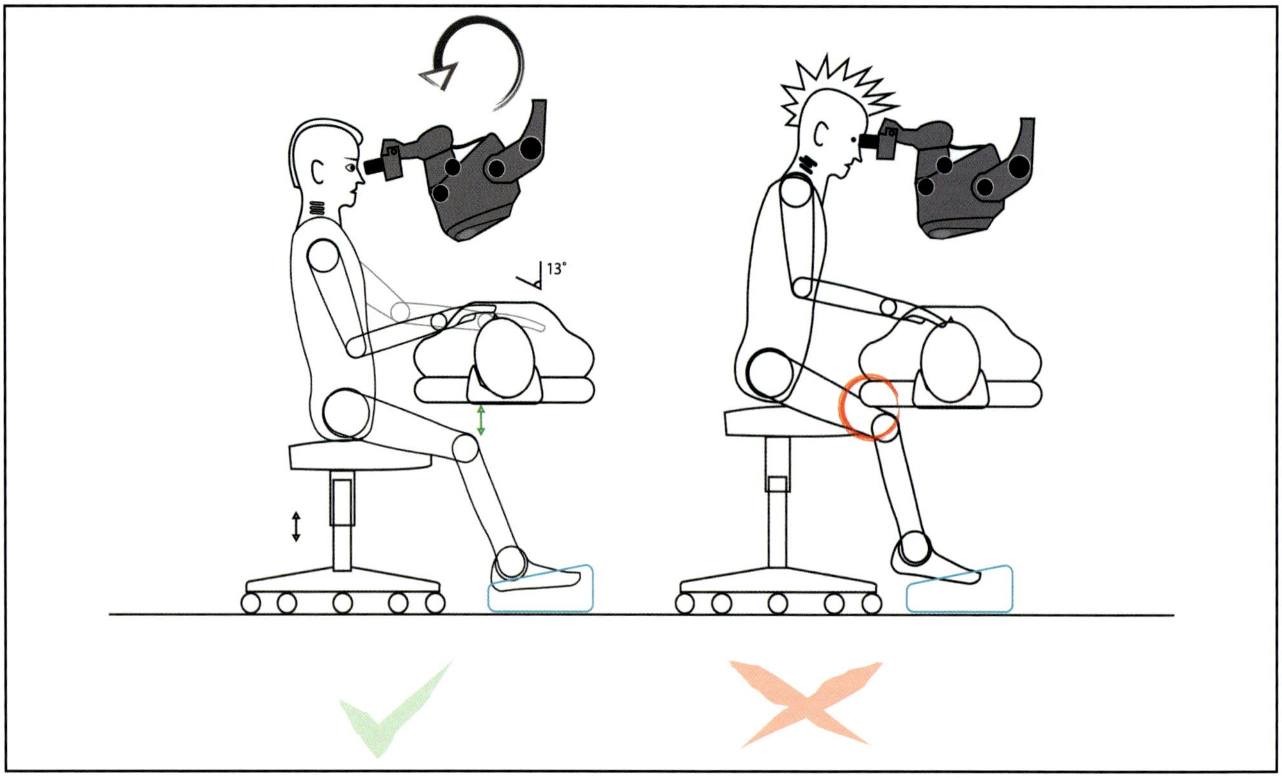

3. If your seat is lower, there will be more room for your knees under the patient's head.
4. A lower seat height also allows for a natural foot position, which translates into more control over the phaco and microscope pedals. Sitting too high forces you to put weight on your feet for support, thus reducing precision and control.

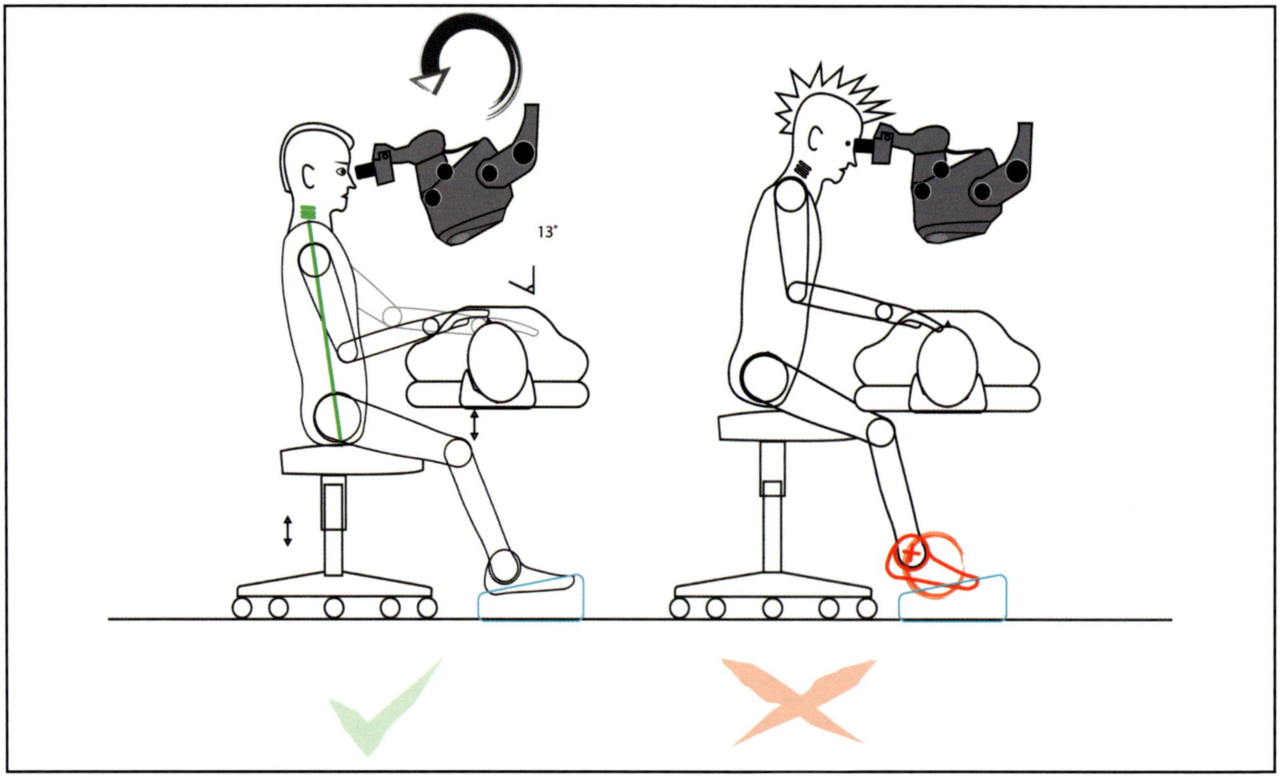

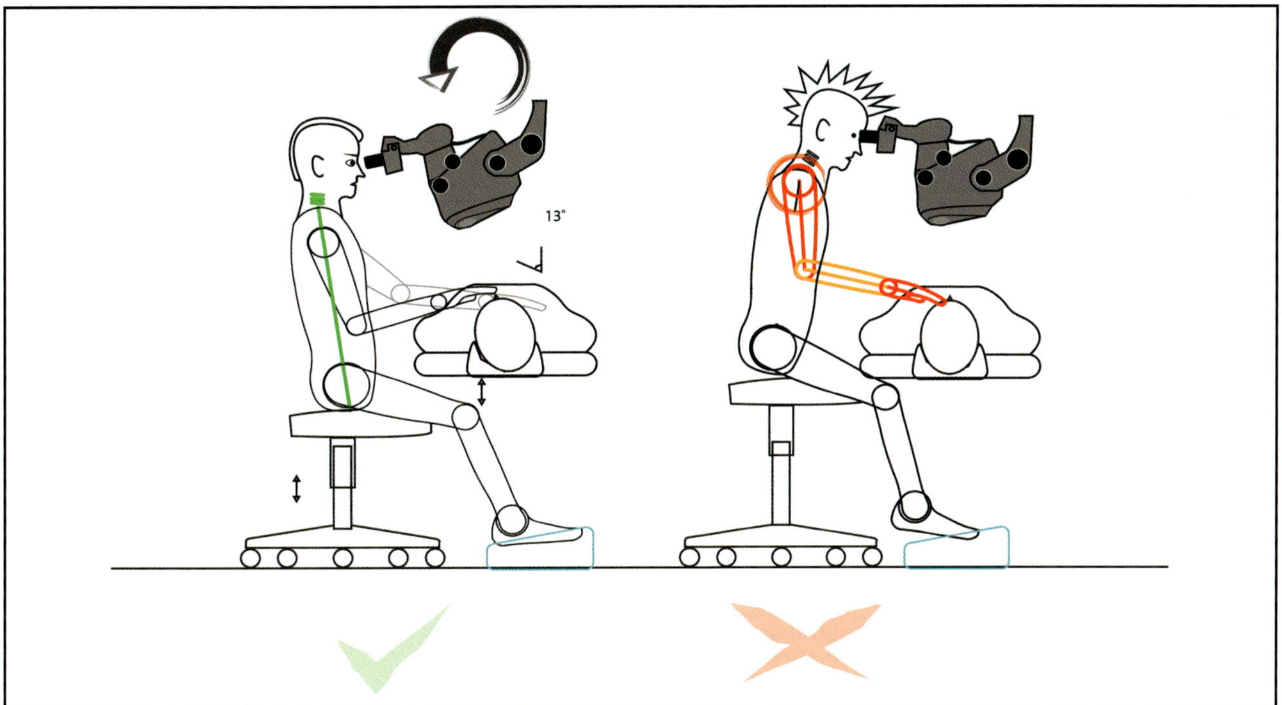

5. Relax the shoulders. This allows for the elbows to adopt a normal position and reduces tremor. Tired muscles shake and your arms/hands are no exception.
6. Tilt the microscope toward you, approximately 13 degrees. This brings the oculars closer toward you and allows you to sit more upright, instead of having to lean over the patient. There are many benefits to this: better "stacking" of the cervical vertebrae (reducing the risk of neck pain or a slipped cervical vertebra); easier to maintain an erect spine without having to bend over to reach the patient; more room to maneuver when your body is further away from the patient's head instead of crammed up against it; and more control over the eye when the hands are free to move up and down, instead of being forced down onto the eye by an excessively bent over posture.

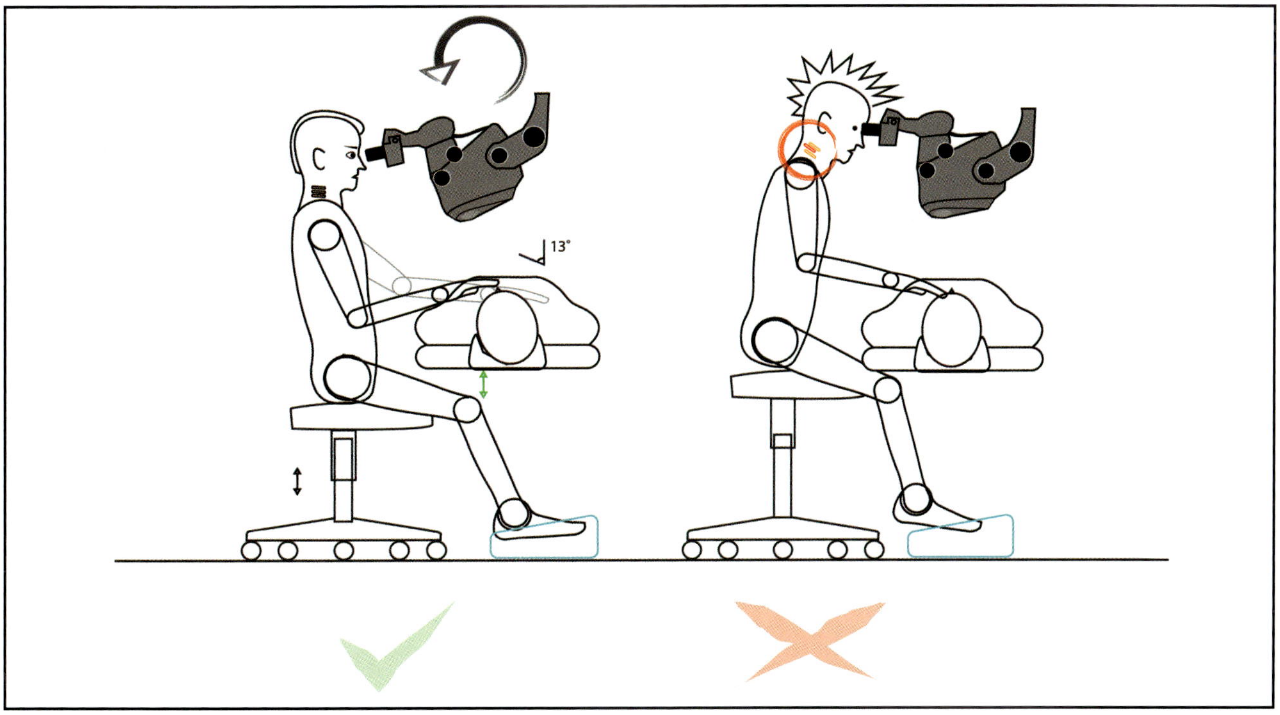

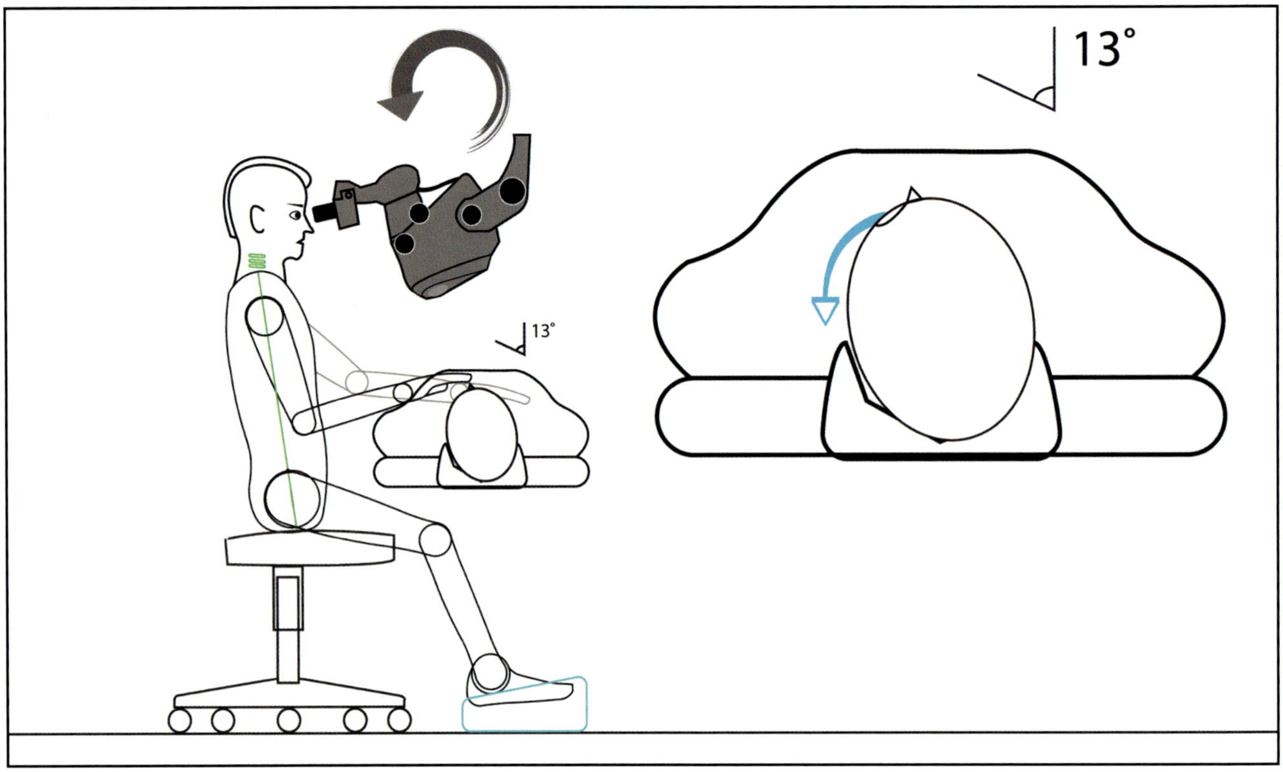

7. Tilting the patient's head slightly toward you (10 degrees) also has the advantage of allowing for balanced salt solution to flow out of the orbit and reduce pooling, thus improving visualization.

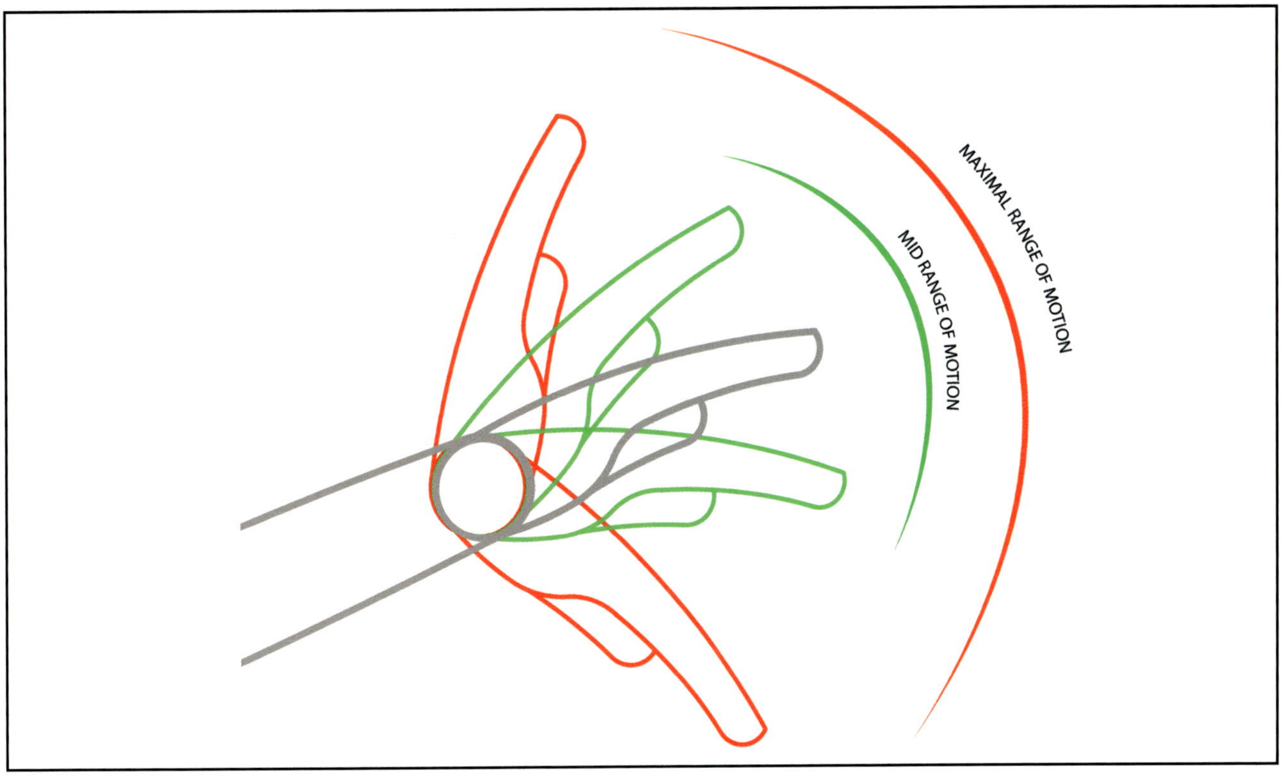

Range of motion (ROM) is "the full movement potential of a joint, usually its range of flexion and extension." It is an indicator of a joint's health. ROM is limited by poor flexibility (tight muscles/soft tissues) and arthropathy.

ROM is important because it not only determines how we move our instruments inside the eye, but also with what precision. Every joint has proprioceptors that give us the ability to understand a specific joint's position in space, and mechanoreceptors that give us sensitivity to movement, resistance, pressure, etc. The sensitivity of these receptors is highest during mid-ROM. The movement of a joint is smoother and more controlled during mid-ROM. Conversely, shaking and tremor are exacerbated by bringing an articulation to extremes of its ROM. The importance of these concepts as eye surgeons lies in that the way we position our bodies and hands determine the precision with which intraocular maneuvers are performed. It is therefore important that the motions we intend to perform with an instrument are within our joints' ROMs (especially the wrist), ideally within the mid-range.

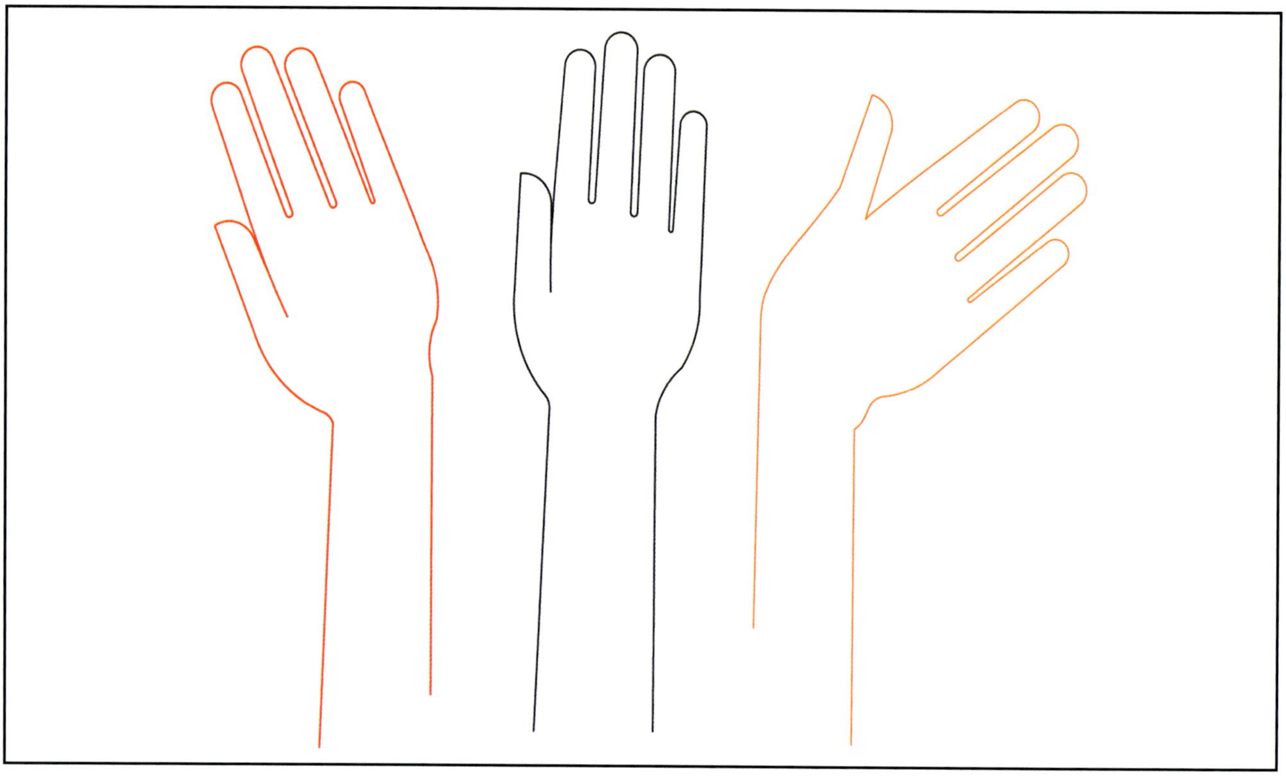

Wrist movements outlined above: Ulnar flexion (right), radial flexion (left), flexion and extension.

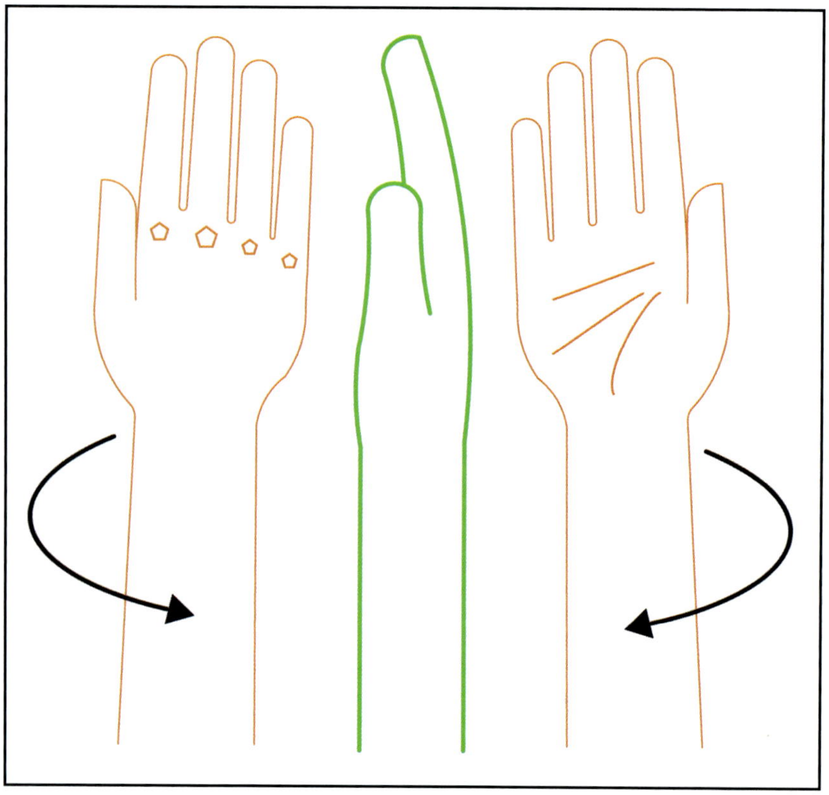

Pronation (left).
Supination (right).

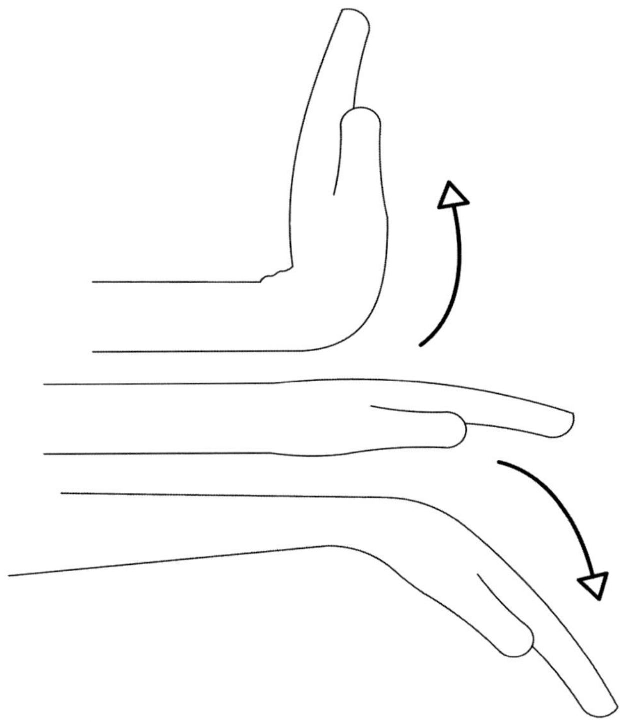

Wrist extension (above), neutral (center), wrist flexion (below).

HAND GRIPS

How we hold our instruments is paramount. Different grips set the wrist up to move in specific patterns. A given hand grip will facilitate a specific arc of motion (eg, ulnar flexion) while limiting another arc. The way we hold our instruments should make intraocular maneuvers natural, smooth, and easy while preventing other undesired movements.

We have identified 5 hand grips that we most commonly use. We encourage the reader to become familiar with these grips, experimenting with which arcs of motion they facilitate or preclude. Every person is different and so are joints, so rather than defining which hand grips are universally best for each maneuver, we suggest that surgeons invest some time to think about hand grips during preoperative planning and before each step of surgery. Furthermore, incision location and characteristics should be in accordance with the hand grips that will be used.

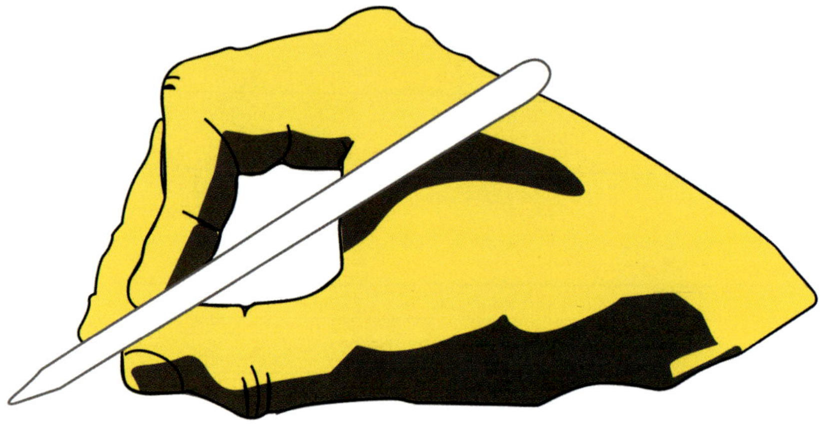

The Pencil Grip

This is the grip that the majority of surgeons are most comfortable with, for obvious reasons. It provides very good control of instruments given the sensitivity and mobility provided by the flexion of the fingers. An important consideration when using this grip is that it tends to aim instruments down (posteriorly into the eye). Another consideration is that this grip can feel unnatural when entering through a temporal incision (surgeon's view 6 o'clock) as these locations force the wrists into extreme flexion.

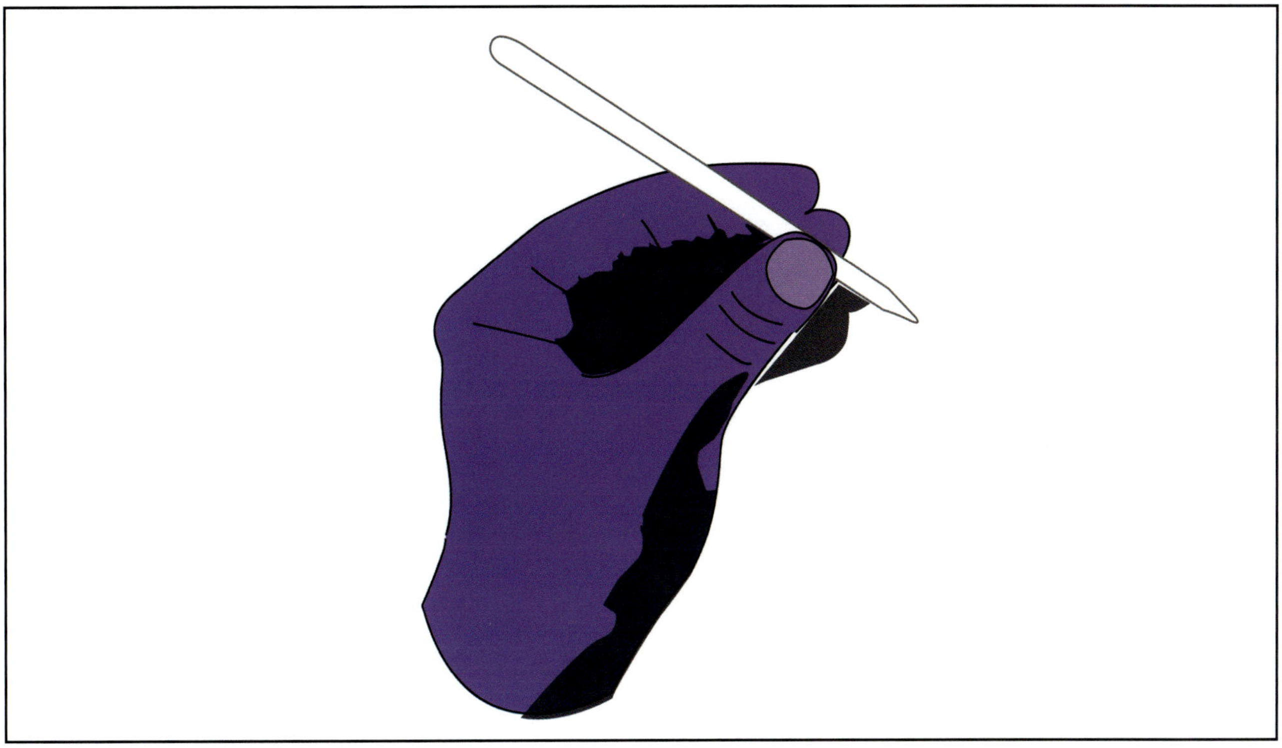

The Dart Thrower Grip

This is, in a way, a combination of the pencil grip and the underhand grip. This is a grip that allows for a light grip on instruments and permits rolling instrument shafts between the thumb and the rest of the fingers.

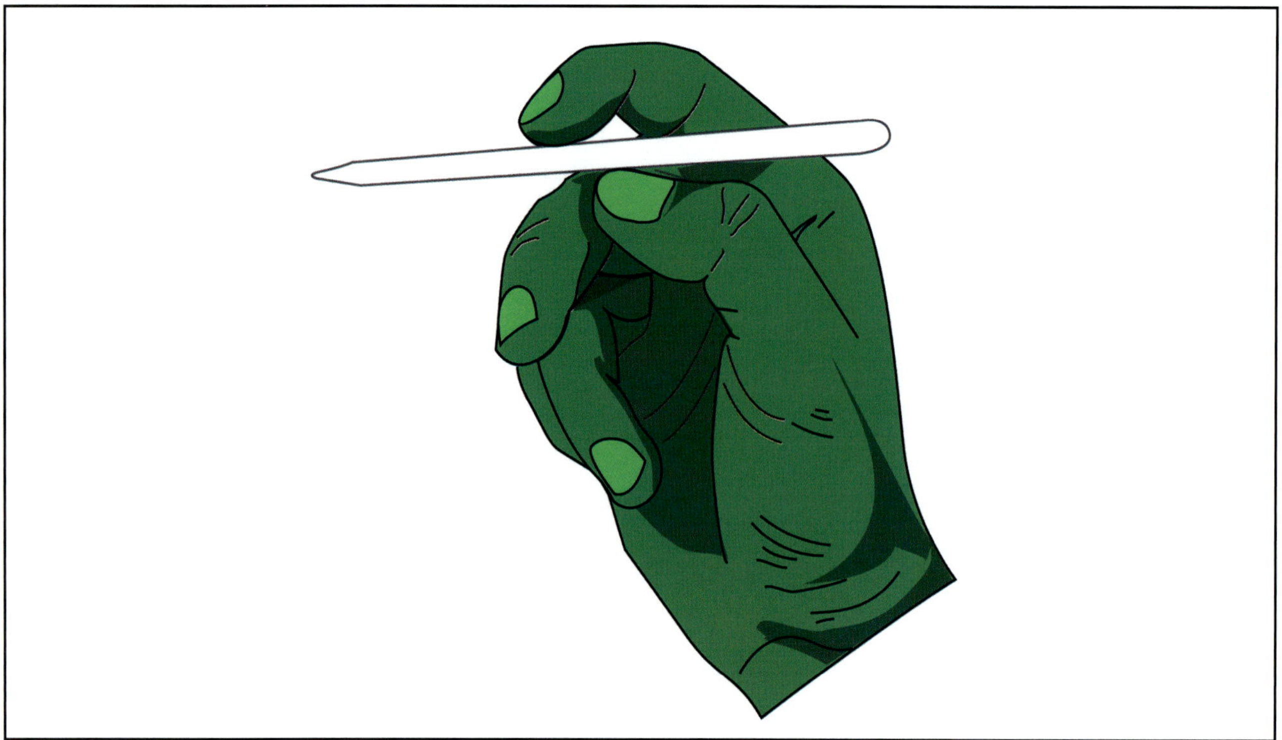

The Cigar Grip

This grip promotes keeping wrists low and instruments at PEL. It also comes in handy when requiring instruments to stay parallel to the iris plane.

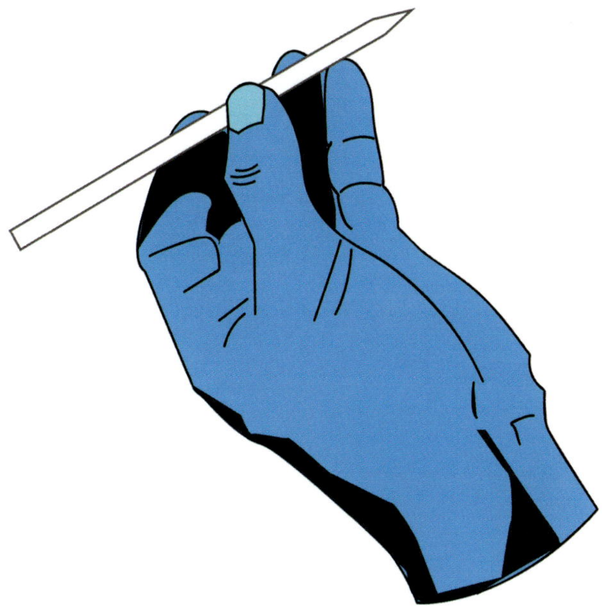

The Underhand Grip

Holding instruments in full supination allows for a good ulnar flexion and extension arc of motion. The knuckles can be rested on the patient's forehead or cheekbone to allow for precise, controlled motion.

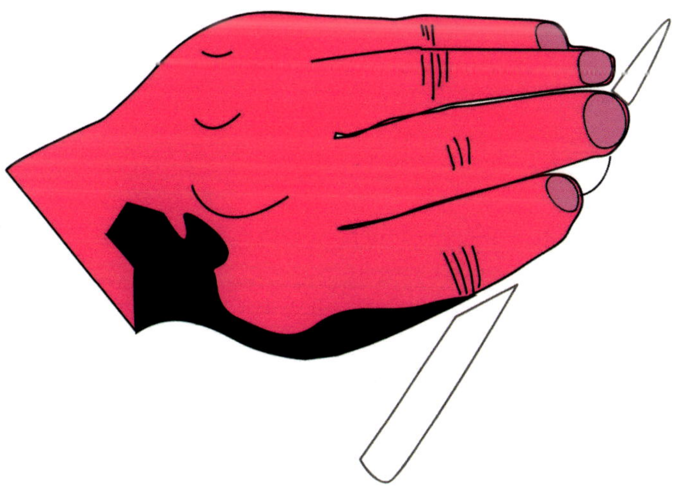

The Overhand Grip

In this grip, the instruments are held in full pronation. The key to this grip is to use the whole arm and abduct the elbow away from the torso (like having a "chicken wing"). The fifth finger (pinkie) can be used to stabilize the hand against the patient's head. This maneuver is useful when desiring a ROM that is parallel to the iris plane, and to hold instruments still inside the eye, as when docking a needle into a cannula.

CHAPTER 3

INCISIONS

INTRODUCTION

Incisions are the port of entry for our instruments, our access to the delicate structures within the eye. Usually one of the first steps in surgery, their importance cannot be overemphasized.

Incision construction, location, and direction will facilitate or hinder intraocular procedures. Incisions should be thoroughly thought over and constructed carefully.

Following are some key concepts regarding incisions.

Ahmed IK, Campos-Möller X, Shah M, Sheybani A. *Illustrated Advanced Anterior Segment Surgery: A Step-by-Step Guide for Challenging Cases* (pp 21-26).

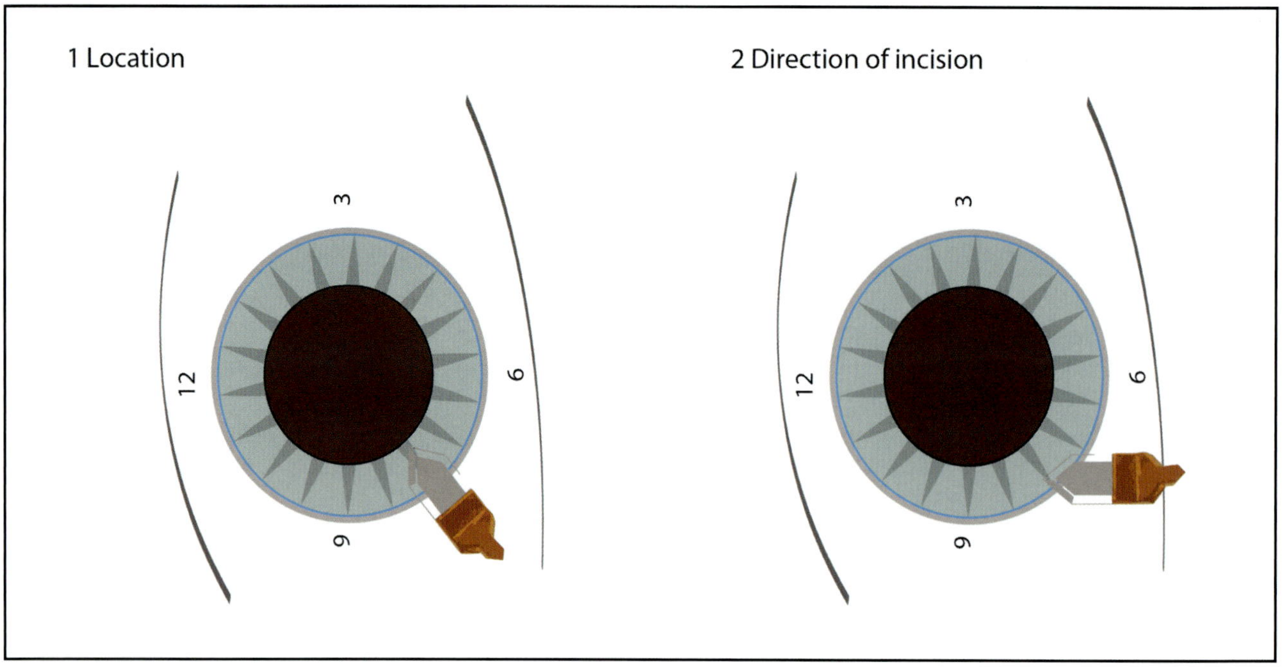

1. Clock hour location. This is perhaps the most straight-forward concept, but it is the foundation for a good incision. Location should provide easy access to the intraocular structures that the surgeon will work with while staying away from other structures and instruments. Important considerations are the orbital anatomy and instrument size. Incisions location must maximize comfort and range of motion.

2. Direction of incision. An incision at a specific clock hour can have multiple directions. It can be radial (pointing toward the visual axis) or tangential (more parallel to the limbus). Direction of incisions is key when working with tissues in the periphery of the eye, such as iris suturing. Ideally, an instrument's trajectory should follow the natural direction of the incision. Forcing a range of motion can torque the incision, generating corneal folds that hinder visibility and allowing for exit of ophthalmic viscosurgical device and, hence, anterior chamber shallowing.

3 Incision orientation

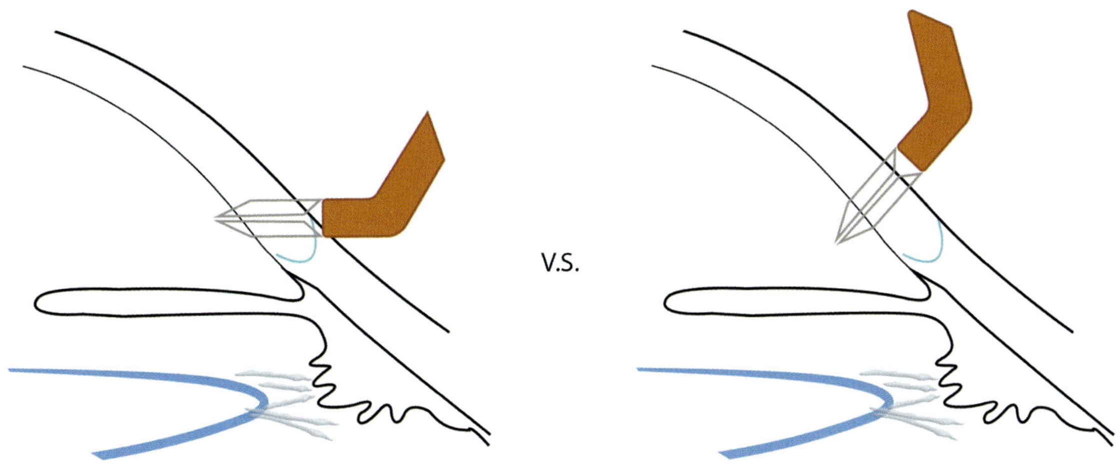

3. Incision orientation. This concept refers to the anterior or posterior trajectory of an incision. Similar to incision direction, incision orientation should seek the trajectory of an instrument that will facilitate access to the ocular structures that will be addressed. More limbal incisions generally allow for a trajectory that is parallel to the iris plane, whereas more clear corneal incisions will have a tendency to point more posteriorly (perpendicular to the iris plane).

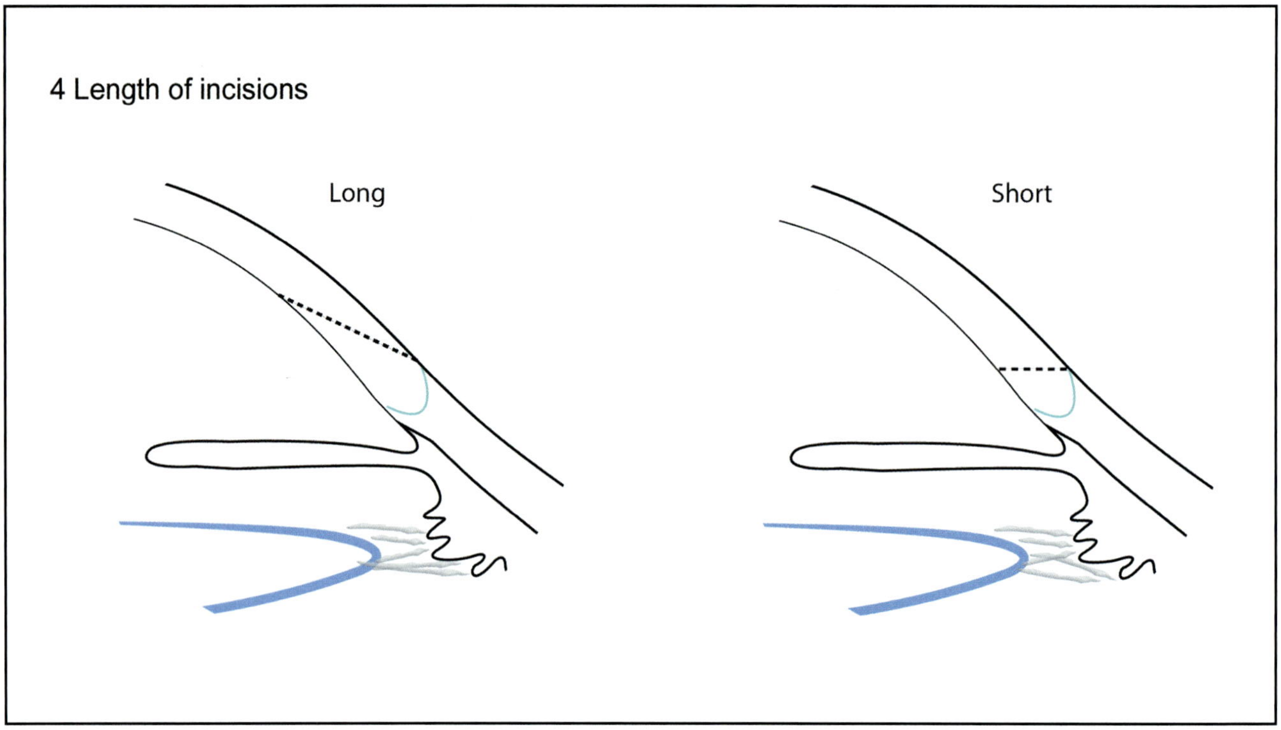

4. Length of incisions. The more perpendicular to the corneal plane, the shorter an incision will be. It is important to consider this as shorter incisions tend to leak more, and incisions that are too long tend to be difficult to enter. Short incisions are generally acceptable for narrow (< 1 mm) paracenteses, whereas wider incisions should be constructed longer, or even triplanar.

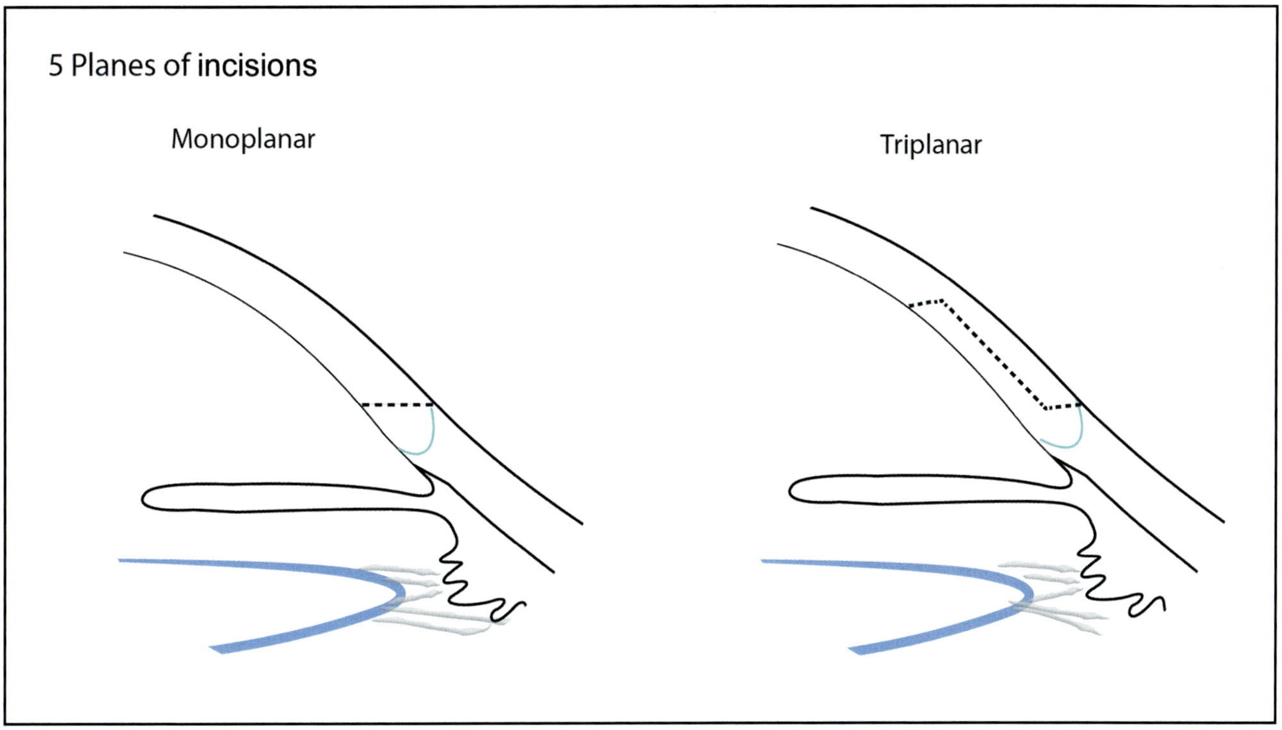

5. Planes of incisions. This refers to the number of steps (or trajectory changes) within the incision's construction. Monoplanar incisions leak more but are easier to enter. This construction should be exclusively for narrow incisions. Triplanar incisions are more watertight but can be harder to access. Most incisions larger than 2 mm should have a bi- or triplanar construction to reduce wound leak.

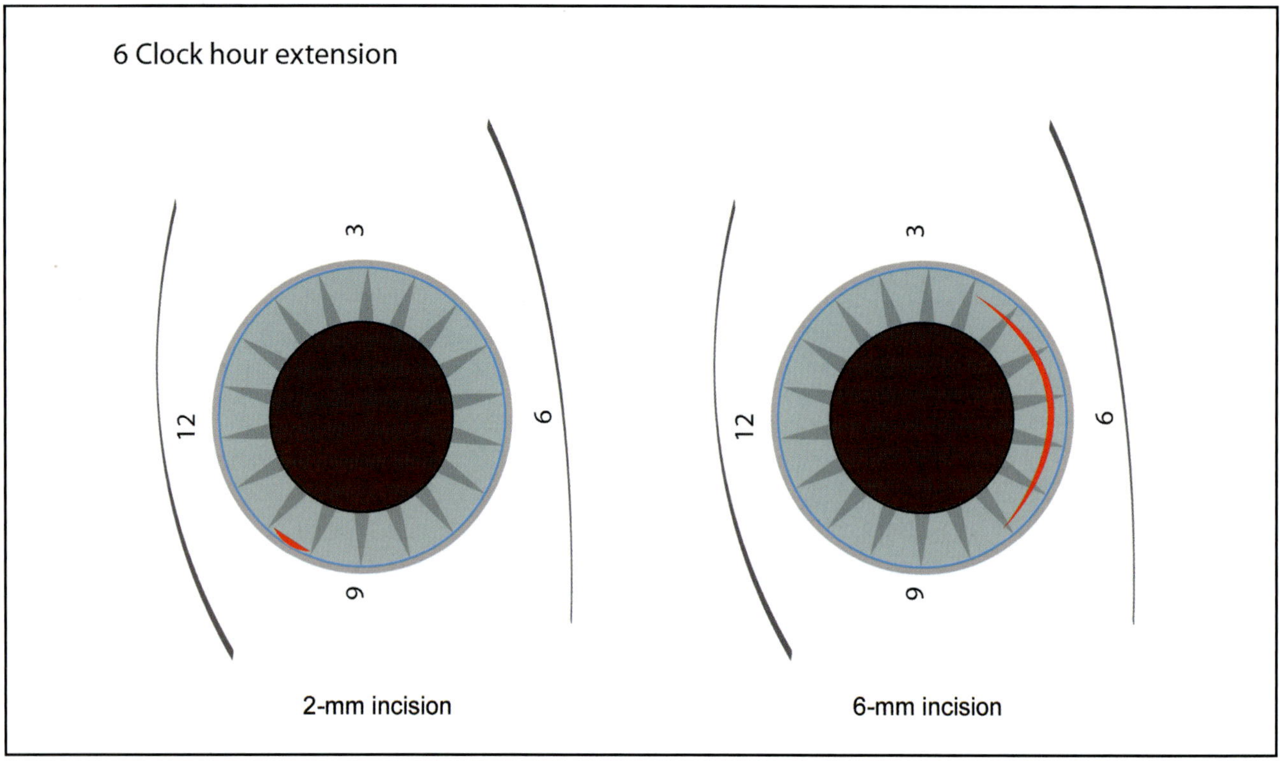

6. Clock hour extension (incision width). This refers to the number of clock hours that an incision covers. This will be determined by the size of the instruments or devices that are intended to go through the incision. Generally, incisions up to 3 mm can be sealed with hydration alone (when adequately constructed). Incisions over 3 mm should be sutured. The larger the clock hour extension, the more a wound will affect postoperative corneal cylinder (this can be both an advantage and a disadvantage).

CHAPTER 4

HOW TO PERFOM A CAPSULORRHEXIS THROUGH A SMALL PUPIL

INTRODUCTION

Cataract surgery in the presence of a small pupil is challenging but can be managed in several ways.

There are multiple causes for a small intraoperative pupil that can all be managed similarly. In the presence of posterior synechiae, these must be freed from the anterior capsule before the capsulorrhexis is initiated.

In this chapter, we discuss how to free synechiae and perform a capsulorrhexis without the use of additional pupil-expanding devices.

KEY POINTS

- Gentle blunt dissection is typically sufficient to lyse posterior synechiae, but care must be taken to avoid damaging the anterior capsule.
- If 360 degrees of synechiae are present, a patent peripheral iridotomy can be used to inject cohesive ophthalmic viscosurgical device (OVD), helping to separate the iris from the anterior capsule.
- Create multiple paracenteses as needed to complete the synechiolysis.
- After successful synechiolysis, iris retractor devices (hooks or rings) can help to expand the pupil. Another option is to use the "under the blankets" technique.
- Utilize high magnification and appropriate illumination to ensure that there is no trauma to the anterior capsule during this technique.
- Although rare, capsule runouts can occur in areas of prior iridocapsular adhesions.

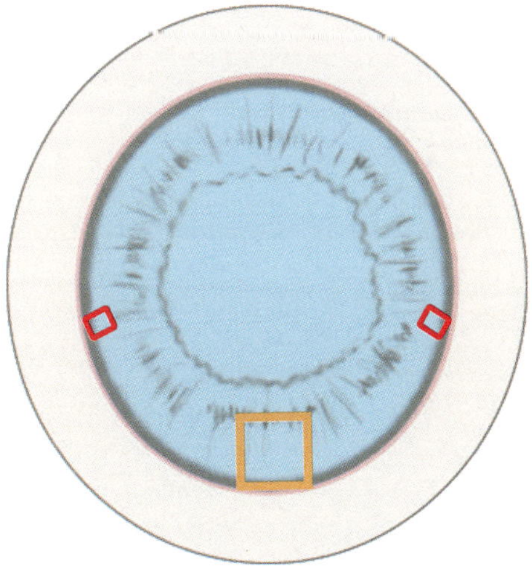

- Standard phaco with knife and fork

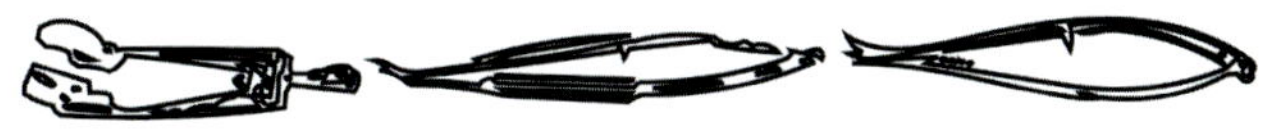

- Angled Kuglen hook
- Cohesive OVD on a 27-g blunt cannula

Ahmed IK, Campos-Möller X, Shah M, Sheybani A. *Illustrated Advanced Anterior Segment Surgery: A Step-by-Step Guide for Challenging Cases* (pp 27-29).

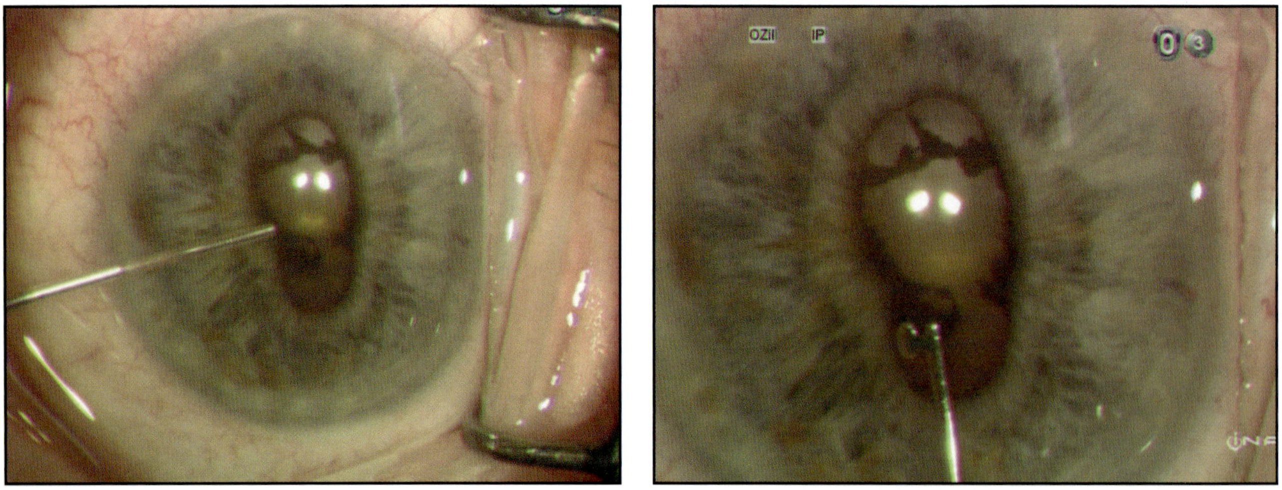

Cohesive OVD injected under the iris through an area where there are no synechiae can be used to viscodissect iris from anterior capsule. A Kuglen hook can then be used to lift the pupil margin upward and peripherally. Avoid touching the anterior capsule when possible. Ensure a 360-degree synechiae liberation. Light, one-instrument stretching can aid in dilating the pupil. We prefer not to use a 2-handed stretch to avoid iris trauma and inflammation. Pupillary membranes should be carefully removed or cut from the pupillary sphincter. If membranes are not removed, iris expansion with hooks can cause radial iris tears.

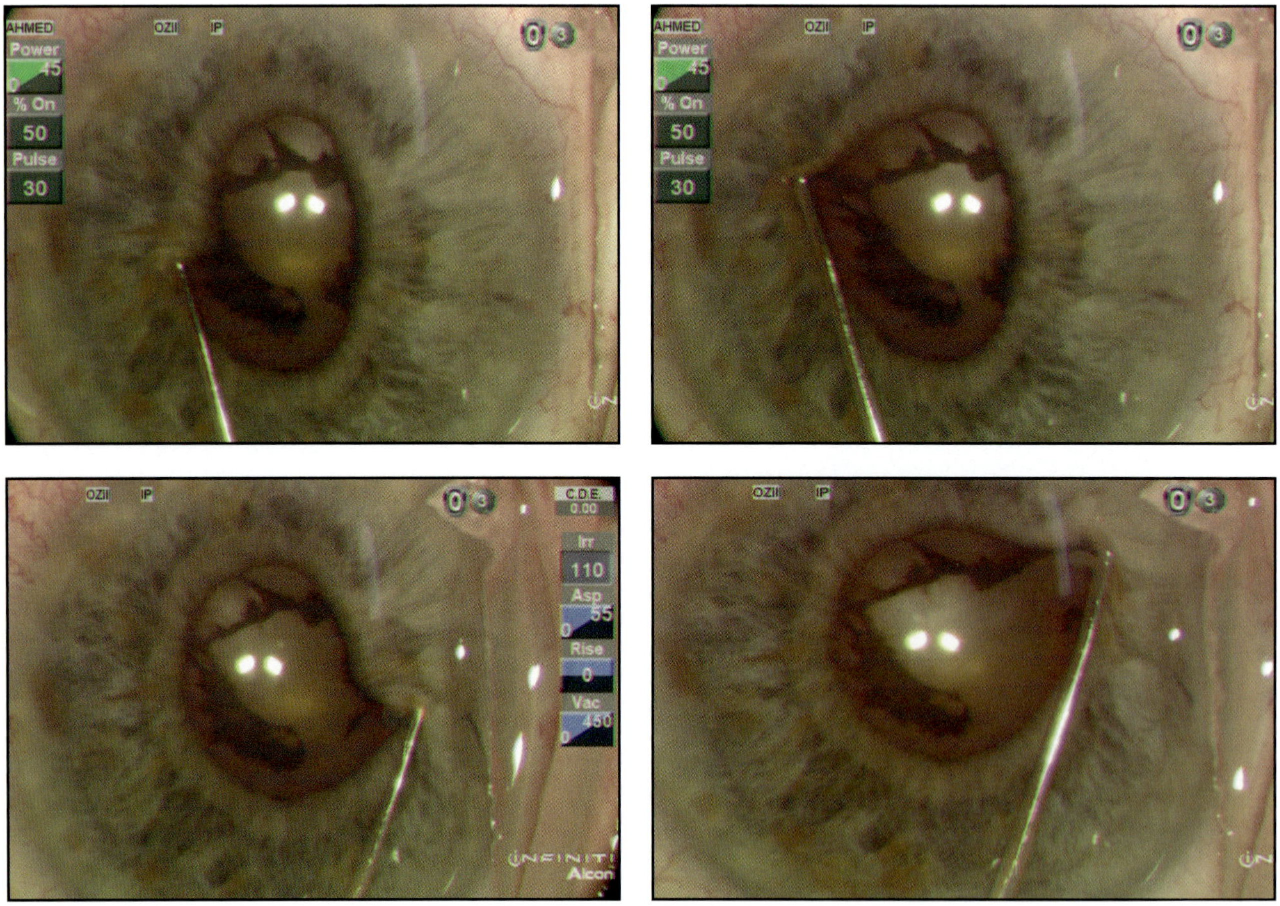

Often, one can achieve nearly 360 degrees of dissection through an incision, but additional incisions may be created as needed to fully release all synechiae.

UNDER THE COVERS CAPSULORRHEXIS

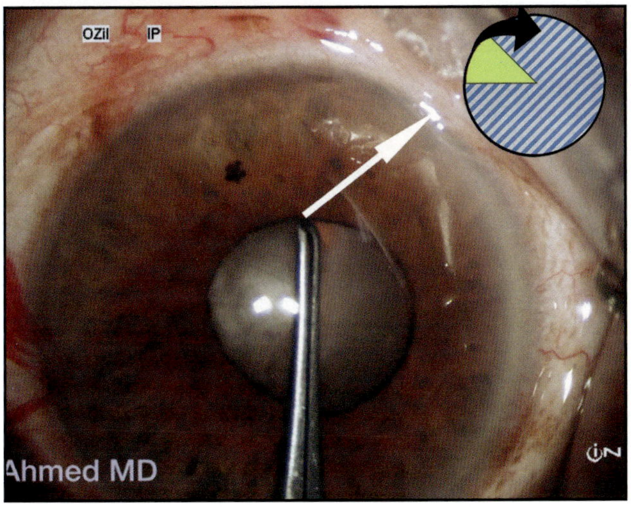

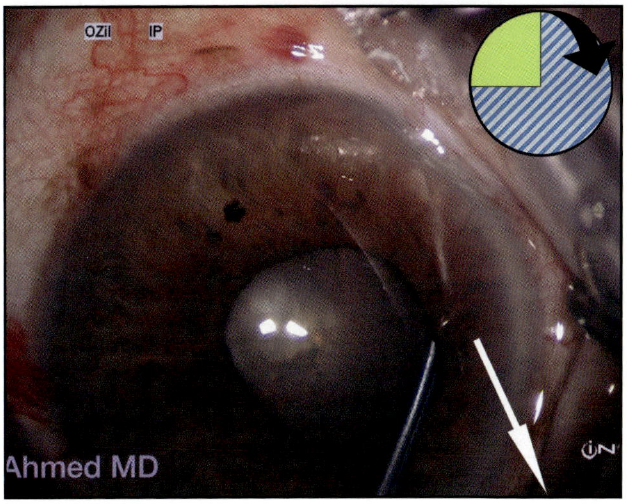

The "under the covers" rhexis is a blind capsulorrhexis maneuver. If the correct concepts are applied, it is actually easier than it seems. The angle of the capsulorrhexis fold is indicative of the direction of travel of the rhexis edge. The capsulorrhexis forceps can even be used under the iris (top right image). Notice how the capsule fold is always perpendicular to the rhexis edge. This is a good indicator that the edge is running circularly. Think of the hands of a clock—they always point radially at the clock hour—so should this fold. White arrows indicate the direction of movement of the capsulorrhexis forceps, and the black arrows indicate the resulting vector of rhexis tear. Circle inserts aid in localization of rhexis edge within each image.

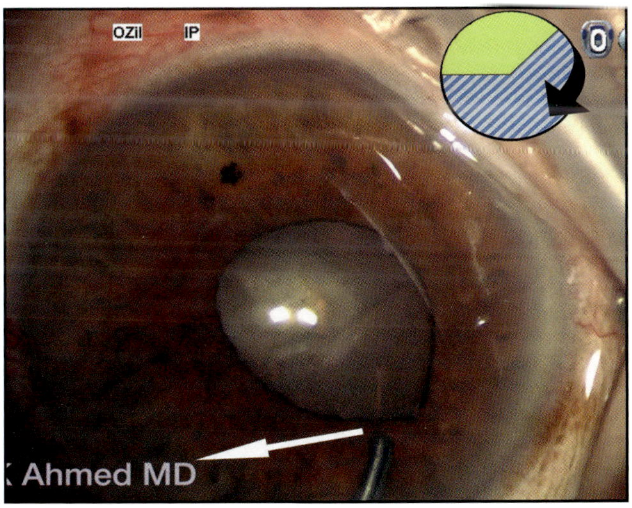

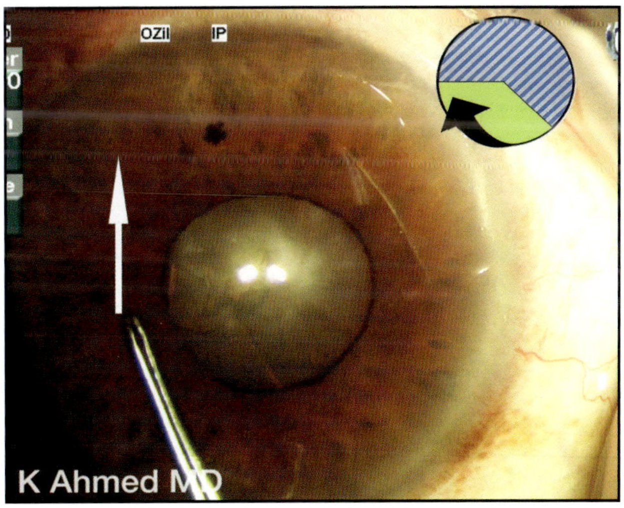

CHAPTER 5

HOW TO INSERT AND REMOVE IRIS HOOKS

INTRODUCTION

Iris hooks can be very useful in the management of small pupil cases or just to increase visualization of the peripheral posterior chamber. In more advanced cases, as you will see in chapters to come, iris hooks can be utilized to stabilize a capsulorrhexis edge in the setting of zonular laxity, and they can be used to secure capsule tension devices for intraoperative stabilization.

KEY POINTS

- Hook insertion is a 2-handed job. You must be comfortable switching between left and right hands for the various steps as needed based on which side of the limbus you are working on.
- Insert all of your hooks and just engage iris before tightening one down.
- It is best to be gentle and work symmetrically, tightening them after all have been placed.
- Create incisions just posterior to the limbus—NOT clear corneal!
- Large stab incisions will leak during the case; since iris hooks can fit through very small incisions, it is preferable to keep these incisions narrow.
- Aim the stab incisions posteriorly toward the mid-iris, not parallel to the iris plane. This will prevent the pupil from being pulled up too far toward the cornea.
- Be cautious not to engage or tear the anterior capsule with the hook tips.
- Think of the hooks as you would an oar on a rowboat: if you want the hook end to go down toward the pupil, you must lift upon the trailing, external end. The incision acts as a fulcrum.
- With disposable hooks, it may be advisable to trim the external ends of the hooks supporting the superior and inferior pupil after tightening. With patient movement, these hooks can interact with the patient's lids to cause pain and distort the intraocular contents.
- For a small pupil case, typically 4 hooks are adequate. However, for an intraoperative floppy iris syndrome case, an additional fifth hook placed subincisionally can be helpful.

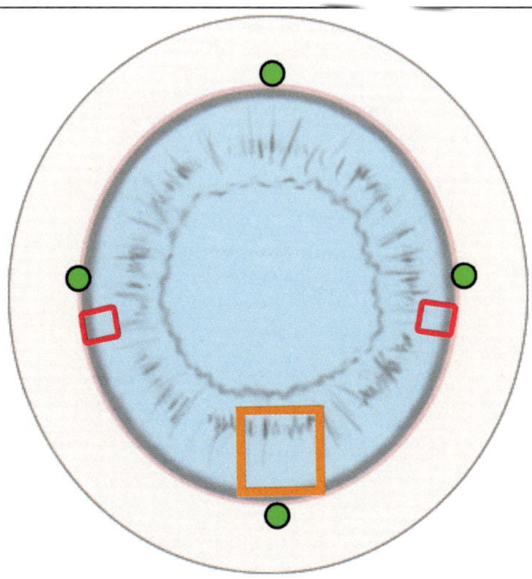

- Standard phaco
- Small stab incisions, limbal, <1 mm width, placed at 4 to 5 points

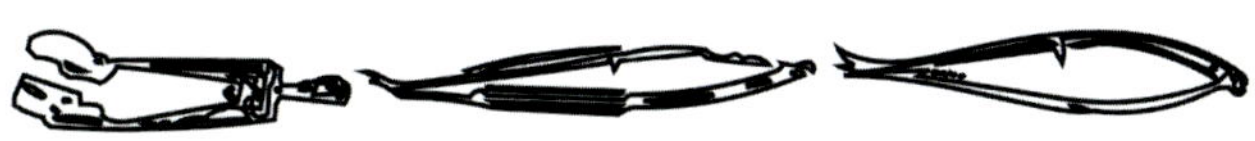

- Side port blade
- Colibri forceps
- Curved or straight tyers
- Iris hooks

Ahmed IK, Campos-Möller X, Shah M, Sheybani A. *Illustrated Advanced Anterior Segment Surgery: A Step-by-Step Guide for Challenging Cases* (pp 31-36).

The first step is to decide what sector(s) of the iris need to be retracted; this will determine the distribution of the iris hooks. If there are specific areas of the posterior chamber that need to be visualized, place hooks accordingly. We prefer a posterior limbal incision to pull the iris more parallel to the iris plane, rather than up toward the cornea. We aim incisions posteriorly toward the pupil margin to facilitate engagement with the hook. Incisions need not be wide; less than 1 mm is usually enough.

More posterior incisions allow for a hook trajectory that is parallel to the iris plane and are more suitable for iris retraction than anterior incisions, which allow for a hook trajectory that is oblique to the iris plane and are more suitable for capsular support.

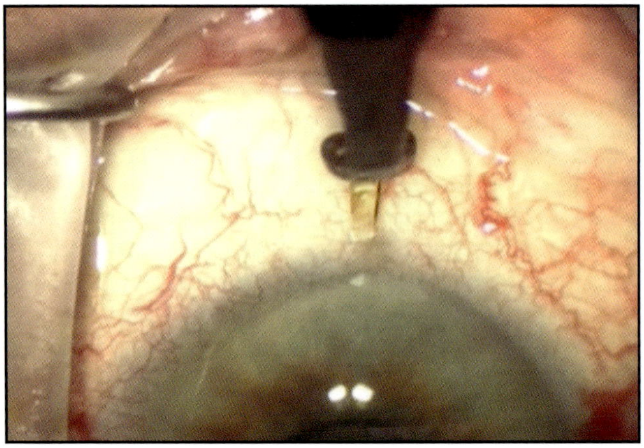

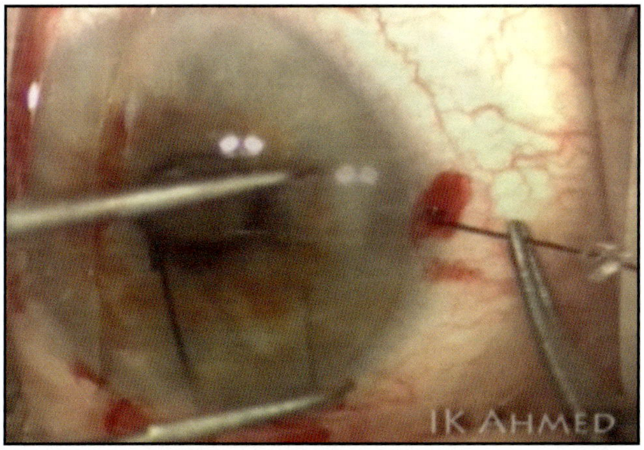

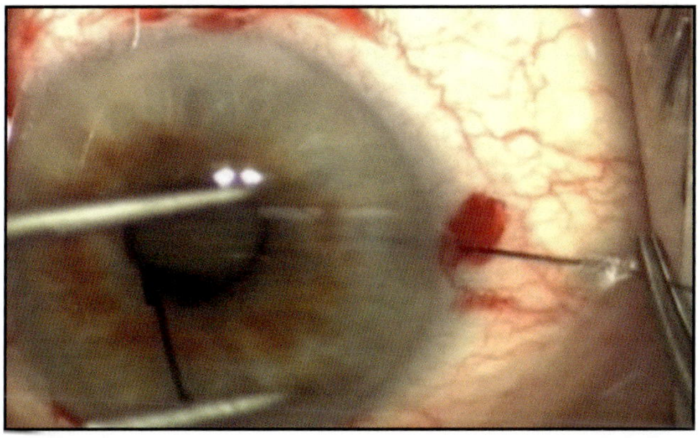

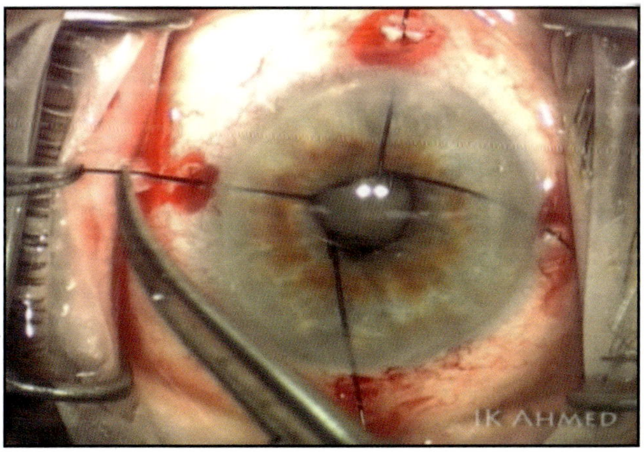

- To make entry easier, use your tying forceps to grab the hook just distal to the hook end, and advance this business end into the anterior chamber.
- Aim the hook toward the pupil margin, remembering to operate the hook like an oar.
- Grasp the distal end of the hook with tyers to stabilize it while advancing the slider to secure the hook in place. Do not fully retract the iris until all hooks have been placed.
- Repeat the above steps as needed until all hooks have been placed.
- Tighten the hooks sequentially after all of them are engaging the pupil.

Rotating the hook from the sleeve will allow for correct orientation of the working end of the hook.

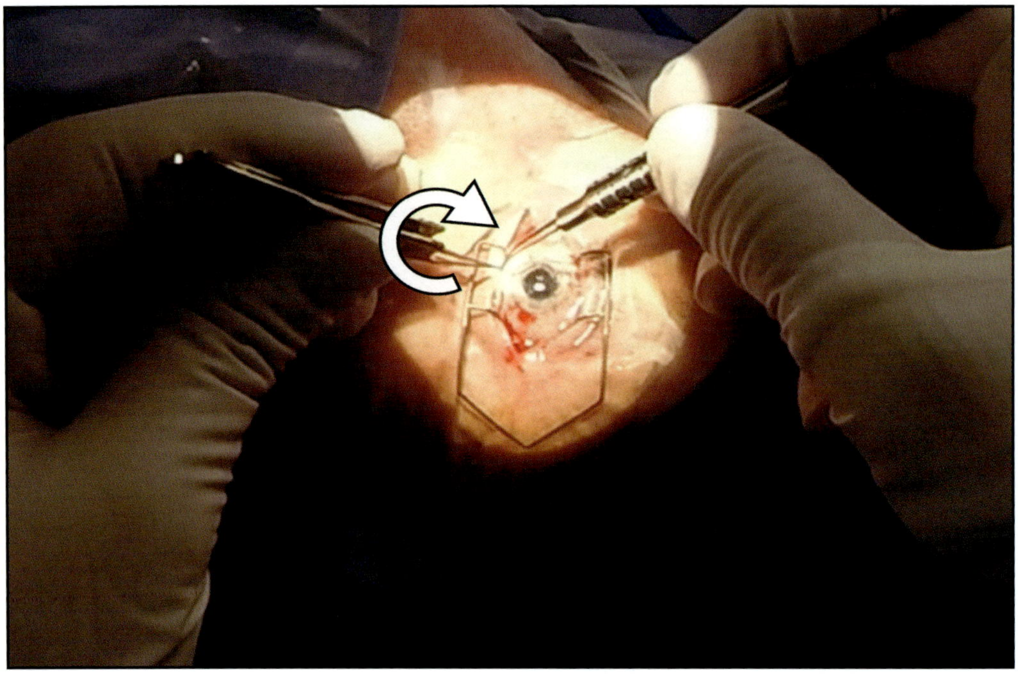

Once the iris has been engaged, the sleeve can be advanced down the shaft of the hook to adjust tension on the pupil margin and degree of dilation.

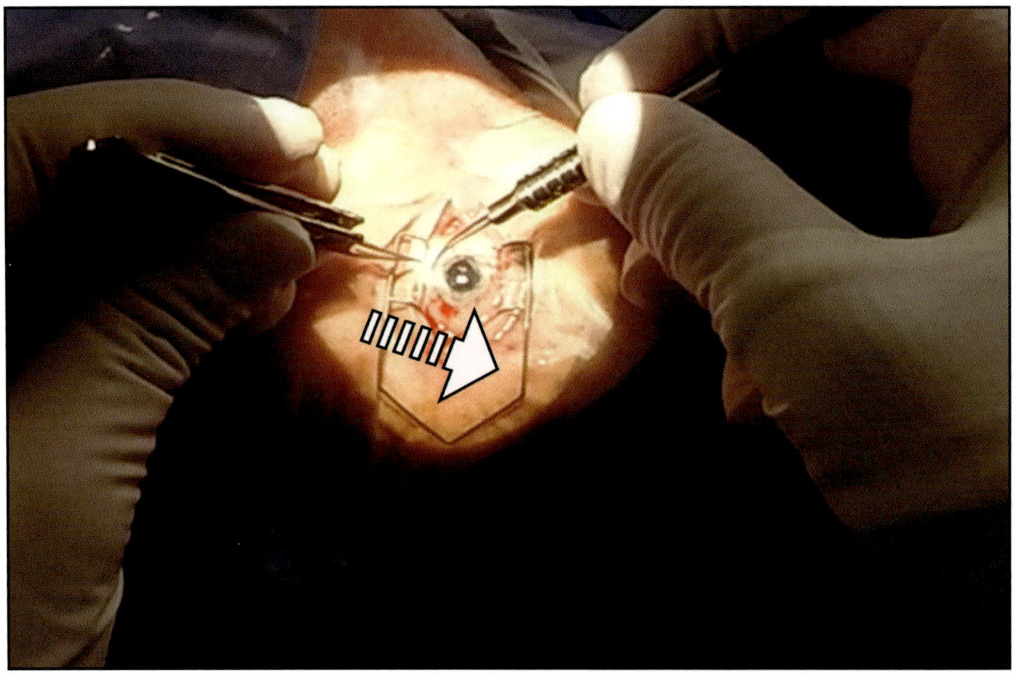

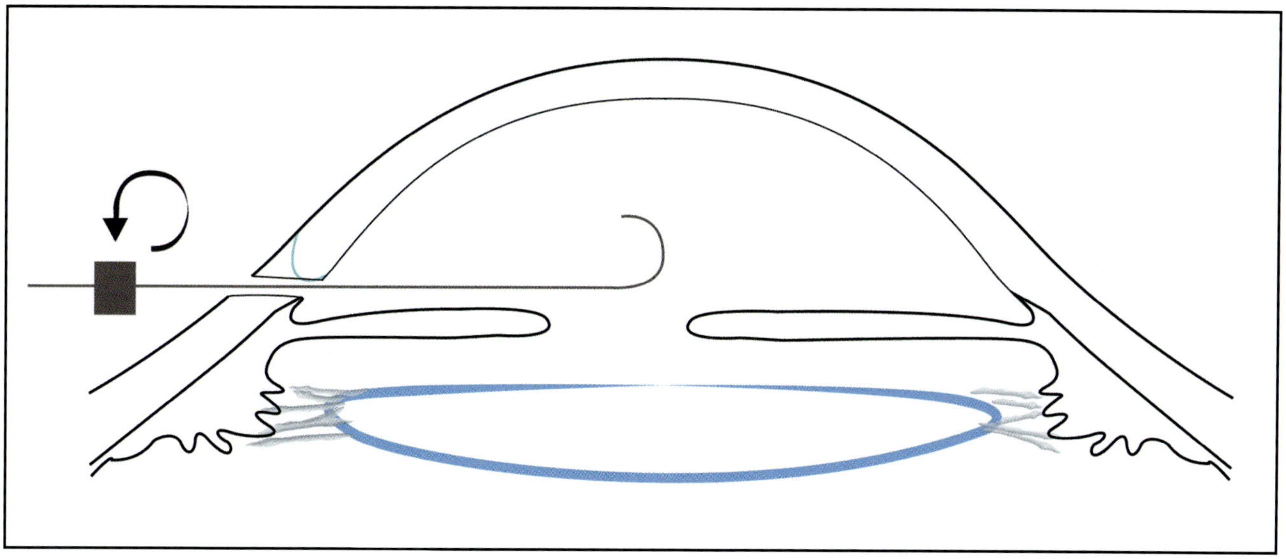

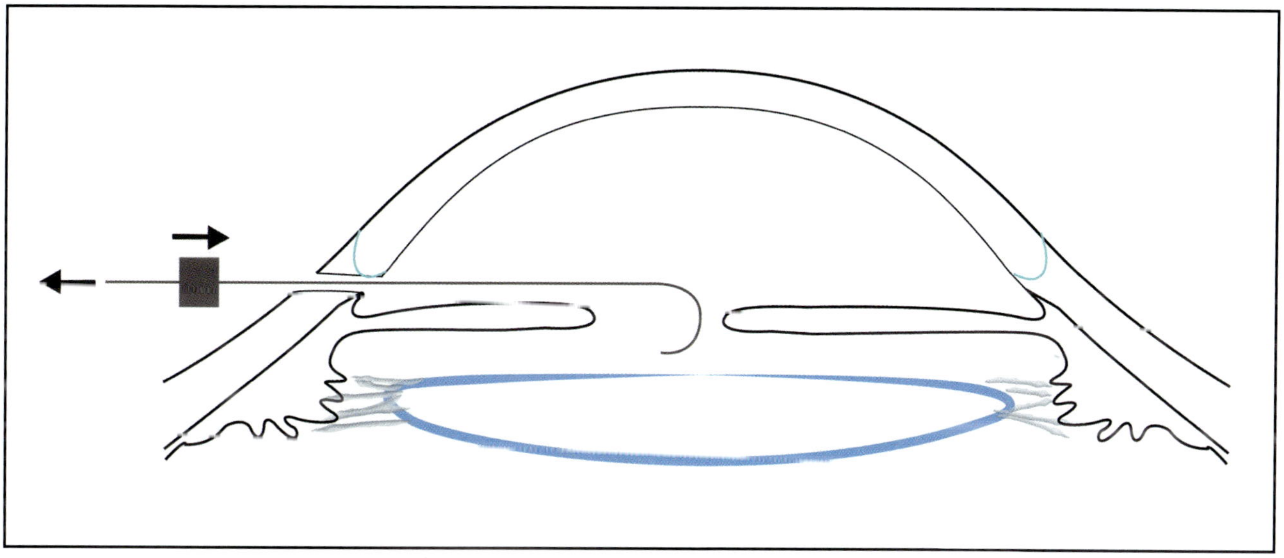

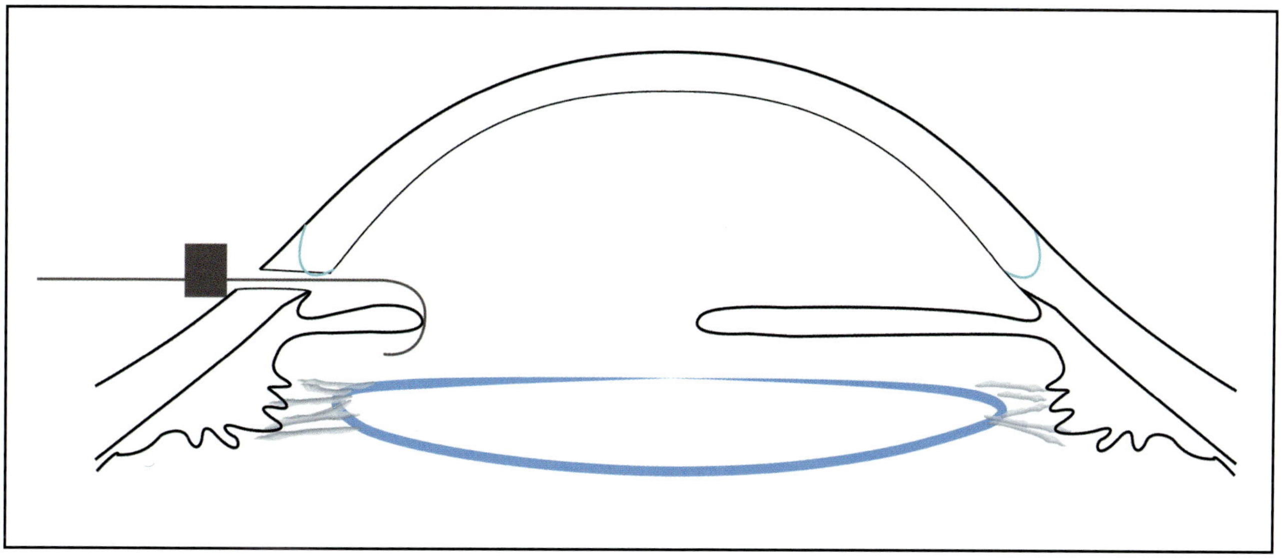

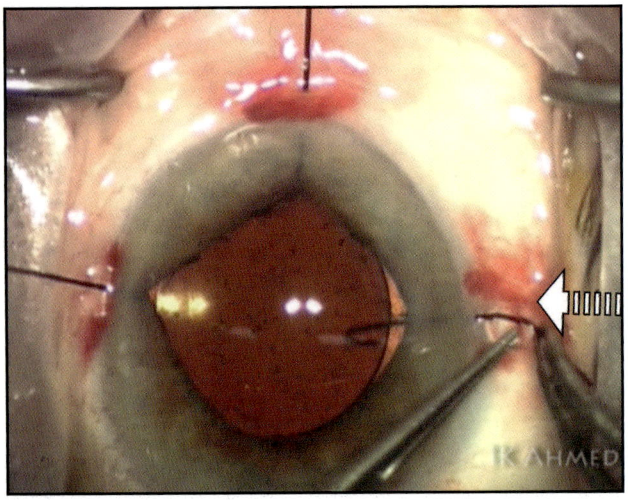

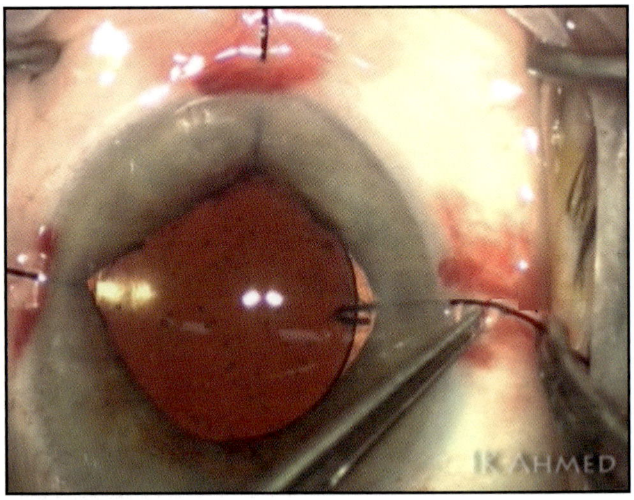

To release the hook from the pupil margin, hold the sleeve with a forceps in 1 hand and slide the shaft of the hook forward with a tyer in the other hand.

To explant, keep the hook parallel to the iris plane and change the angle around 45 degrees to avoid catching the hook on the incision. The movement should follow the shape of the hook tip.

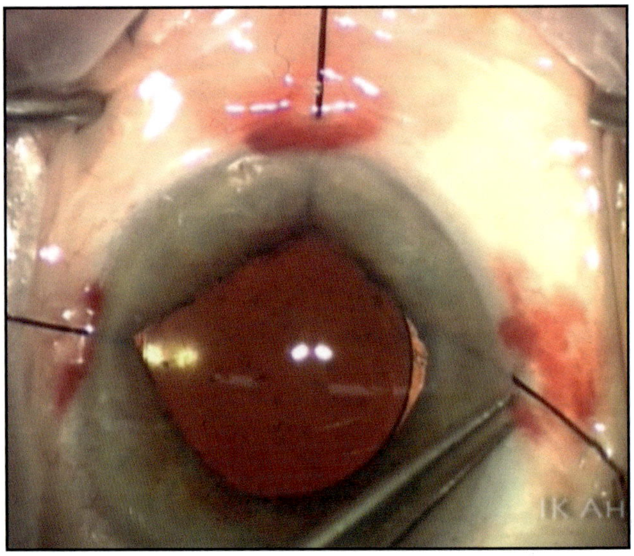

CHAPTER 6

HOW TO INSERT AND REMOVE MALYUGIN RINGS

INTRODUCTION

The Malyugin ring is a one-step pupil expander that is useful in a variety of small pupil and intraoperative floppy iris syndrome cases. The device is easily deployed through a one-handed injector system, and the same injector can be utilized in device retrieval.

With its "diamond" configuration, the ring expands the pupil in a manner that facilitates entry and exit of instruments through a temporal corneal incision and a paracentesis.

KEY POINTS

- While the Malyugin ring can be placed by relying only on the dominant hand, using a second instrument can make insertion more efficient.
- Inject some cohesive ophthalmic viscosurgical device (OVD) under the nasal iris to facilitate engagement with the leading loop.
- While the ring is very easy to use, in combination with its injector, it can be somewhat bulky.
- Be mindful of the device's dimensions. Avoid endothelial trauma and consider an alternative iris retractor in eyes with small anterior chamber depths.
- Avoid Malyugin ring insertion if a capsulotomy has been started as there is risk for capsular tears during insertion.
- During the procedure, avoid inadvertent capture of the capsulotomy edge with potential for zonular injury.

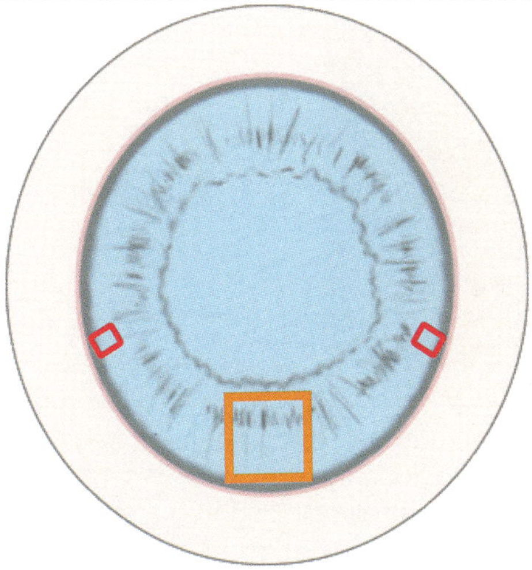

- Standard phaco with knife and fork paracentesis

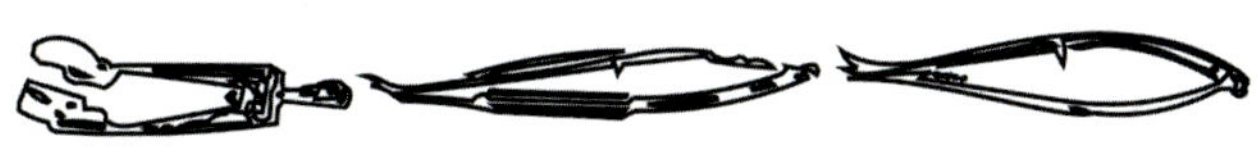

- Cohesive OVD
- Malyugin ring and inserter—the ring comes in 6.25- and 7-mm sizes—choose based on the pre-existing pupil diameter (6.25 mm is adequate in most cases)
- Mini collar button or Kuglen hook

Ahmed IK, Campos-Möller X, Shah M, Sheybani A. *Illustrated Advanced Anterior Segment Surgery: A Step-by-Step Guide for Challenging Cases* (pp 37-42).

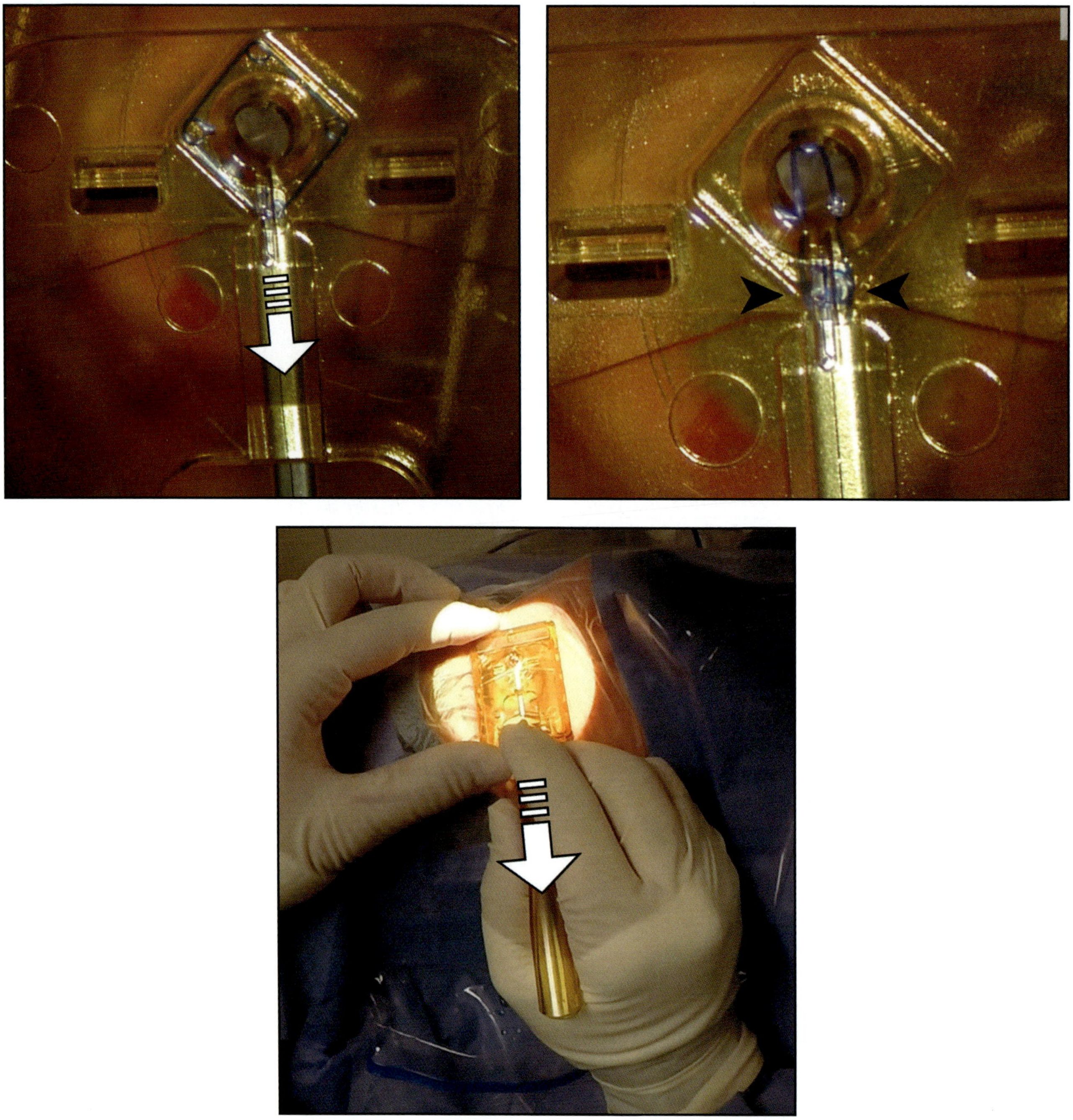

The Malyugin ring comes inside a case that is attached to the injector, but the device needs to be retracted into the injector before uncoupling from the case. To do this, slowly pull back on the sliding knob (white arrow), ensuring that the hook of the injector has engaged with the trailing loop of the Malyugin ring. Pay attention to the 2 central scrolls (black arrows) as they enter the shaft of the injector because they can get entangled. Once the ring is completely inside the injector, it can be separated from the cartridge, and the device is loaded for use.

- Create a temporal clear corneal incision.
- Instill dispersive OVD to protect the corneal endothelium.
- Instill a small amount of viscoelastic under the nasal pupil to gently lift up the pupil margin, being careful not to overfill.
- Insert the injector into the anterior chamber with the aid of a 0.12 or Colibri forceps to open the main incision.

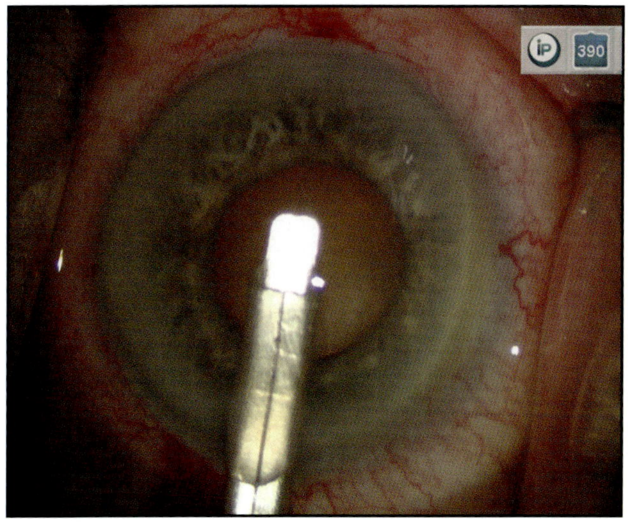

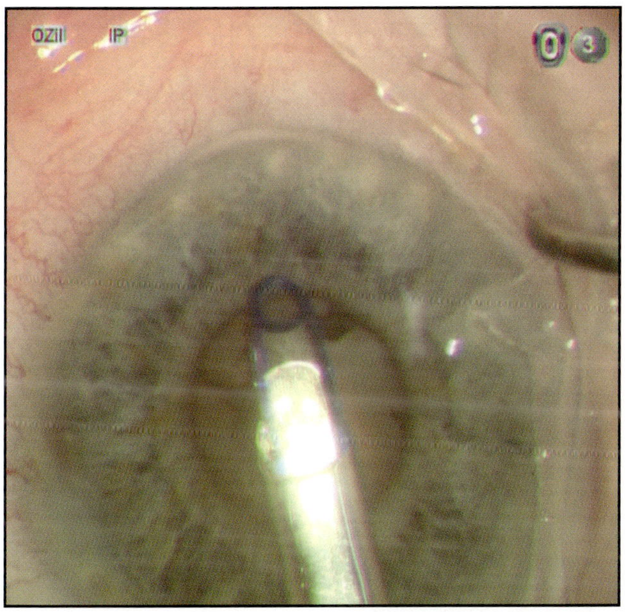

Advance the plunger slightly, to externalize only the leading scroll and engage on the iris directly in front of the injector.

Continue sliding the plunger to deploy the ring while simultaneously pulling the injector back toward the incision. This will prevent the ring from damaging iridocorneal angle structures or causing an iridodialysis.

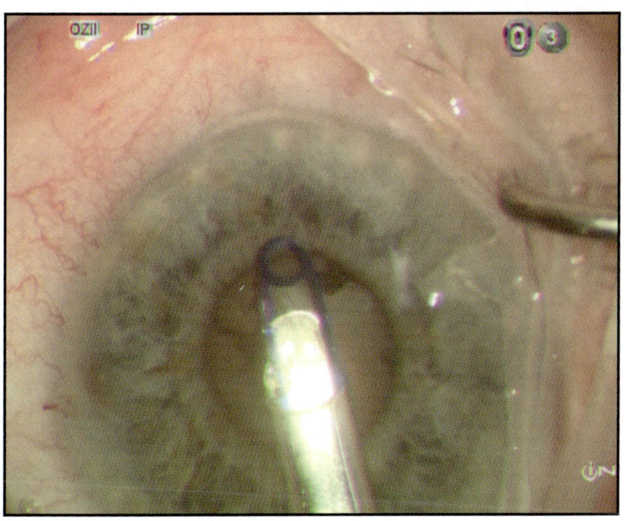

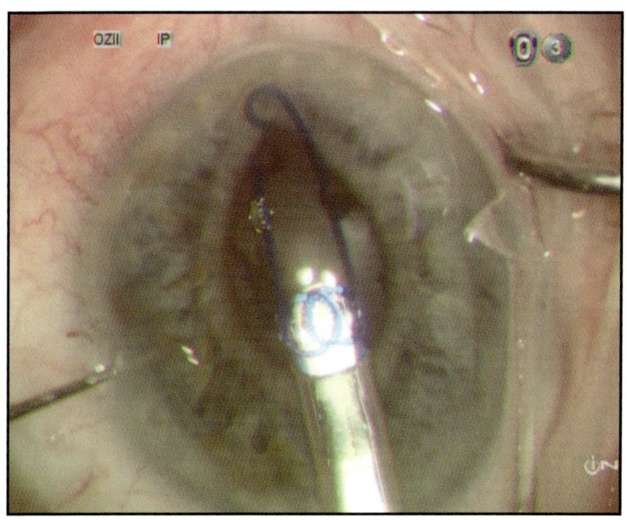

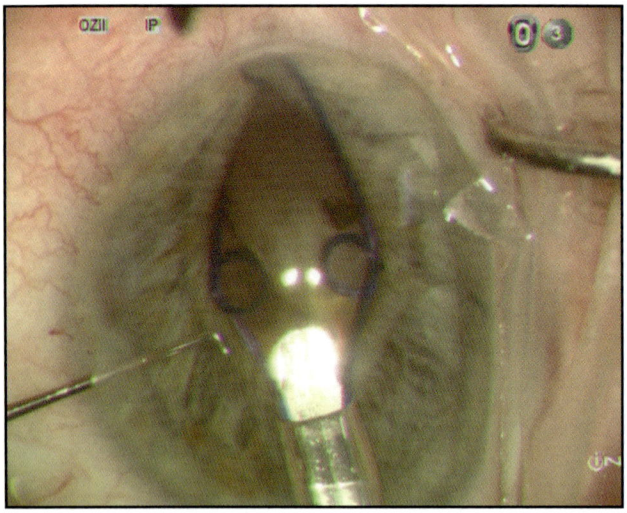

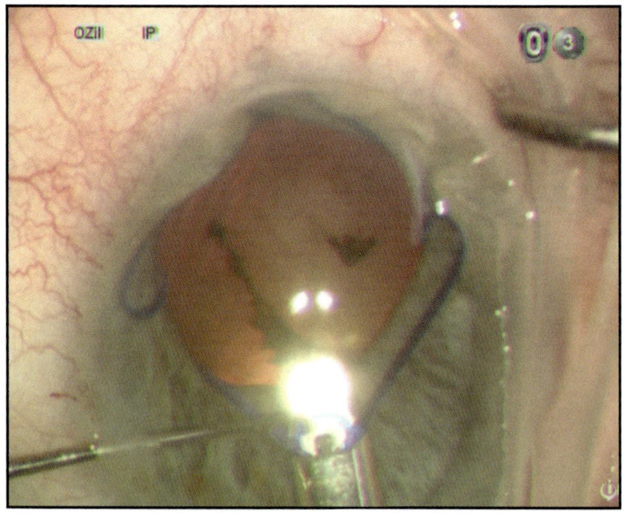

To engage the superior and inferior scrolls, a rocking motion can sometimes be employed. A Sinskey hook through the paracentesis can be used to facilitate adequate engagement. If doing so, it is more effective to hook the bar between the scrolls as opposed to the scrolls themselves. As the device continues to be injected, the trailing scroll will be exposed as the hook of the injector lifts—use the second instrument to position this scroll on the temporal iris. When withdrawing the injector out of the wound, keep the plunger pushed all the way forward; otherwise, it can catch the proximal (temporal) loop and draw the ring out of the eye.

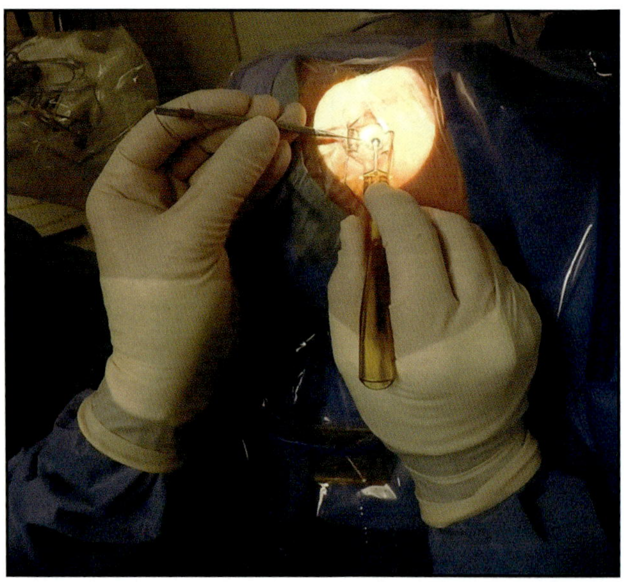

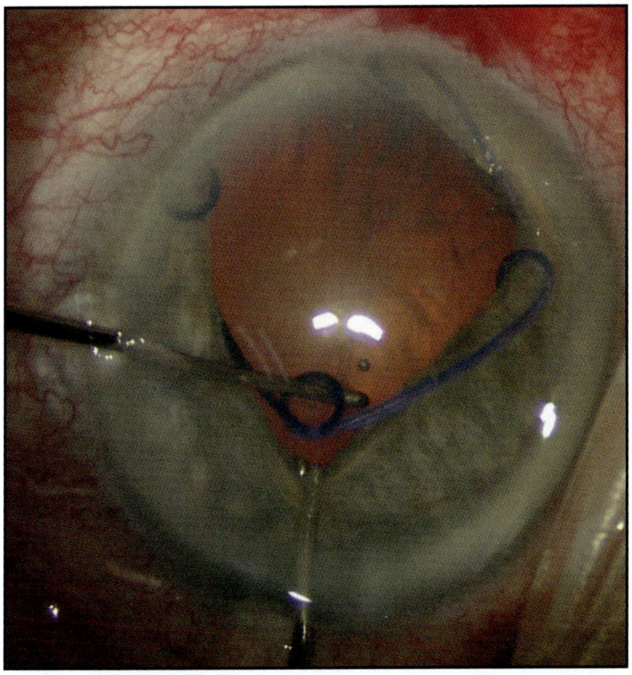

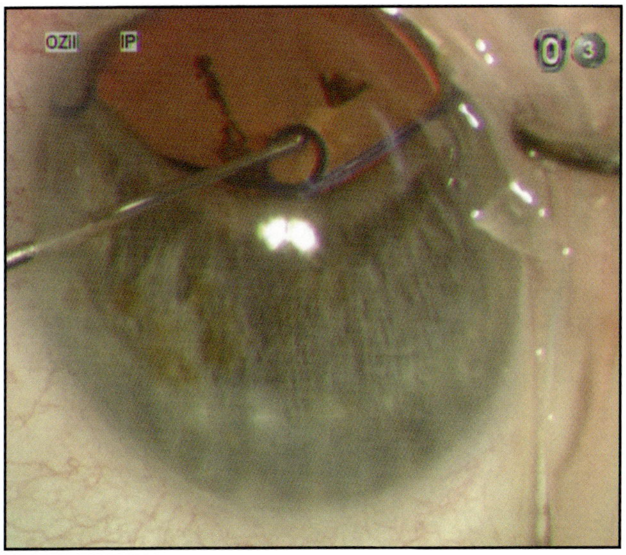

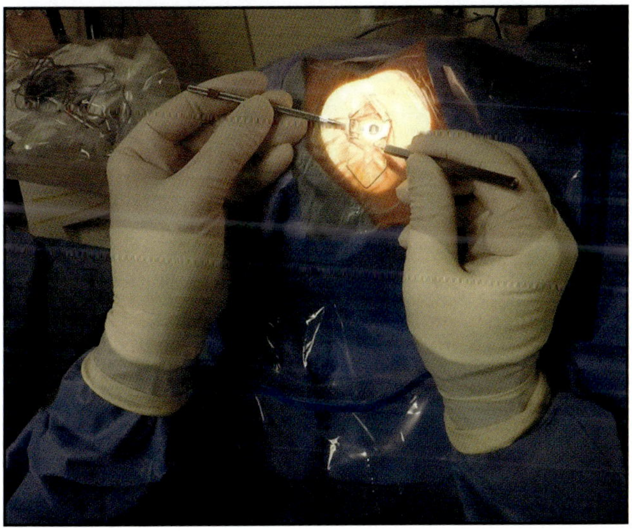

An alternative for engaging the proximal scroll is to use a Kuglen hook to pull the iris peripherally, instead of attempting to push the proximal scroll centrally, which may push the entire ring into the nasal iridocorneal angle. The ring can also be centered on the lens with the use of the Sinskey hook. The capsulorrhexis can now be started.

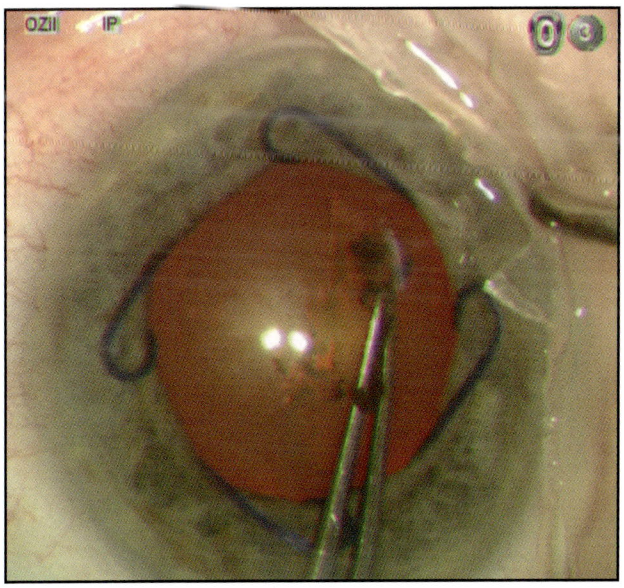

Ring removal. Ensure that the anterior chamber is still formed with OVD. Disengage the distal loop first. With the use of a Sinskey or Kuglen hook, bring it anterior to the iris. Repeat this step for the proximal loop. Insert the injector face down (this allows the hook to be pointed away from the corneal endothelium). Catch the hook on the distal (temporal) loop. Slowly pull back on the sliding button, making sure the superior and inferior loops are no longer attached to the iris, and not twisting. Use the second instrument as needed to release them.

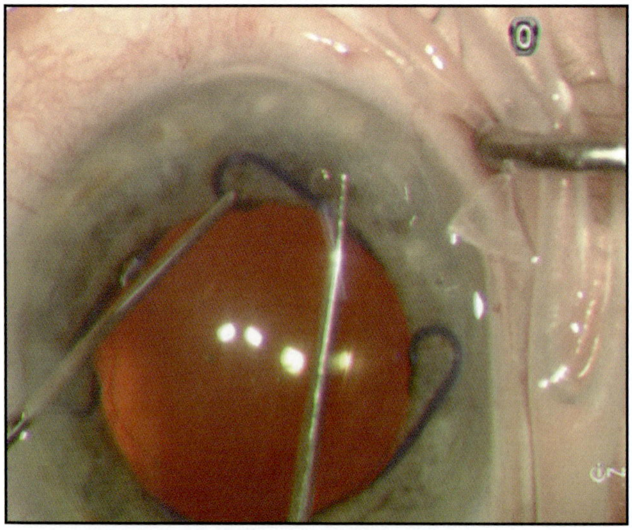

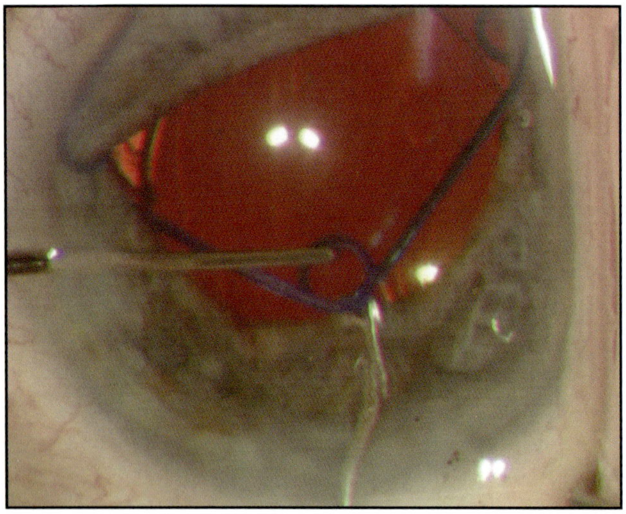

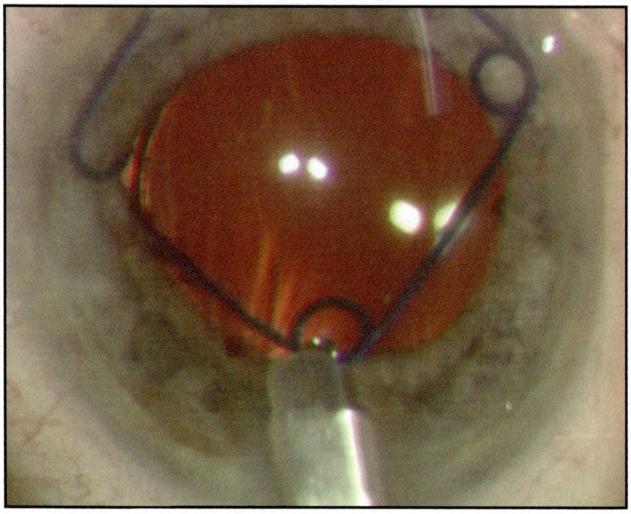

It may be necessary to align the superior and inferior loops inside the injector to facilitate retraction. For this, flip the injector over so that the loops are visible and use a Sinskey hook to feed the loops into the injector shaft. Once the entire ring is inside the shaft of the injector, it can be retrieved from the eye. Sometimes, this is not possible as the scrolls loop around the injector tongue. Bringing the loops to just within the mouth of the injector (below, left) is enough to then remove the device from the eye. The main point with removal is to not force the entire ring into the injector if it catches around a scroll; this may cause the ring to twist and can injure ocular structures.

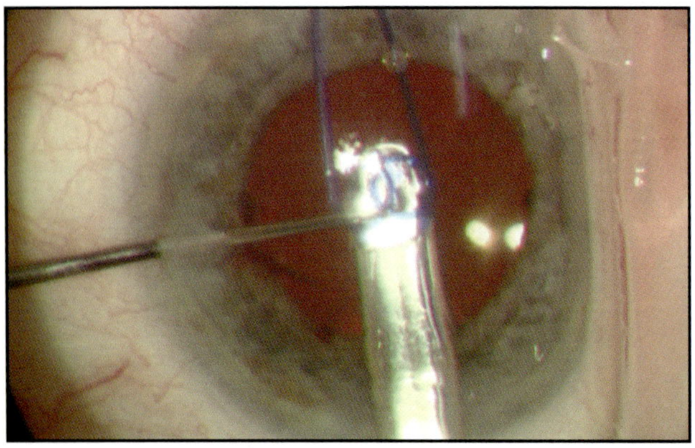

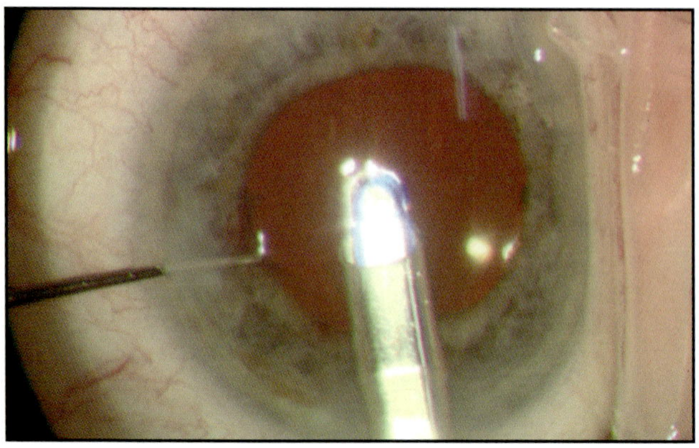

CHAPTER 7

CAPSULORRHEXIS IN THE SETTING OF WEAK ZONULES

INTRODUCTION

Adequate capsulorrhexis creation is pivotal in performing successful phacoemulsification.

However, the act requires countertraction from an intact zonular apparatus. Zonular laxity can make initiation and propagation of the capsulorrhexis a very difficult endeavor.

Additionally, as these cases may rely upon advanced support devices (such as capsule retractors, capsular tension rings, and capsular tension segments), a continuous and curvilinear capsulotomy is of utmost importance.

KEY POINTS

- A successful capsulorrhexis relies on countertraction, so be aware of the areas where zonular support is present, and where it is not.
- Use both the dominant and nondominant hand for propagating the capsulorrhexis.
- Take care not to make the capsulorrhexis too big or too small. Too small, and nuclear mobilization becomes difficult, risking further zonular stress. Too large, and there may be an insufficient anterior capsule shelf for utilization of capsule hooks or capsular support devices.
- Place iris hooks in the anterior chamber before starting the capsulorrhexis.
- Be familiar with intraocular microinstruments (micrograspers, microscissors, microforceps).
- Identify areas of focal zonulopathy by using a Kuglen hook to move the iris out of the way.
- Preoperative imaging, if available, can be very helpful here as well.

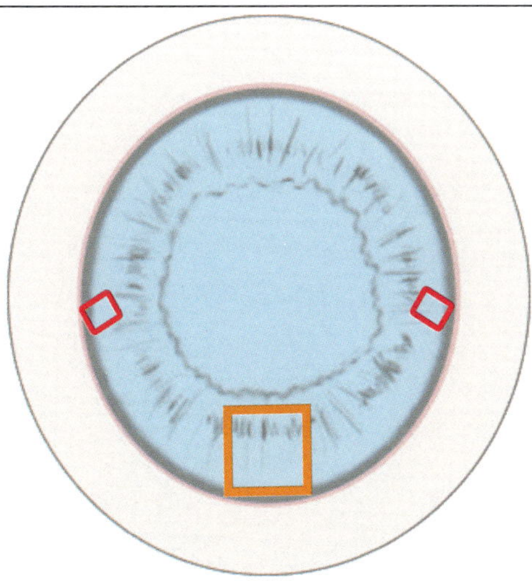

- Standard phaco with knife and fork

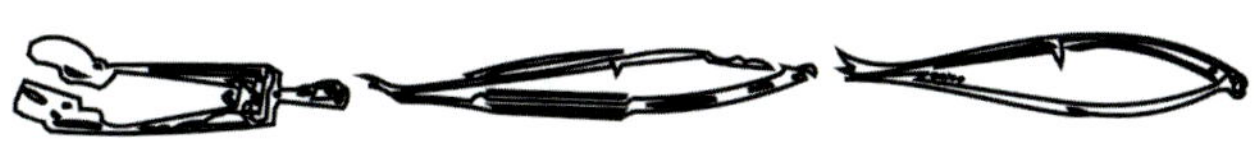

- Capsulorrhexis forceps
- Microsurgical Technology, Inc iris micrograspers
- Iris hooks
- Kuglen hook

Ahmed IK, Campos-Möller X, Shah M, Sheybani A. *Illustrated Advanced Anterior Segment Surgery: A Step-by-Step Guide for Challenging Cases* (pp 43-48).

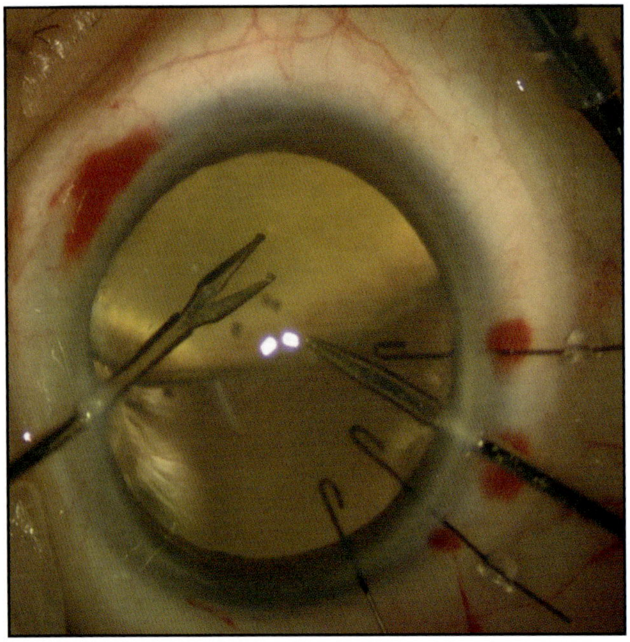

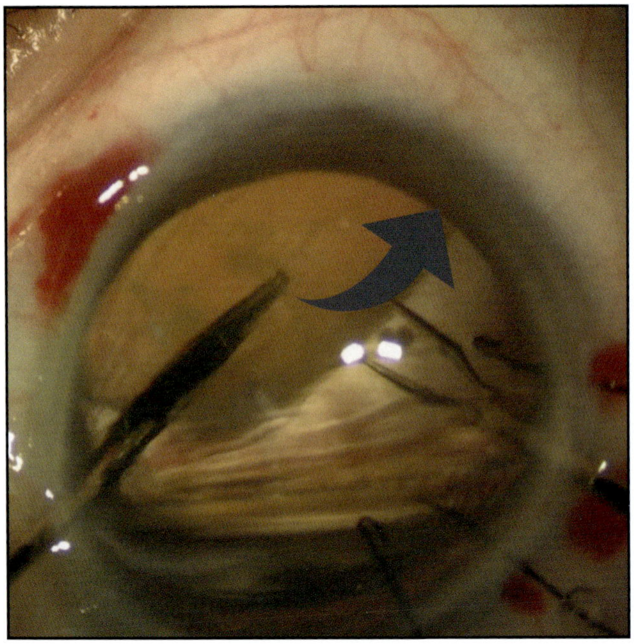

Initiate the capsulorrhexis as you would a routine case, by puncturing the anterior capsule centrally. A high-velocity, low-amplitude movement is necessary. In cases with significant zonular laxity, you may not be able to successfully puncture through with a sharp forceps, for which a cystotome may be useful.

In the setting of severe lens subluxation, an iris micrograsper can be useful for centering the lens and initiating the capsulorrhexis. Use the iris micrograsper to pinch the center of the lens and bring it toward its normal anatomical position. Use a second iris micrograsper to pinch and tear the beginning of a capsulorrhexis. Be prepared to alternate hands as needed, using one hand to stabilize the lens by grabbing capsulorrhexis edge while using the other hand to further propagate the tear. The principle of countertraction is important here—go toward focal zonulopathy in order to recruit the intact zonules on the opposite side. If the zonulopathy is diffuse, you may need to utilize other means of countertraction. A Kuglen hook can be used to provide countertraction on the capsulorrhexis edge as well.

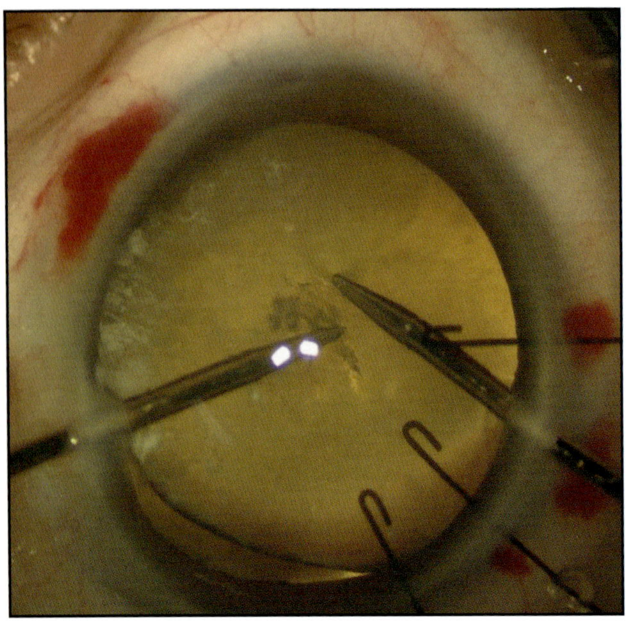

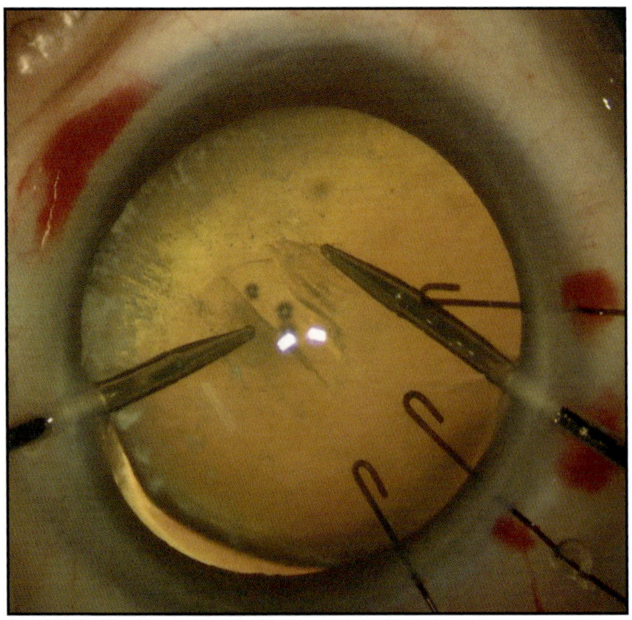

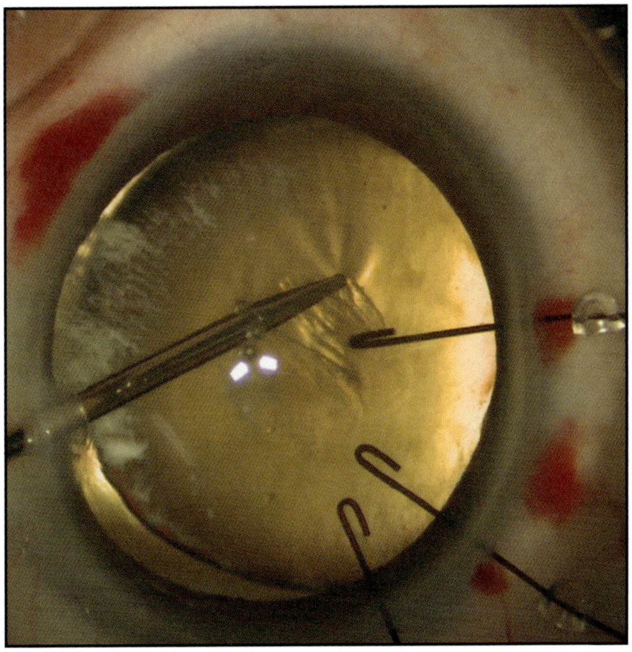

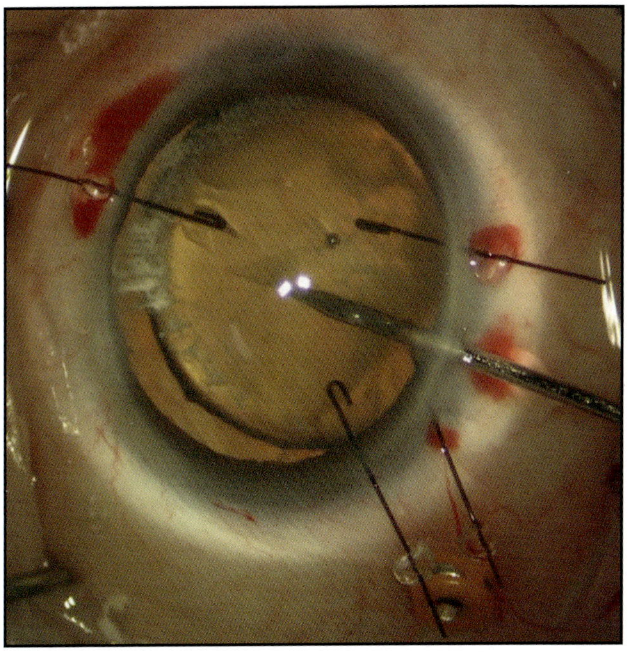

Be prepared to switch hands as needed as you proceed:

- Iris hooks here serve a dual purpose: providing countertraction for capsulorrhexis propagation and maintaining centration and levitation of a severely subluxed lens.

Be very specific about where hooks are inserted:

- Hooks should be placed AWAY from the direction of the capsulorrhexis propagation, such that they provide countertraction.
- As you proceed around the clock, you will need to remove some hooks and place others in new places such that you have countertraction at all times.
- When the capsulorrhexis starts heading in the direction of a hook, that hook must be removed. Failure to do so could result in a runout.
- Place additional hooks to provide countertraction as you continue to propagate the circular capsulorrhexis.
- Take care not to put too much traction on the hooks as this, too, can result in a radial tear.

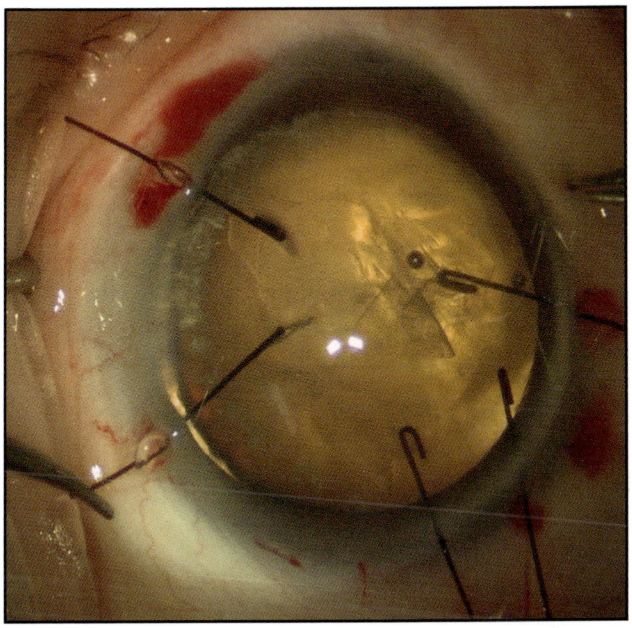

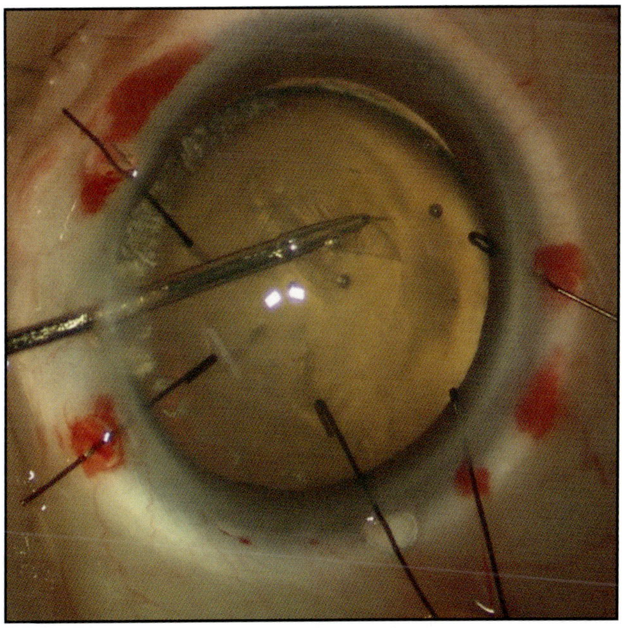

Once the rhexis has been successfully completed, phacoemulsification of the lens can be carried out with the support from the hooks alone, but additional capsular support devices will be required for intraocular lens fixation. The choice of a capsular tension ring, a modified capsular tension ring, or a capsular tension segment will depend on the degree of zonulopathy and surgeon preference. For the case shown in this chapter, we opted for 2 capsular tension segments and a capsular tension ring.

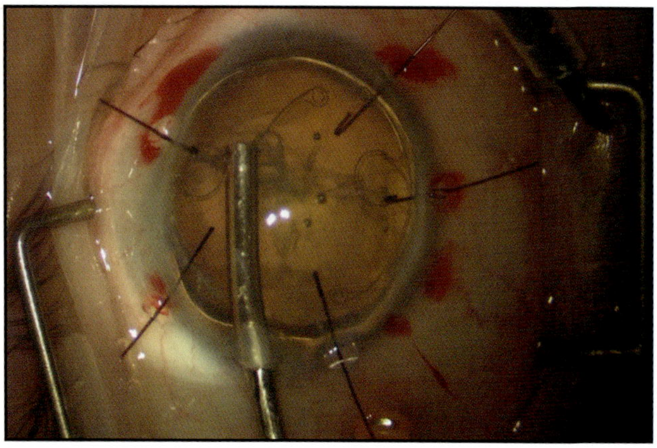

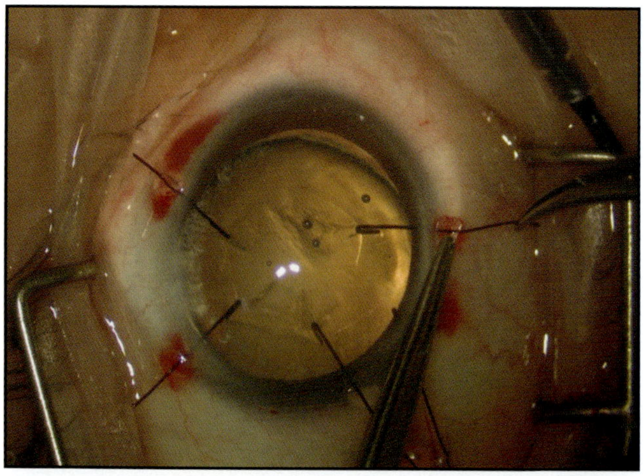

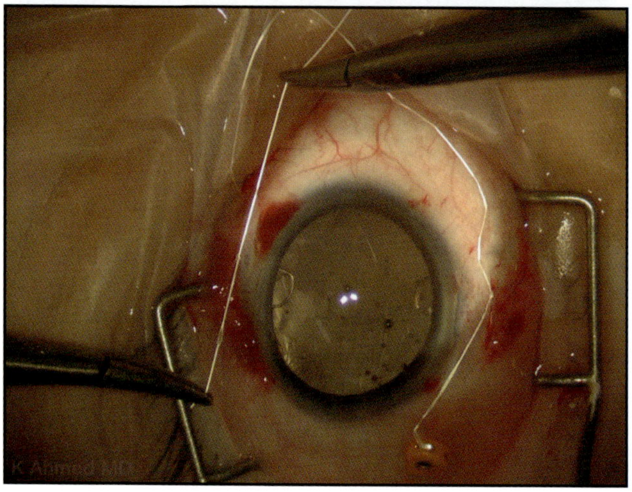

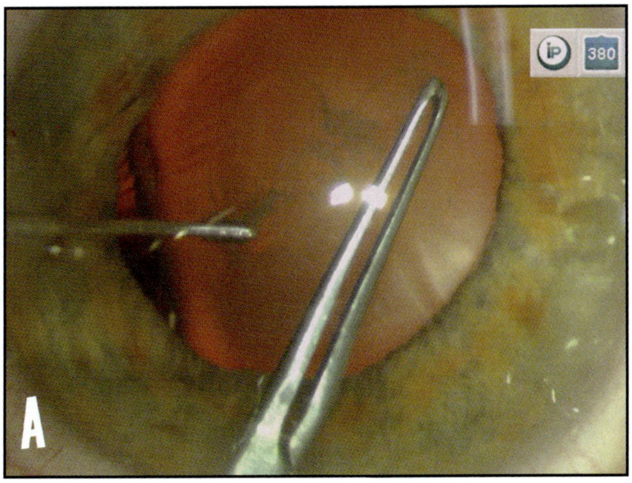

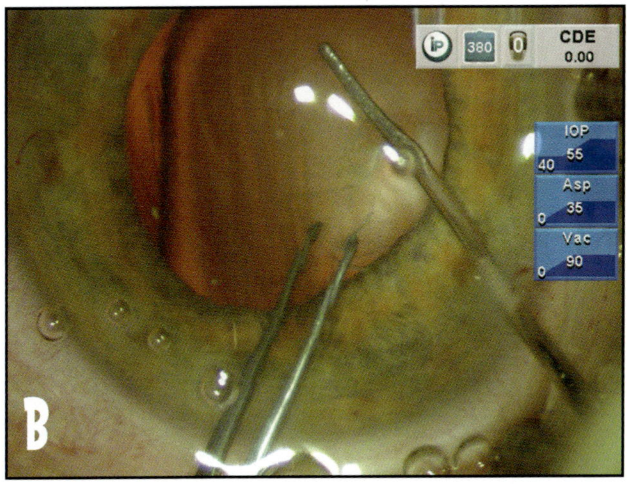

Images A and B are taken from a separate case with less severe zonulopathy, where the Kuglen hook was enough to provide countertraction and the entire rhexis was completed without support from iris hooks or capsule retractors. This is also an option.

Notice how stab incisions for iris hooks are more anterior when their purpose is to support the capsule rather than retract the iris. The more anterior incision placement facilitates a more posterior direction of the iris hook, thus making it easier to engage the capsulorrhexis edge.

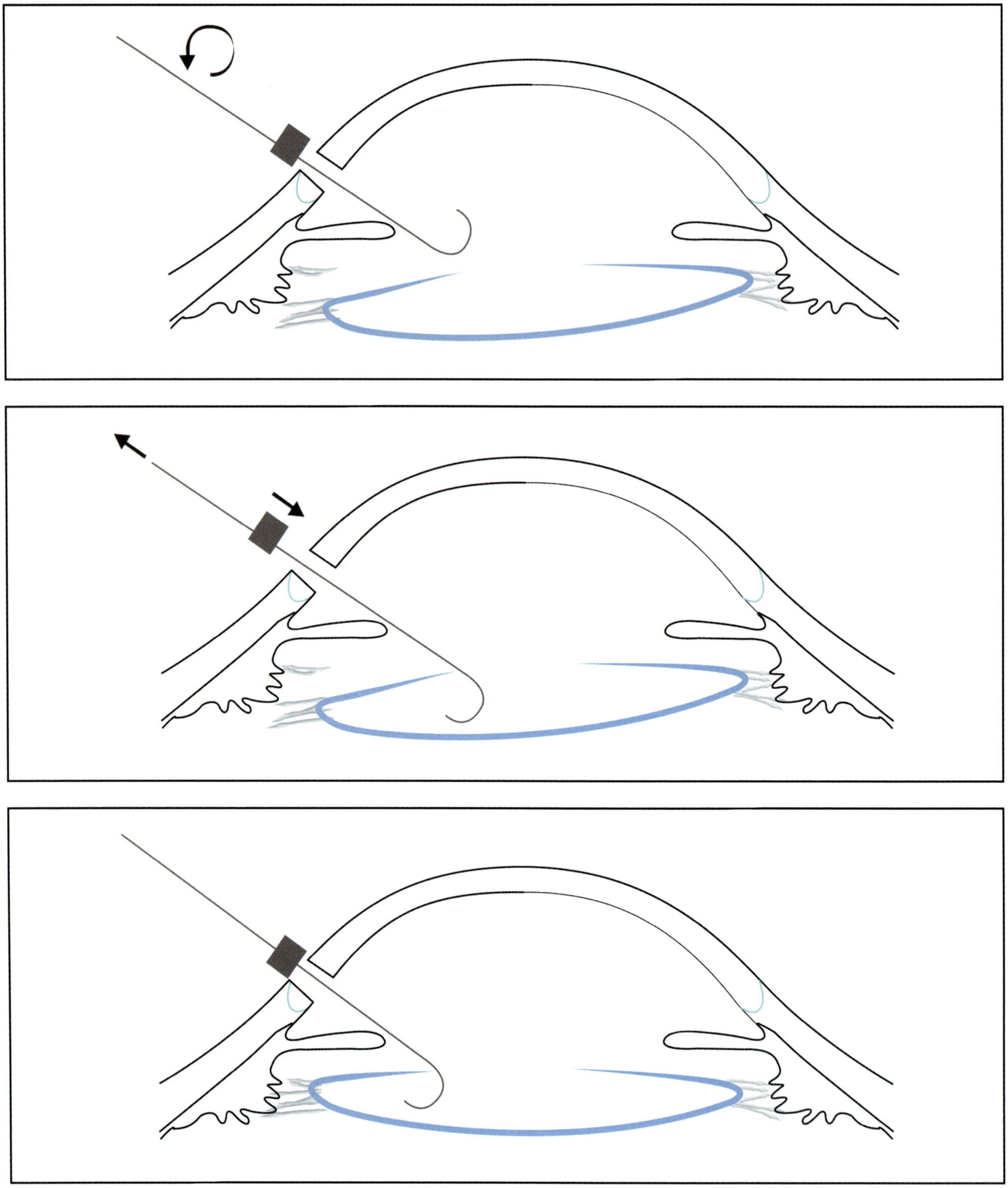

Iris retractor hooks can be used to hold the capsular bag in place during surgery. The key point is to make the incisions in clear cornea, which will naturally direct the hooks posteriorly, instead of parallel to the iris plane. Avoid overtightening of the sleeves as this may cause further zonular damage. Capsule-specific retractors can be implanted similarly and have the advantage of being polished and less prone to causing capsule tears.

CHAPTER 8

OTHER CHALLENGING CAPSULORRHEXIS SITUATIONS

INTRODUCTION

Intumescent cataracts present their own challenges. Often, these cataracts have relatively high intracapsular pressures, which can result in rapid radialization of the capsulorrhexis, also known as the dreaded *Argentinian flag sign*. Furthermore, the anterior capsules in these patients can often have areas of irregular fibrosis or thickening, further complicating the creation of a continuous curvilinear capsulorrhexis.

KEY POINTS

- A careful preoperative exam can often reveal areas of anterior capsule fibrosis or irregularity, as well as fluid-filled clefts within the lens that can be suggestive of increased intracapsular pressure.
- Be prepared for zonulopathy, comorbid pupil defects, or other challenges that might require surgical management.
- Trypan blue is often necessary to visualize the anterior capsule and highlight areas of fibrosis or capsular irregularity.

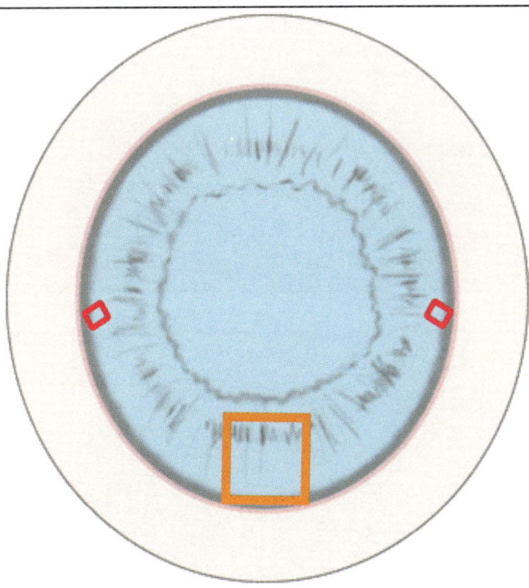

- Standard phaco with knife and fork

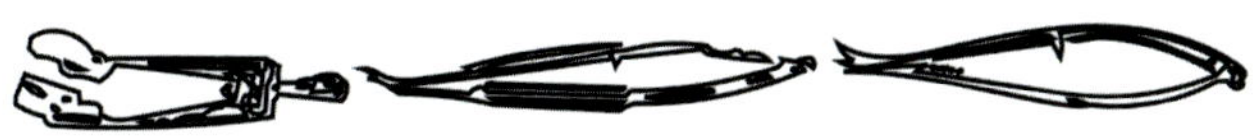

- Trypan blue capsular dye
- 25-g needle on balanced salt solution (BSS) syringe
- Utrata forceps
- Microscissors
- Iris microforceps
- Superviscous ophthalmic viscosurgical device (OVD) such as Healon5 (hyaluronic acid)

Ahmed IK, Campos-Möller X, Shah M, Sheybani A. *Illustrated Advanced Anterior Segment Surgery: A Step-by-Step Guide for Challenging Cases* (pp 49-54).

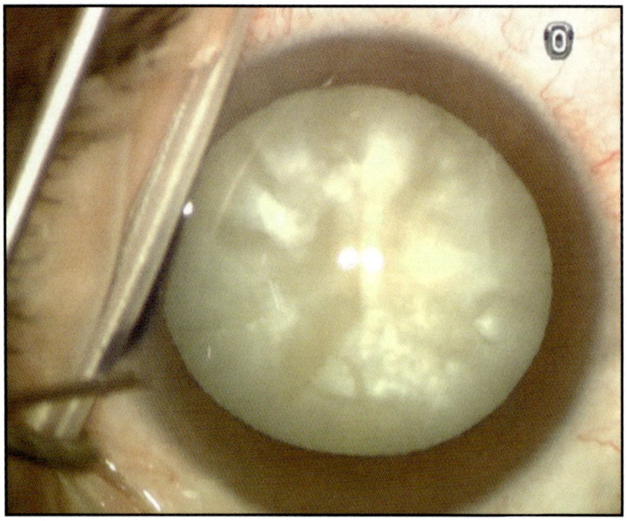

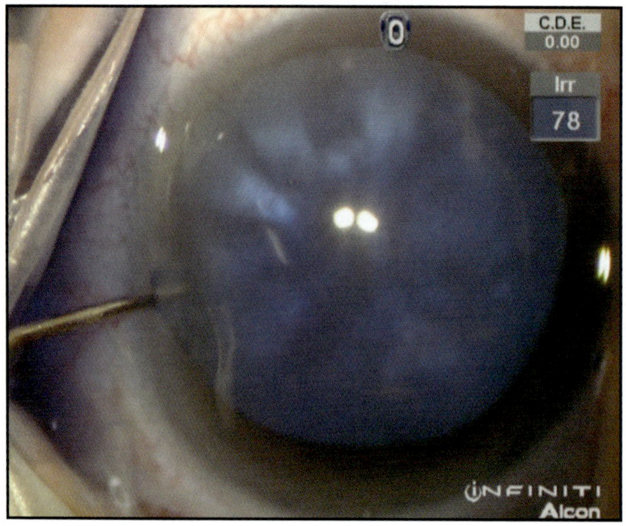

Instill trypan blue to stain the anterior capsule. While this can be done by simply filling the anterior chamber with the stain, there can be some migration posterior to the lens if there is a zonular defect. As such, it may be better to "paint" the anterior capsule under OVD by swiping with the 27-g cannula. Consider the use of a super-cohesive viscoelastic to flatten the anterior capsule.

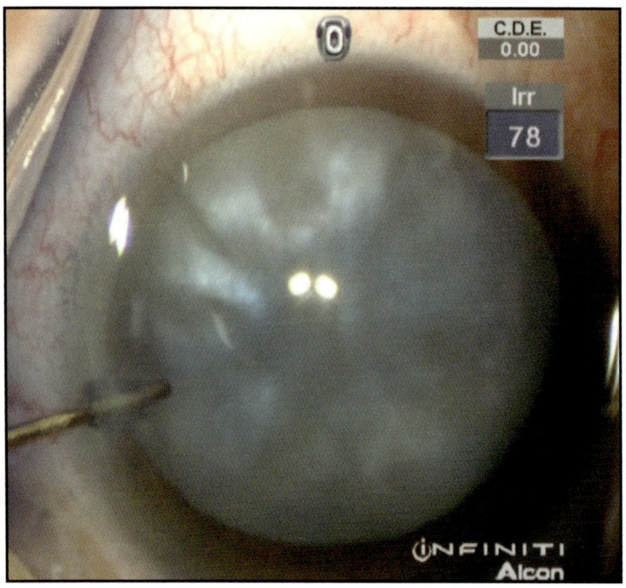

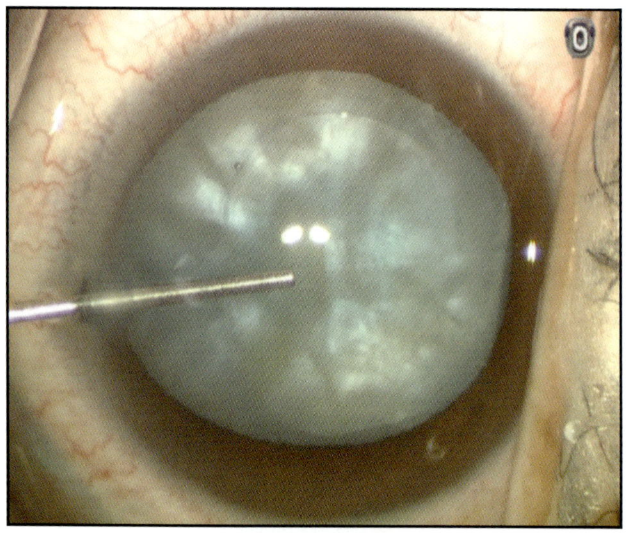

Identify areas of capsular fibrosis. Avoid initiating the capsulorrhexis at that spot if it can be avoided.

To decompress the lens and reduce intracapsular pressure, place a 25-g needle of BSS through the main incision and incise the anterior capsule centrally. Gently aspirate the liquefied lens contents while taking care to avoid any lateral movement of the needle as this may propagate the capsule tear.

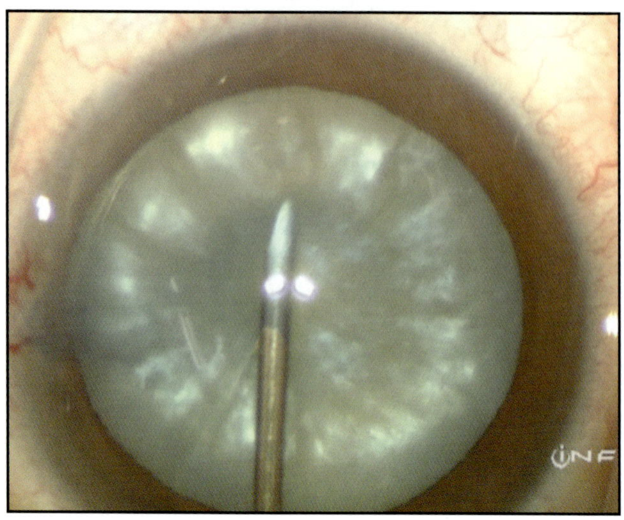

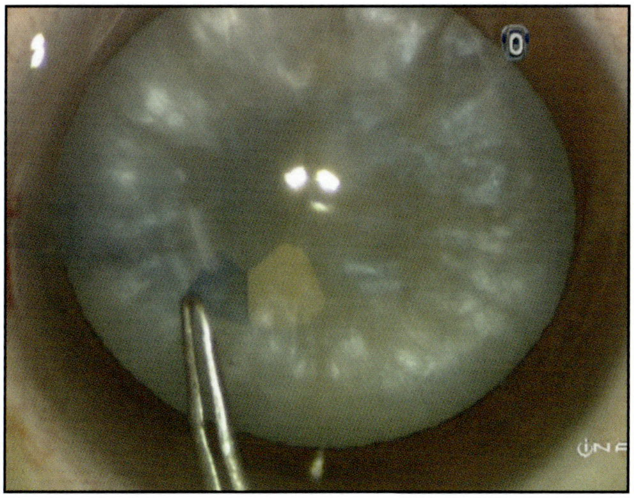

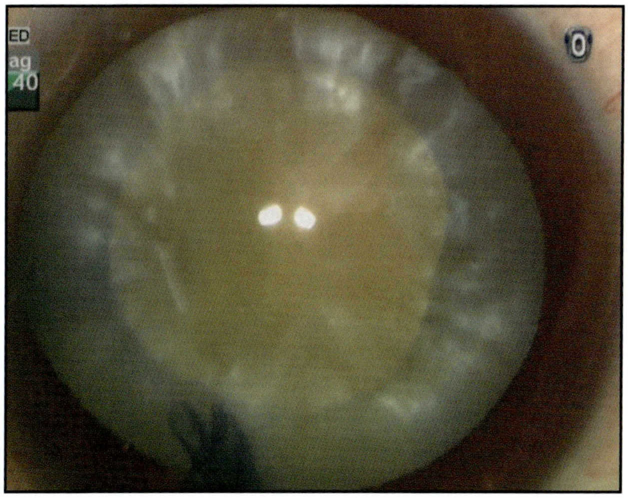

Proceed with the usual capsulorrhexis maneuver. Avoid areas of capsular fibrosis, planning a rhexis trajectory that avoids these areas.

Utilize microscissors to restart the capsulorrhexis if needed to avoid the fibrotic areas. Once left with areas of capsular fibrosis, grasp the fibrotic area with iris microforceps and use microscissors to cut the fibrotic area. Take care to follow the contour of the surrounding capsulorrhexis to ensure continuity.

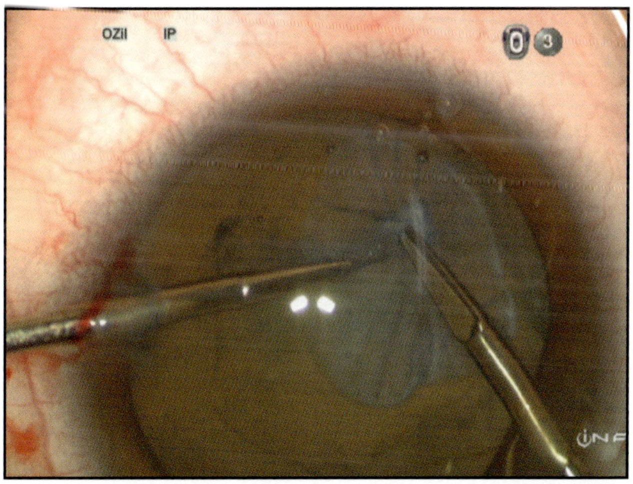

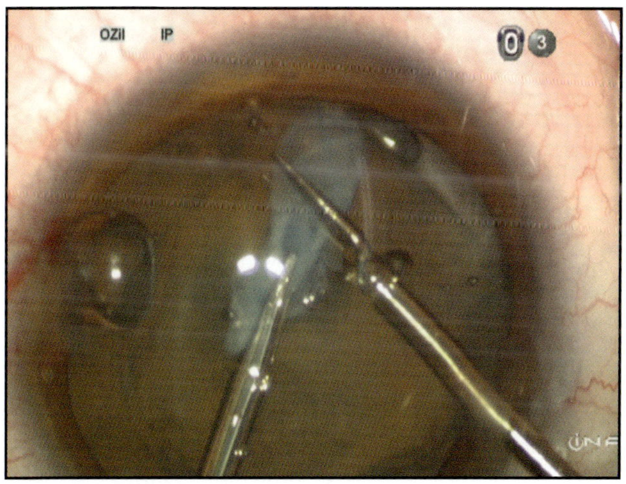

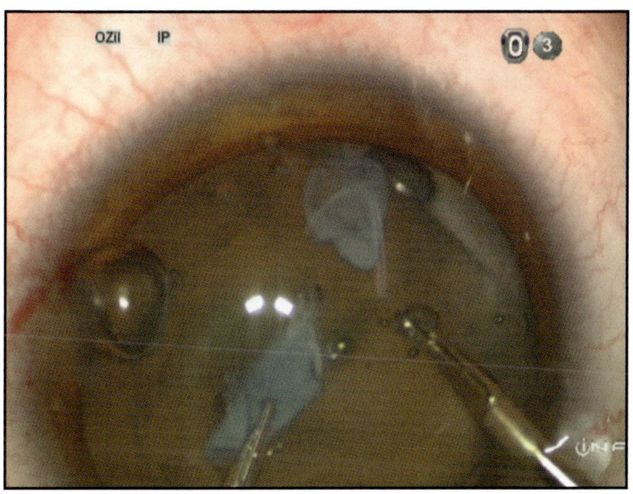

The cut area of the rhexis is weaker and prone to runout, so care must be taken not to exercise traction in these clock hours (eg, as with a capsule retractor).

HOW TO RECOVER AN ANTERIOR CAPSULE RUNOUT

Every once in a while, a capsulorrhexis can go awry. With intact zonules, there can be a tendency for radialization of the anterior capsulotomy. Prompt recognition and management of a capsulorrhexis runout can make the difference between an otherwise routine cataract extraction and a disaster.

- Preventative action is key! Recognize when the capsule is starting to misbehave and be proactive.
- Think about your vector forces in 3 dimensions to understand why the capsule is running out.
- Think about your vector forces in 2 dimensions to redirect the capsulorrhexis from the periphery.

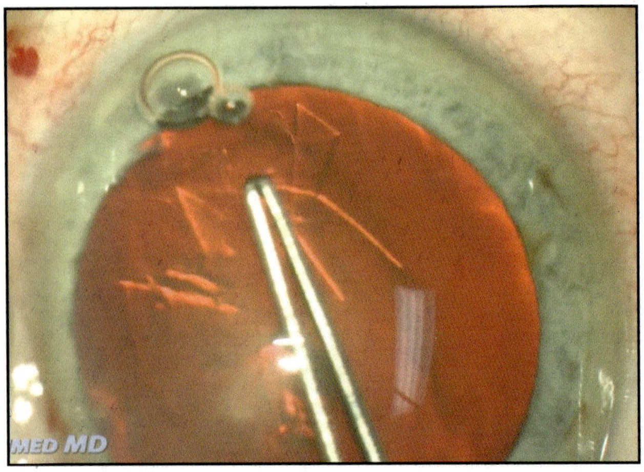

Completely unfold the capsulorrhexis.

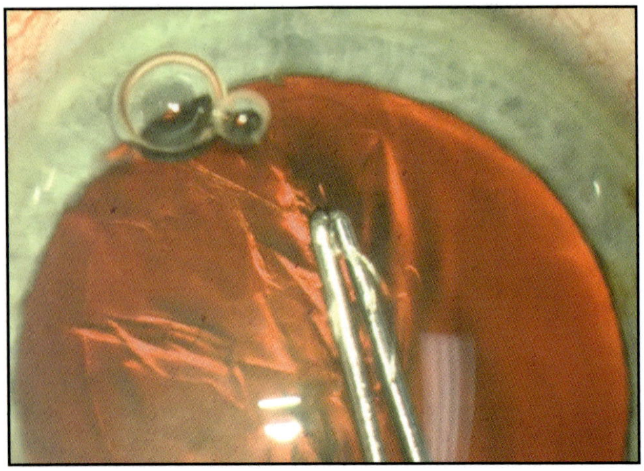

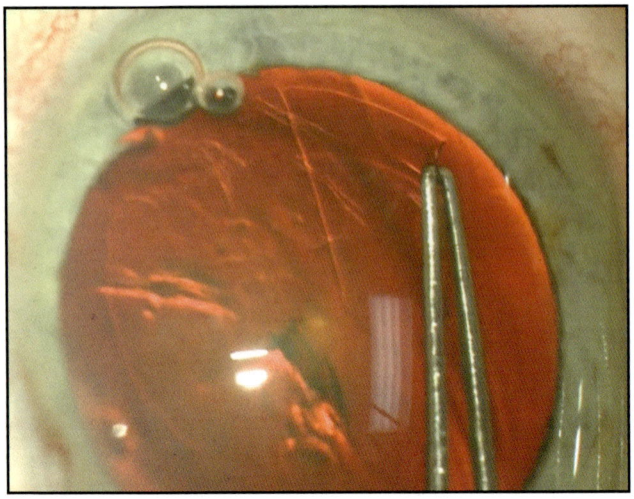

At the earliest sign of radialization of the anterior capsule, transition from a traditional shearing technique to a stretching technique.

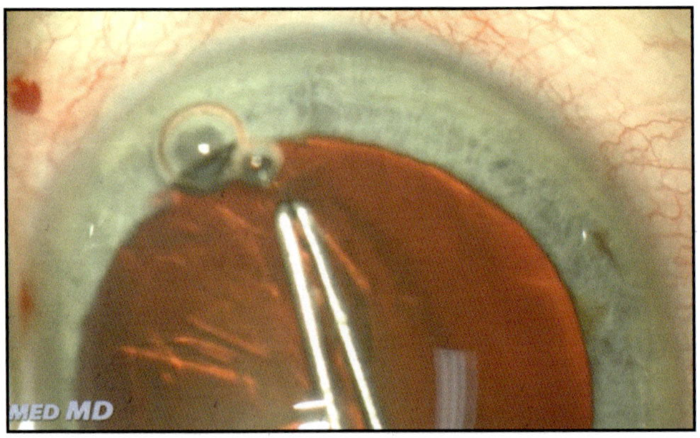

Grasp the unfolded capsulotomy edge about 1 mm from where it inserts into the rest of the anterior capsule.

- Pull gently 90 degrees away from the desired direction of the capsulorrhexis tear propagation.
- Once the capsulotomy edge has moved back toward the center, refold the capsule and return to the shearing technique.
- Use additional cohesive viscoelastic to flatten the anterior capsule; minimizing the domed architecture can reduce the propensity for the capsulorrhexis to run "downhill."

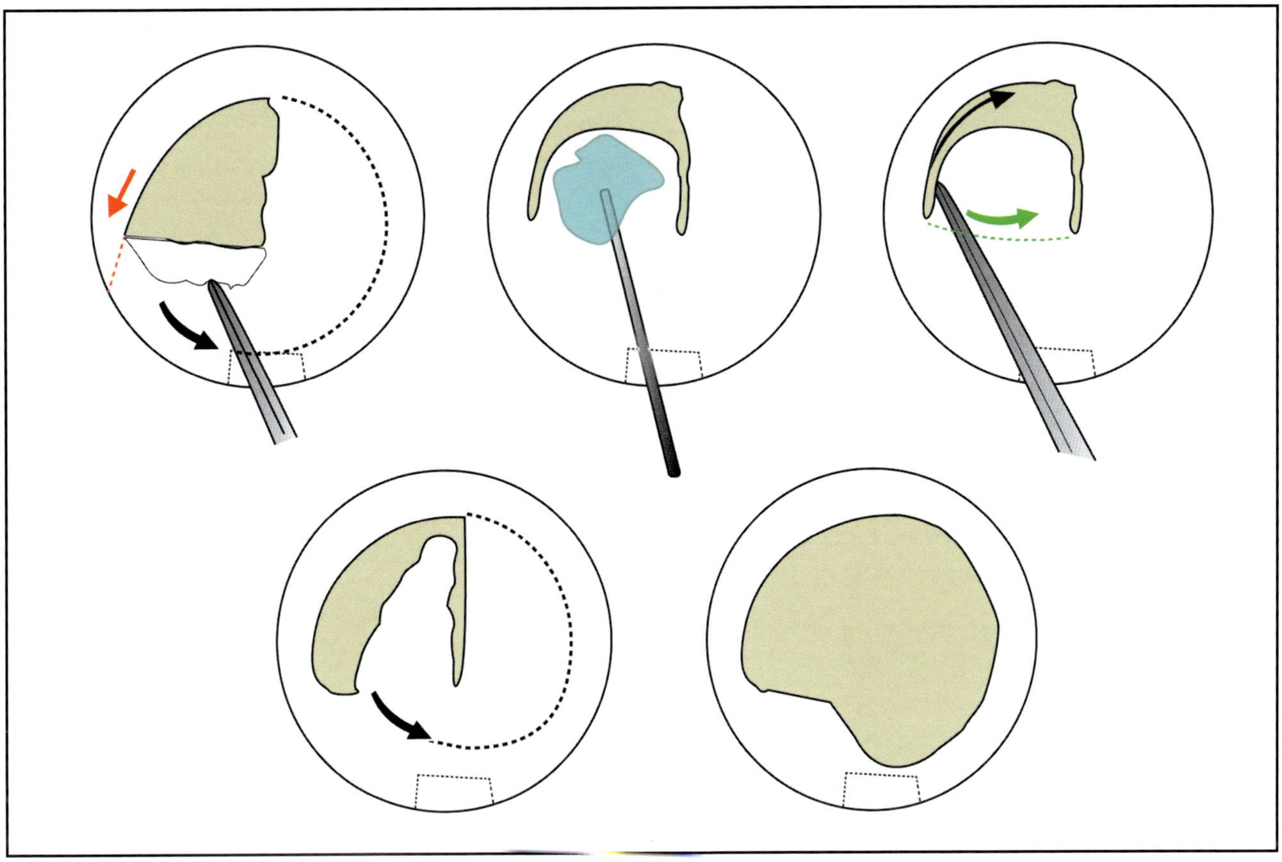

The Little maneuver explained above:

1. The red arrow indicates the direction of the tear runout if the surgeon were to continue traction in the direction of the black arrow.
2. In order to correct the direction of tear, refold the rhexis flap back onto the lens and instill a small amount of cohesive OVD over the flap. Be careful not to inject under the flap as this may propagate the tear.
3. In order to correct the direction of the tear, traction must be applied in exactly the opposite direction as that which initially caused the runout (black arrow). This will now cause the tear to run toward the center of the lens (green arrow). Think about "retracing" the contour of the rhexis that has already been created (black arrow).
4. This figure shows the corrected direction, which usually looks like a small "step" in the rhexis. The capsulorrhexis can now be completed as if no runout had occurred.
5. It is common to have a step or a break in the circularity of the rhexis. Care must be taken to avoid overcorrecting the runout, causing the "step" to come close to the visual axis.

PHACOEMULSIFICATION IN THE PRESENCE OF AN ANTERIOR CAPSULE RUNOUT

Sometimes, despite our best efforts, the anterior capsulotomy can radialize. Typically, this radialization will not extend to the posterior capsule, so standard phacoemulsification can continue with some technique modifications.

While hydrodissection should be avoided, hydrodelineation should be performed to facilitate nuclear disassembly. When addressing the nucleus, avoid excessive lateral separation of nuclear fragments and avoid nucleus rotation. One can consider a cross chop or a V-groove technique to remove the nucleus without rotating it.

Maintain anterior chamber pressurization and depth when removing the phaco or irrigation/aspiration handpiece, as collapse of the anterior chamber can cause the radial tear to extend further. Use OVD or BSS to maintain the chamber.

In removing cortical material, use automated irrigation/aspiration in a tangential stripping manner, moving toward the area of radialization. Address the cortex in the area of radialization last, and consider using a dry aspiration technique with a cannula for better control.

Unless the posterior capsule has been compromised, an intraocular lens can be placed in the capsular bag with haptics oriented 90 degrees away from the radialization. Sulcus placement of an appropriate intraocular lens is an acceptable alternative.

CHAPTER 9

HOW TO USE CAPSULE RETRACTORS

INTRODUCTION

Stabilizing the lens during phacoemulsification is the first key to successful management of subluxated cataracts. Capsular retractors are a practical tool for stabilizing the capsular bag. They have the advantage of having a longer working end that reaches into the capsular fornix. Their rounded, polished finish is also less prone to tearing anterior capsule than are iris hooks, which can be used for capsular support but were not designed for this purpose.

KEY POINTS

- As with iris hooks, take care to ensure symmetry of forces when ratcheting up tension on the capsule hooks.
- These hooks do not need to be tightened excessively.
- Refer to Chapter 5 as another reference on the use of 2 hands for hook insertion and retrieval.

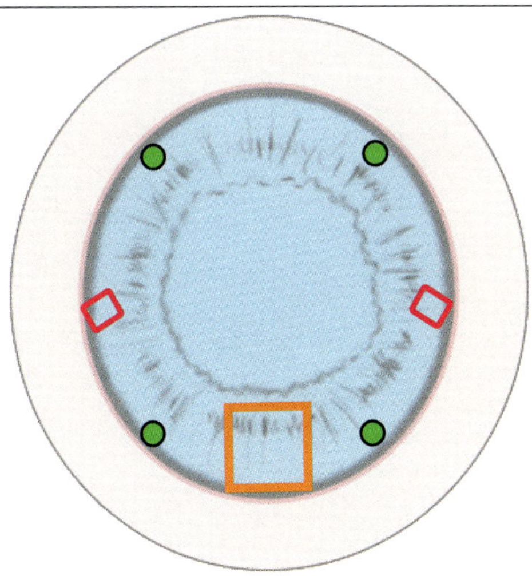

- Standard phaco + knife and fork + 4 paracenteses (anterior limbal-clear corneal, pointing posteriorly)

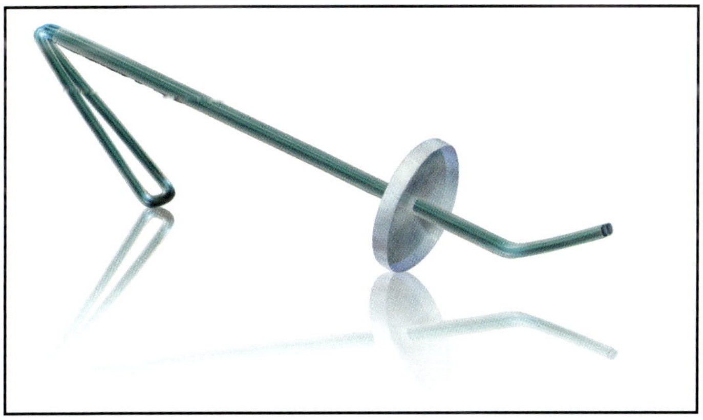

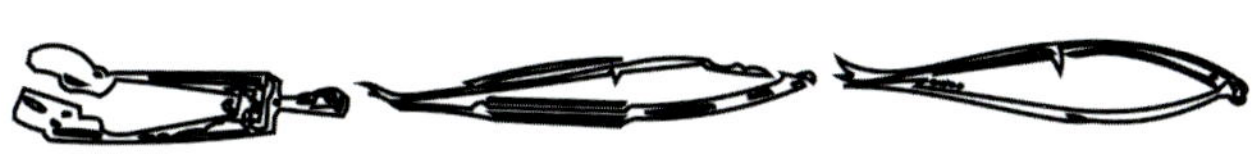

- Side port blade
- Colibri forceps
- Straight or curved tying forceps
- Microsurgical Technology, Inc capsule retractors

Ahmed IK, Campos-Möller X, Shah M, Sheybani A. *Illustrated Advanced Anterior Segment Surgery: A Step-by-Step Guide for Challenging Cases* (pp 55-58).

Typically, 4 paracenteses symmetrically placed around the eye are ideal. The incisions must be anterior limbal or clear corneal, approximately 1 mm in width and aiming posteriorly, given the angled profile of the capsule retractor (this is a key difference from iris hook incisions, which are parallel to the iris plane).

Use cohesive ophthalmic viscosurgical device to expand the plane between the cortex and the anterior capsule at the capsular fornix; this will facilitate insertion of retractors and allow for easier and more zonule-friendly cortical removal later.

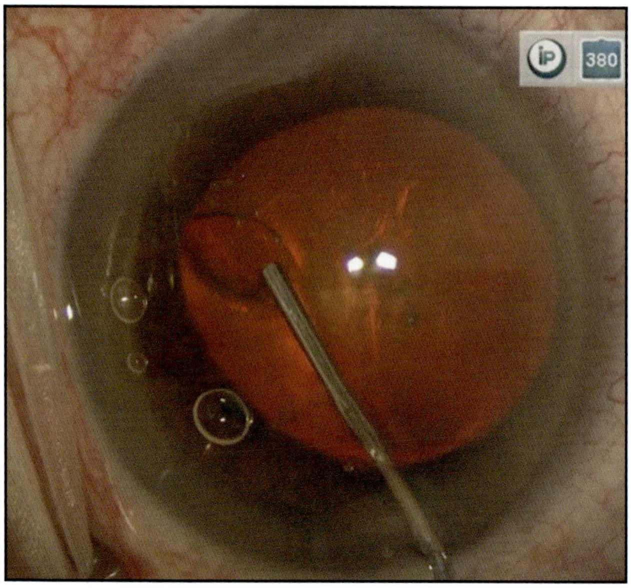

To best control the insertion of the retractor, grasp it with a tying forceps close to the distal or "working" end. This will reduce flexion of the retractor shaft when inserting. Once the tip of the retractor is inside the eye, switch the grip to the distal end of the shaft.

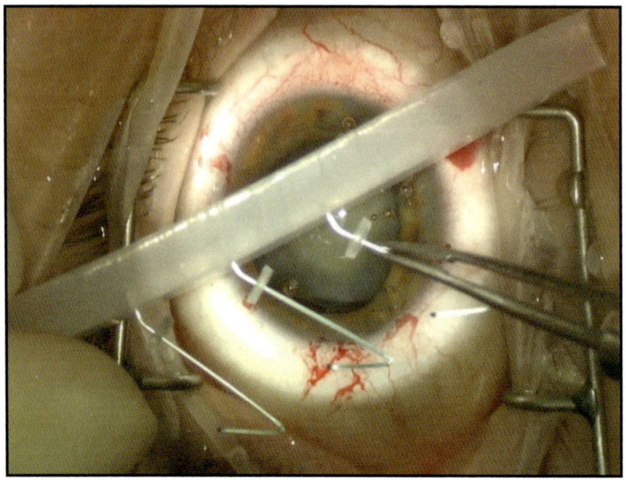

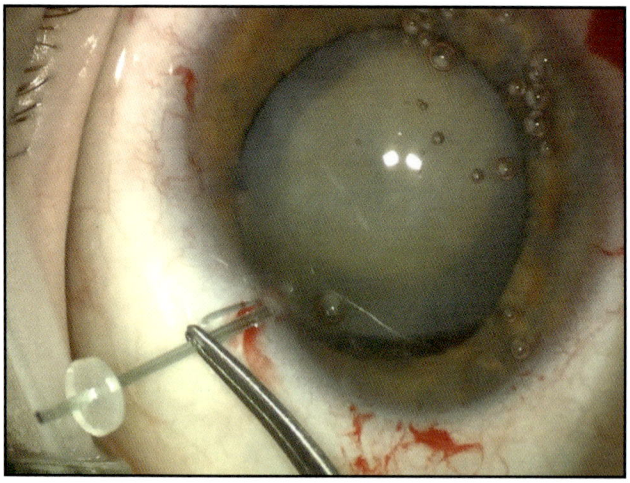

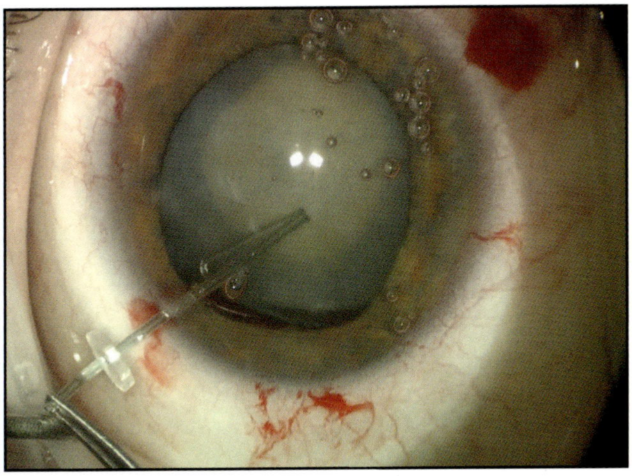

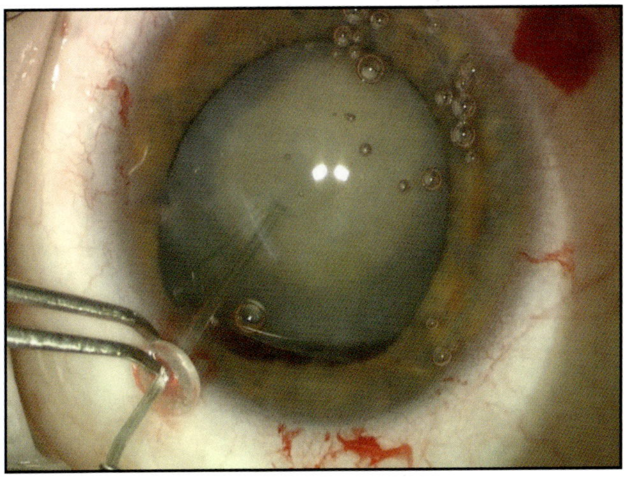

As with the iris hooks chapter, think of the hooks as oars. Pronation of the hand will help engage the hook end underneath the anterior capsular leaflet. Ensure that the hooks are fully supporting the capsule all the way to the fornix. Using a Colibri forceps in your other hand, gently slide the silicone stopper until it reaches the cornea. There is no need to overtighten as the desired goal is for the anterior capsule to just rest on these hooks, rather than pulling the entire lens anteriorly with overtightening.

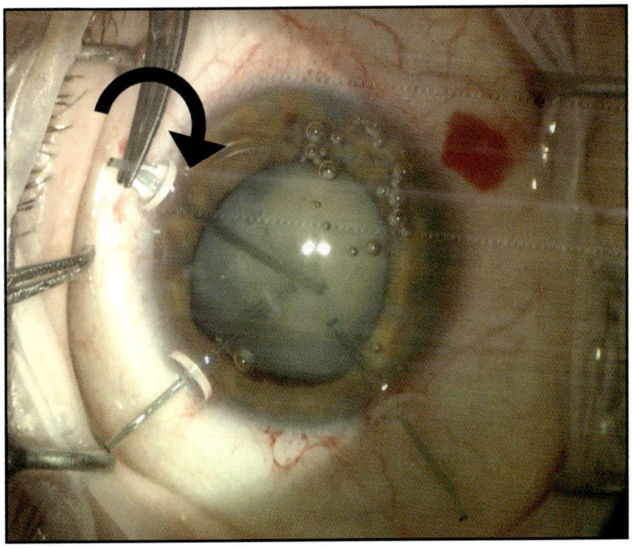

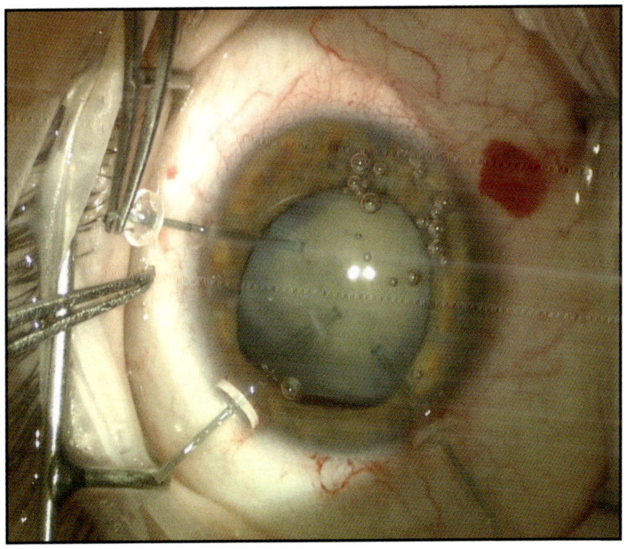

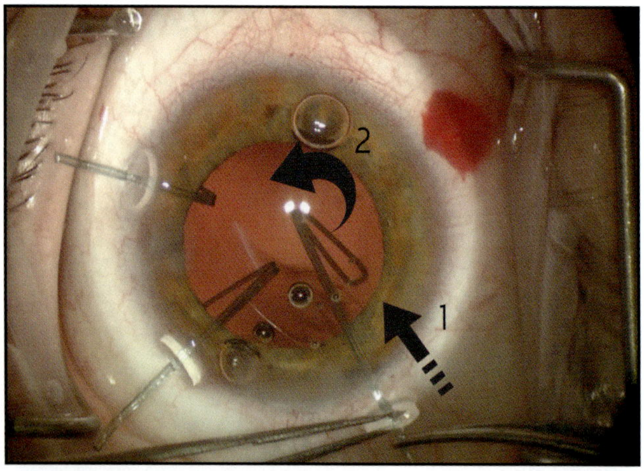

To remove the retractors, slide the silicone stopper back by grasping the shaft of the retractor with the tyer in one hand, while pulling back on the stopper with a Colibri forceps in the other hand.

Disengage the retractor from the capsulorrhexis by inserting the retractor further into the eye, then rotating 180 degrees on its axis so that the tip of the working end is now pointing toward the cornea instead of toward the capsular bag.

As you gently withdraw it from the paracentesis, follow the curve of the retractor once the "shoulder" of the hook approaches the inner ostium of the paracentesis—the end of the hook should be pointing toward the center of the anterior chamber and away from the angle to avoid angle trauma.

As the shoulder starts to exit the eye, change the direction in which you are pulling from horizontally and toward the limbus to vertical and toward the corneal apex (see arrows for direction of each step).

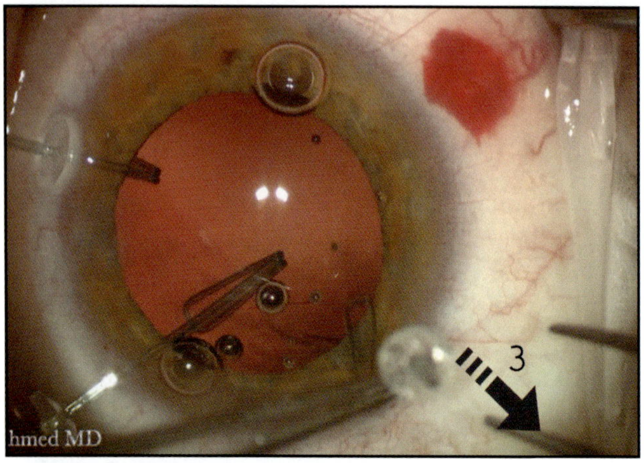

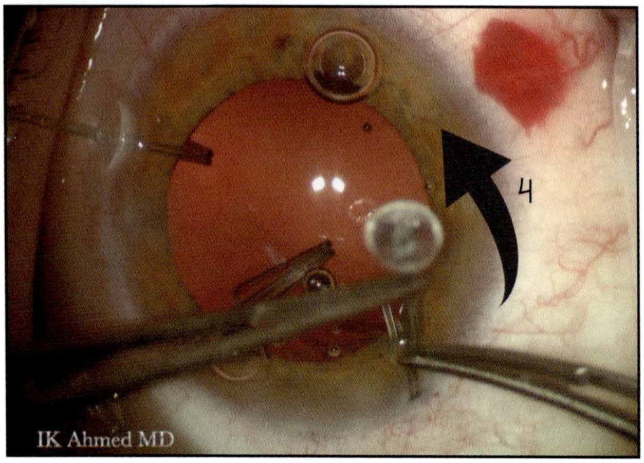

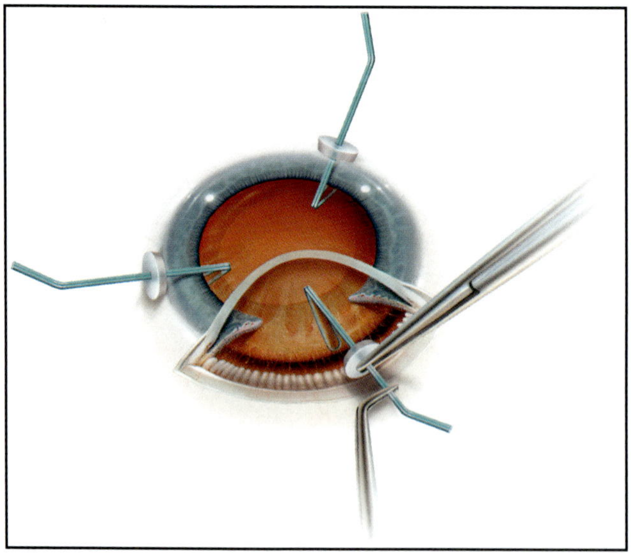

CHAPTER 10

HOW TO INSERT A CAPSULAR TENSION RING

INTRODUCTION

A capsular tension ring (CTR) can be used to address various degrees of zonulopathy.

Typically, a CTR can be used on its own for focal zonulopathy (less than 4 clock hours) when the rest of the zonules are functional, or in the setting of mild to moderate diffuse zonulopathy.

Furthermore, CTRs can be used in combination with other capsule support devices, such as capsular tension segments.

KEY POINTS

- Insert the CTR as late as possible to avoid encountering any issues with cortical removal, but as soon as it is required to prevent capsular collapse or worsening of zonulopathy!
- When inserting a CTR, always have a second instrument ready to help ease the ring off of its injector.
- When inserting the CTR, direct the leading edge toward the area of zonulopathy in order to recruit the intact zonules.
- When in doubt, choose an oversized CTR rather than undersized, as a minimal amount of CTR overlap is not a problem.
- Do not insert CTRs when there is anterior capsule compromise. In posterior capsule openings, conversion to a small continuous curvilinear posterior capsulorrhexis should be performed prior to CTR insertion. Otherwise, small tears can radialize into large ones.

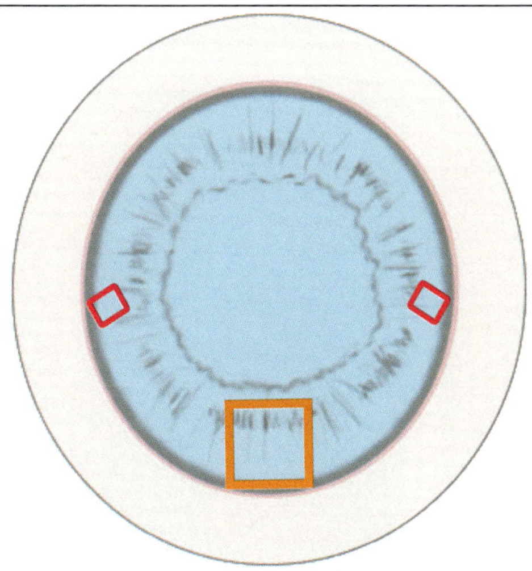

- Standard phaco + knife and fork

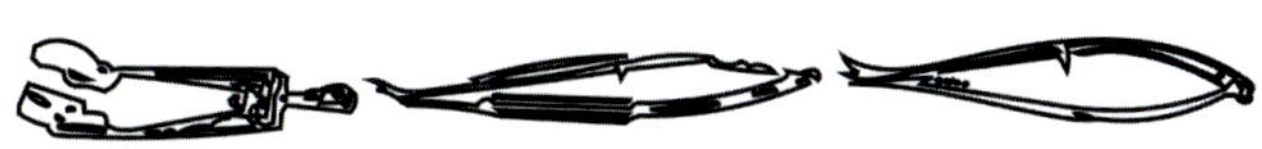

- CTR
- Angled Kuglen hook
- Sinskey hook
- Colibri forceps
- Cohesive viscoelastic

Ahmed IK, Campos-Möller X, Shah M, Sheybani A. *Illustrated Advanced Anterior Segment Surgery: A Step-by-Step Guide for Challenging Cases* (pp 59-63).

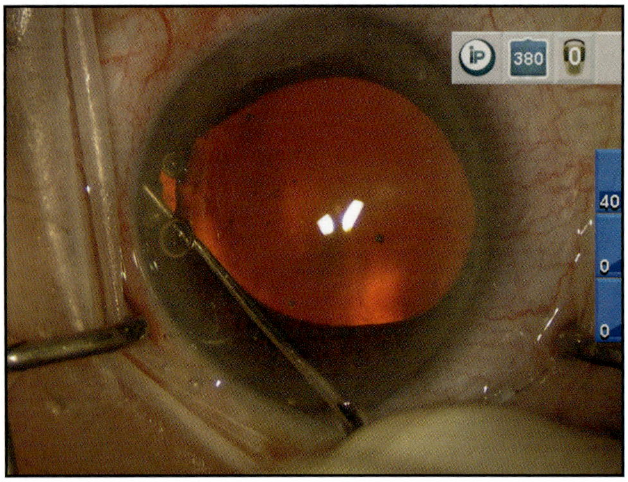

Early insertion:

- After successful completion of the capsulorrhexis, use cohesive viscoelastic to create a plane between the capsule and cortex.
- An easy way to achieve this plane is to inject ophthalmic viscosurgical device (OVD) at the capsule edge pointing down toward the lens substance. Some OVD will begin to expand the plane between the cortex and capsule.
- This will open up a plane that you can then enter with the cannula to further viscoexpand.
- Follow this plane 360 degrees by using various incisions.
- Place an additional bolus of OVD in the area where you will first place the CTR.
- During CTR insertion, make sure the cataract and capsule complex does not move excessively.

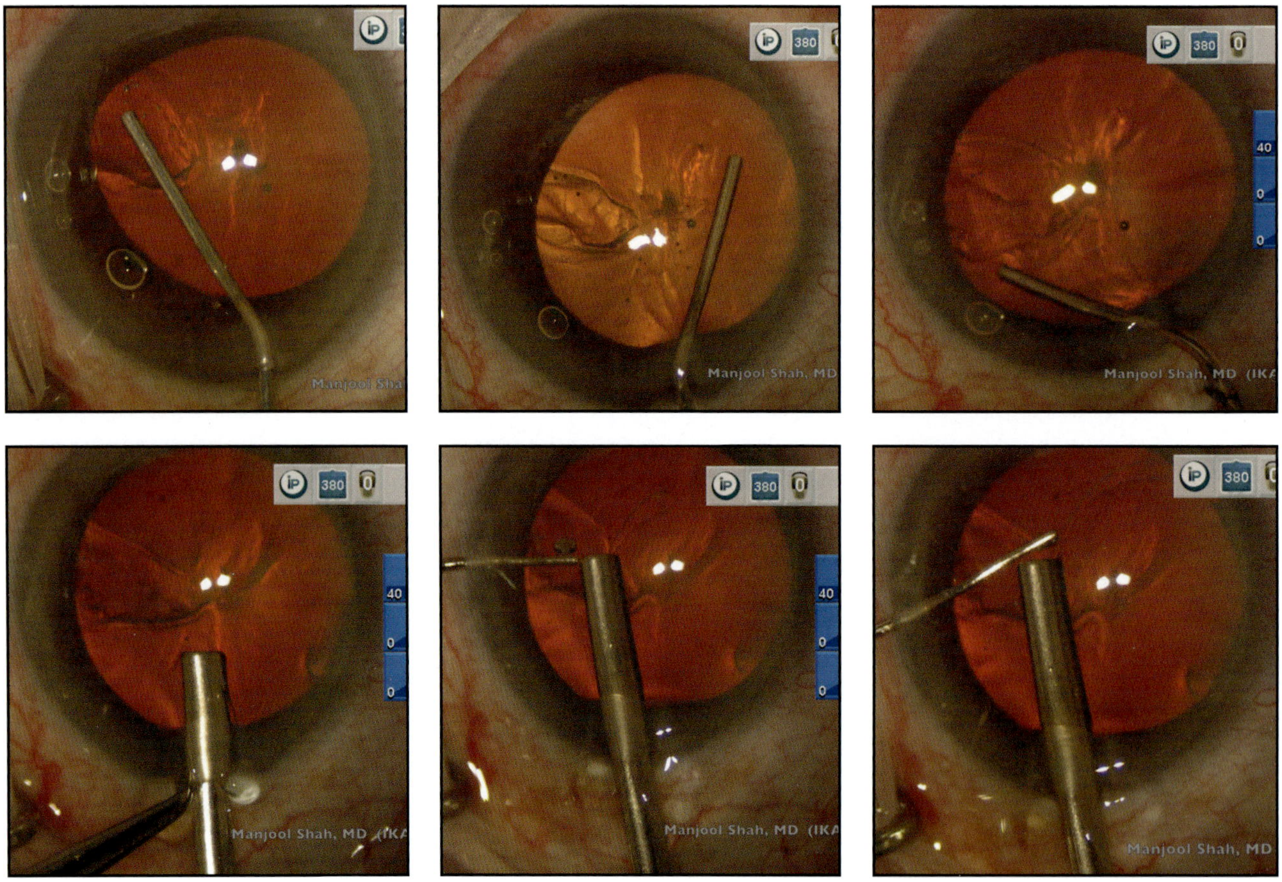

- Insert the CTR injector through the main incision.
- Direct the tip of the injector left (toward the surgeon's 9 o'clock). This will make ring manipulation easier as it will deploy toward the center of the eye. Slowly depress the plunger, making sure the tip of the ring goes under the capsulorrhexis edge.
- A Kuglen hook through the paracentesis can be used to redirect the CTR.

Be observant for excessive capsule movements during CTR insertion as this may indicate that the leading edge of the CTR has gotten ensnared on peripheral capsule. The CTR should advance smoothly; proceeding too aggressively here can result in further zonular trauma. Consider inserting the CTR in the opposite direction if this continues to be a problem.

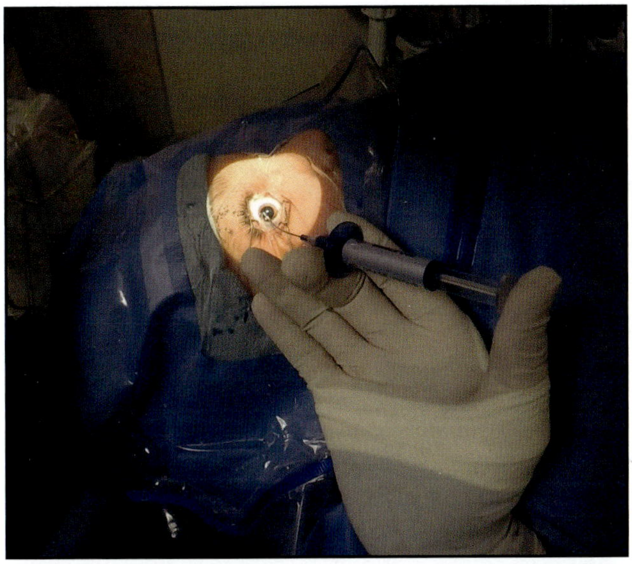

Notice the orientation of injector shaft (curving toward the direction of CTR displacement) during injection. Once the CTR has been completely injected, the injector hand can be pronated to release the injector hook from the CTR. A Sinskey or Kuglen hook can be useful to direct the trailing end of the CTR into the capsular fornix.

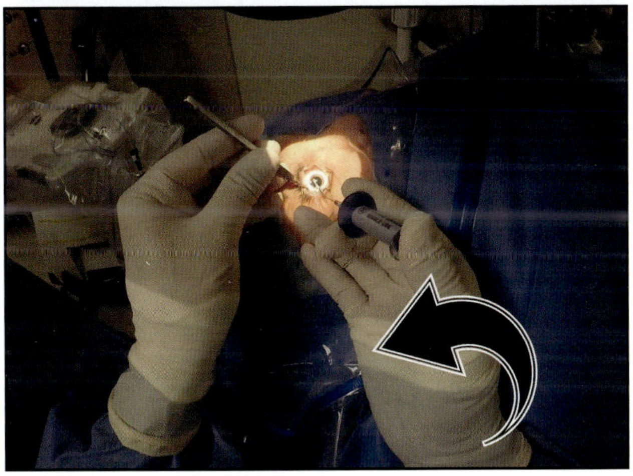

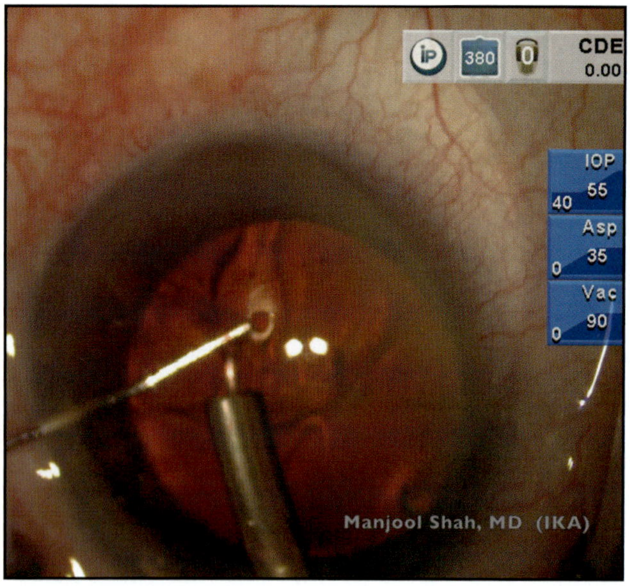

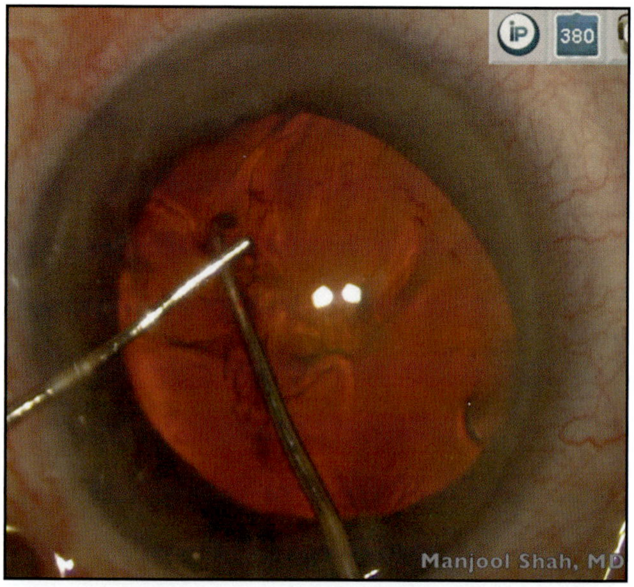

The trailing loop of the CTR is attached to the injector shaft, which has a hook at the tip. The hook can be disengaged from the loop by rotating the wrist counterclockwise. If this does not release the CTR, a Sinskey hook can be used to engage the loop and direct the trailing end of the CTR into the capsular fornix.

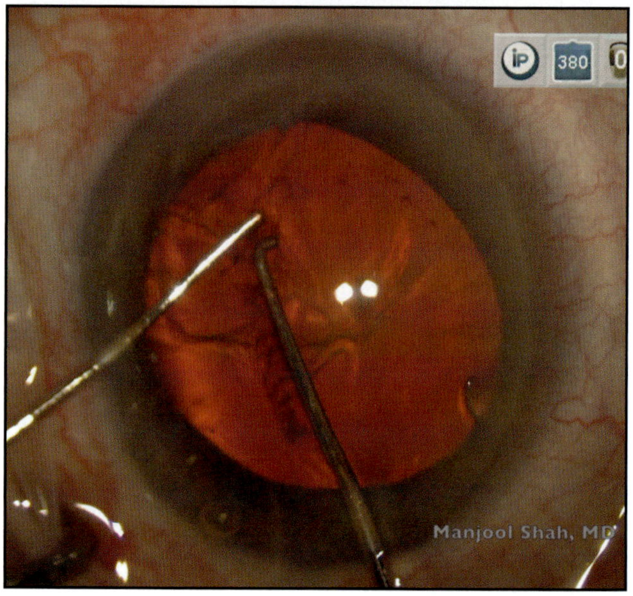

Late insertion:

- After successful nucleus disassembly and cortex removal, make sure the capsular bag is completely filled with cohesive viscoelastic.
- Failure to completely fill the bag can allow the CTR to catch onto a capsular wrinkle, which can cause further zonular trauma and/or a capsule tear.
- Ideally, the leading edge of the CTR should point toward the area of focal zonulopathy.
- At this point, it is important to avoid hitting the posterior capsule. The CTR leading edge should be pointed toward the capsular fornix and at an angle that will allow it to slide parallel to the fornix, to avoid damaging more zonules.
- Similarly, a Kuglen or Sinskey hook through the side port incision can be used to direct the CTR and disengage it from the injector hook.

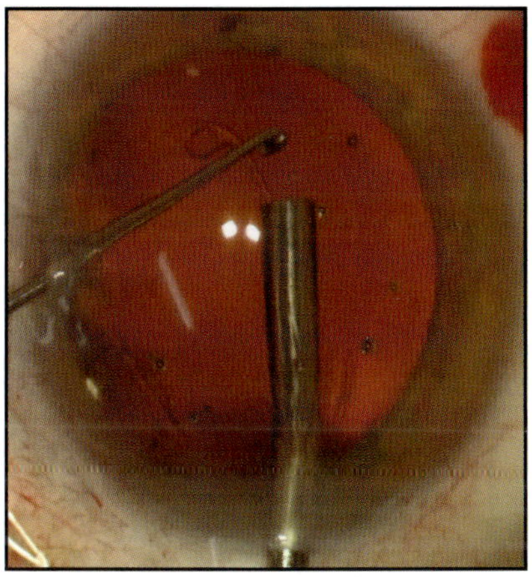

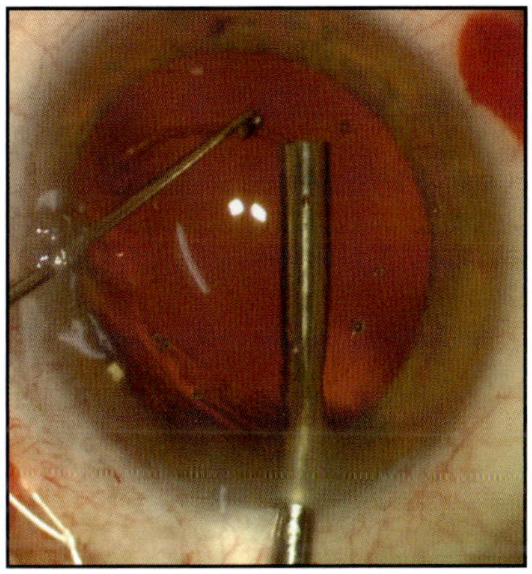

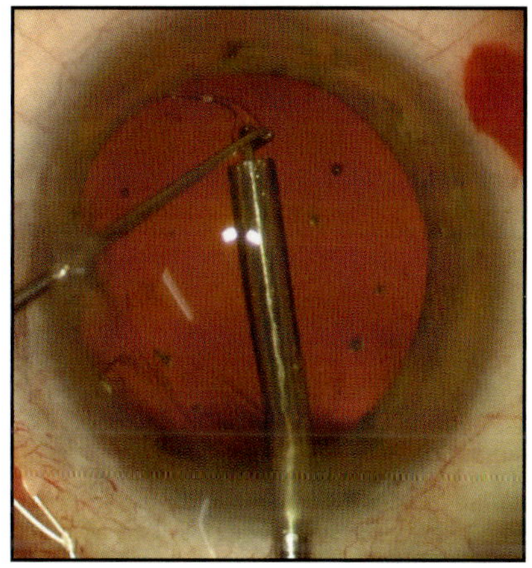

CHAPTER 11

HOW TO IMPLANT CAPSULAR TENSION SEGMENTS

INTRODUCTION

The capsular tension segment (CTS) is a surgical device that can be helpful in the management of crystalline lenses with profound zonulopathy.

Typically, these would be called for in situations of greater than 4 clock hours of focal zonulopathy or severe diffuse zonulopathy. The CTS is a poly(methyl methacrylate) device that has an arc length of 120 degrees and is available in 2 sizes. It has a central fixation eyelet that sits anterior to the plane of the peripheral arc, and is designed to rest anterior to the anterior capsulotomy either intraoperatively or after scleral fixation. There are numerous methods that can be used to utilize the CTS in these complex anterior segment surgeries, but the method presented here demonstrates the facility of the CTS as not only an intraocular lens (IOL)-stabilizing agent, but an intraoperative tool for stabilizing the cataract and capsule complex.

KEY POINTS

- Purposeful incision placement corresponds to areas of zonulopathy.
- Scratch incisions should correspond with the center of the area with zonulopathy.
- Paracentesis for iris hooks corresponds to areas where capsular support will be required.
- Paracentesis for needle docking must be exactly 180 degrees from scratch incisions.
- If placing 2 CTSs, they must be located 180 degrees apart to avoid IOL bag decentration.
- Avoid anterior chamber shallowing to prevent vitreous prolapse.
- Identify areas and degree of zonulopathy with careful preoperative examination and imaging.
- One CTS covers about 90 degrees and is usually sufficient for localized zonulopathy.
- For more diffuse zonular weakness, 2 CTS elements can be placed 180 degrees apart.
- A capsular tension ring (CTR) must always be used in combination with the CTS. The CTS provides fixation and localized support, while the CTR distributes forces and offers circumferential support.

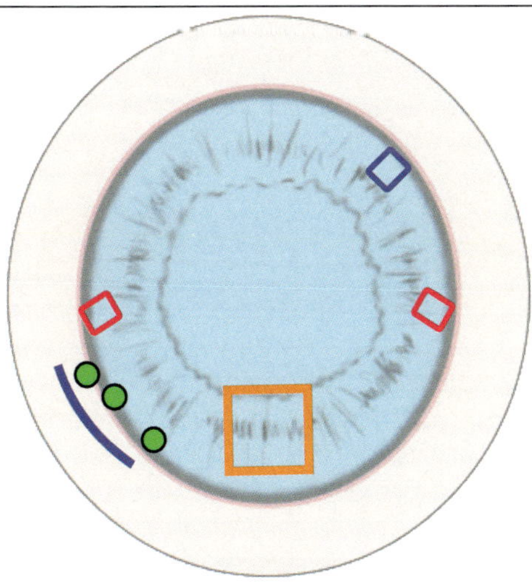

- Standard phaco + knife and fork
- Additional paracentesis approximately 180 degrees from zonular dialysis (site of CTS fixation)
- Partial-thickness scleral scratch incision 1/4 scleral depth 1 mm posterior to the scleral spur, 3 to 4 mm in length in area of planned CTS fixation
- Iris hook incisions in area of planned CTS fixation

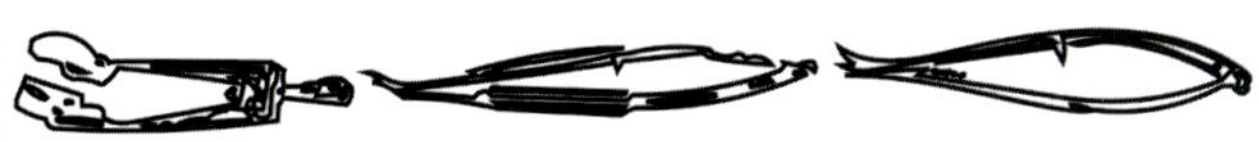

- Sinskey hook
- Iris micrograspers
- Ahmed CTS
- Gore-Tex double-armed suture on CV-8 needle
- Iris hooks
- 25-g sharp hypodermic needle

Ahmed IK, Campos-Möller X, Shah M, Sheybani A. *Illustrated Advanced Anterior Segment Surgery: A Step-by-Step Guide for Challenging Cases* (pp 65-77).

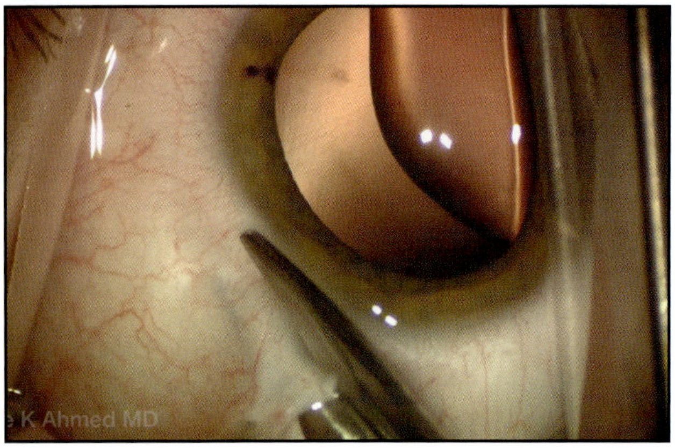

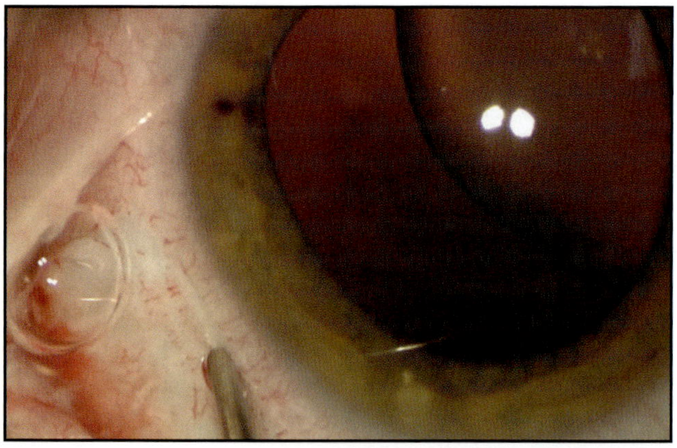

- Create an L-shaped conjunctival peritomy in the area of planned CTS suture fixation.
- Cauterize the scleral bed with wet-field bipolar cautery. Only light hemostasis is required.
- Create a 1/4 scleral depth (300 μm) groove, approximately 4 mm in length and parallel to the limbus, 1 mm posterior to the scleral spur.
- The scleral spur can be identified as the end of the gray zone (which corresponds to the corneal wedge), where the blue/gray zone meets the scleral white. Scleral fibers transition from more haphazard arrangement near limbus to parallel to limbus at the spur. Use this landmark instead of measuring from the limbus because the limbus-sulcus distance varies considerably between eyes, whereas the spur-sulcus distance does not.

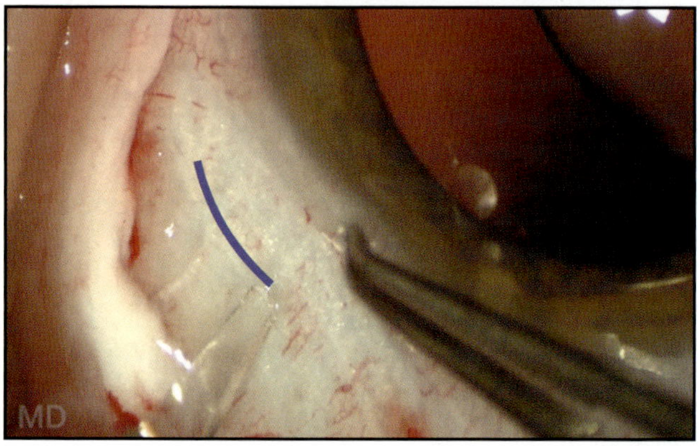

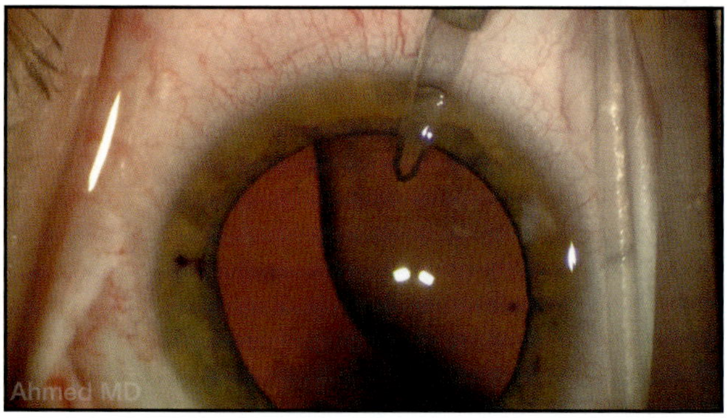

Place knife and fork paracentesis incisions with an extra incision 180 degrees away from planned CTS placement to facilitate scleral suture passage. Instill dispersive ophthalmic viscosurgical device (OVD) and tamponade any areas of visible anterior hyaloid to prevent vitreous prolapse. Consider instillation of a superviscous OVD to flatten the anterior capsule, with care not to overpressurize the anterior chamber as this may cause vitreous prolapse.

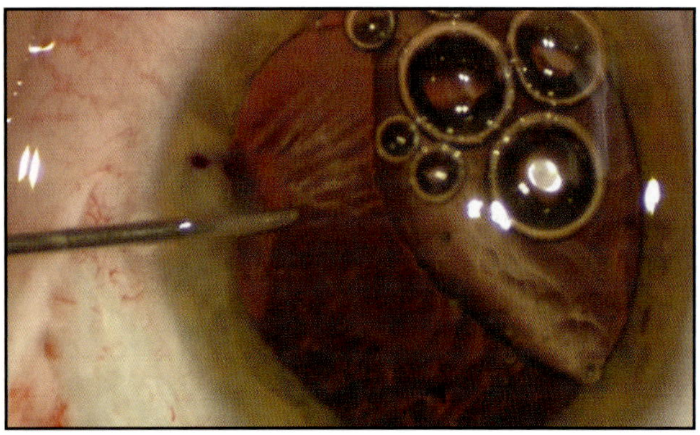

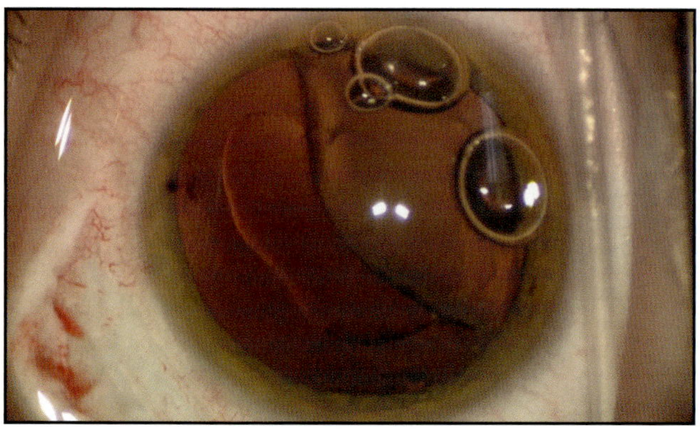

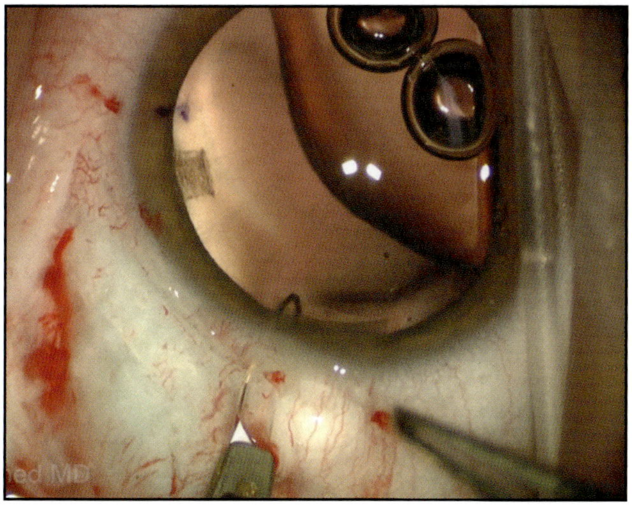

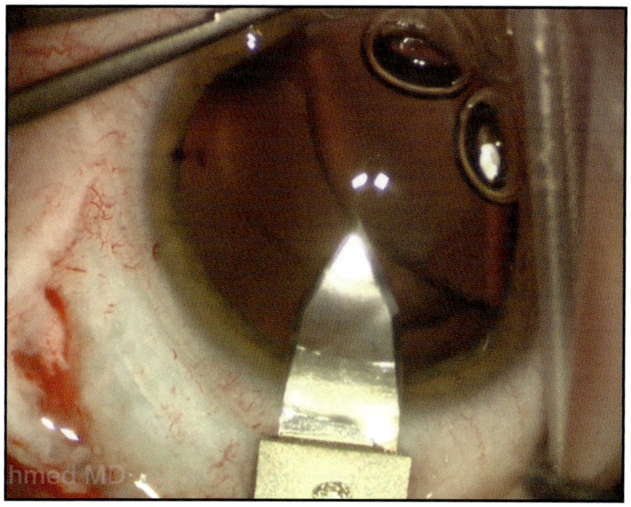

Create incisions for iris hook insertion (usually 3 for a single CTS, but more may be required to support the capsular bag). Create a temporal clear corneal incision for the phacoemulsification needle (2.2 to 2.75 mm), which may be enlarged later in the case. Initiate a capsulorrhexis either with the use of a cystotome, or by using micrograspers for countertraction (refer to Chapter 7).

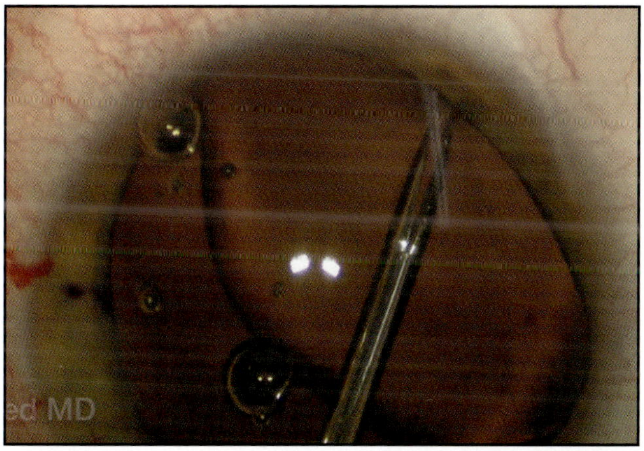

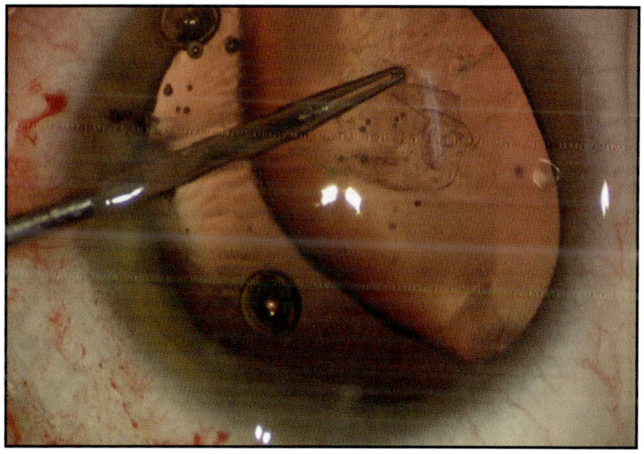

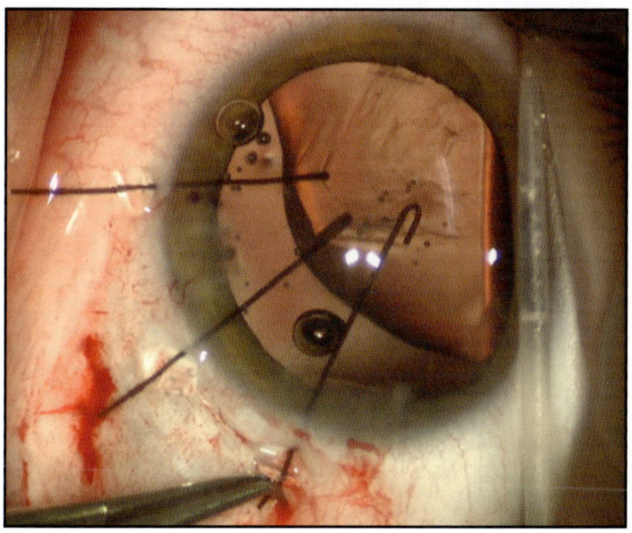

Hook the capsulorrhexis edge to provide countertraction. One of these hooks will ultimately be used to stabilize the CTS during phacoemulsification.

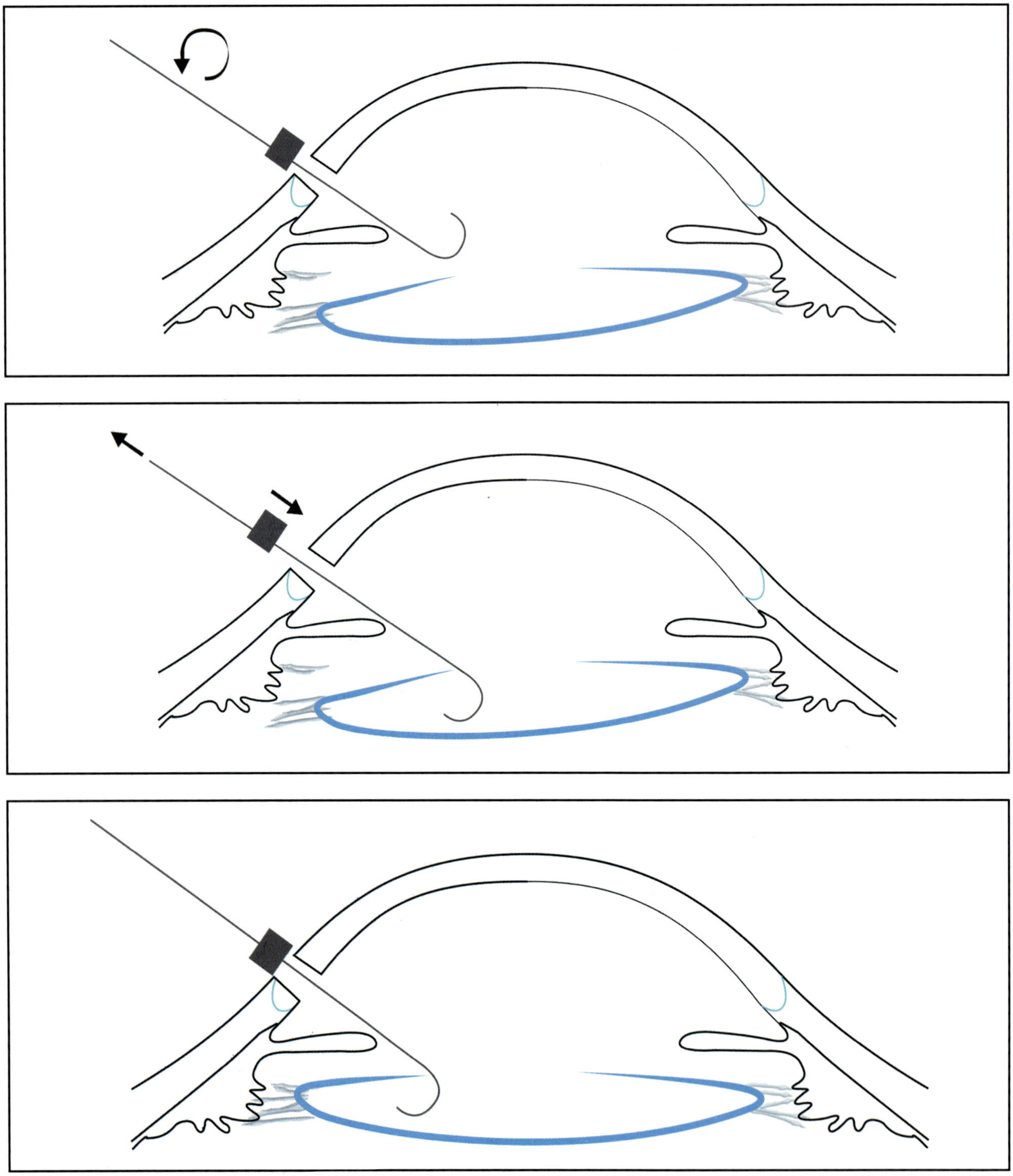

Iris retractor hooks can be used to hold the capsular bag in place during surgery. The key point is to make the incisions in clear cornea, which will naturally direct the hooks posteriorly, instead of parallel to the iris plane. Avoid overtightening of the sleeves as this may cause further zonular damage. Capsule-specific retractors can be implanted similarly and have the advantage of being polished and less prone to causing capsule tears.

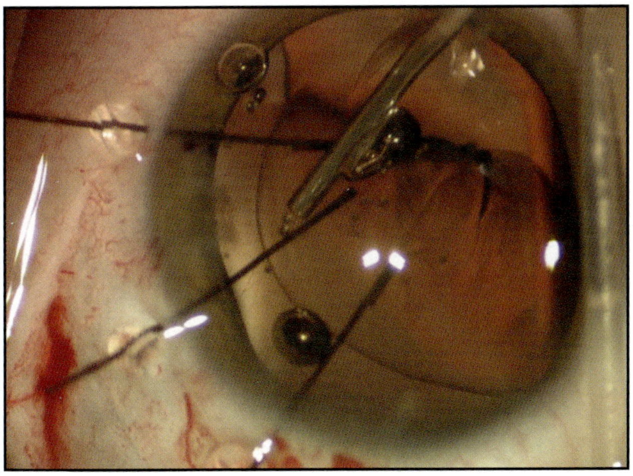

Perform a limited viscodissection in the area of planned CTS implantation. To create space for CTS implantation, refer to the CTR implantation chapter for more pearls.

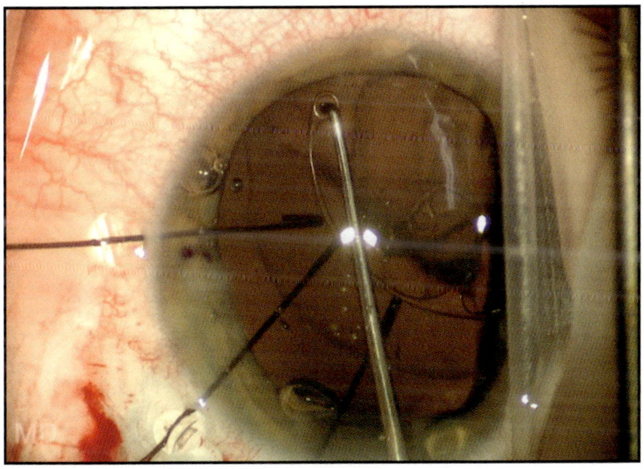

- Use a Sinskey hook to position the CTS in the bag. Ensure that the central fixation eyelet is anterior to the capsulorrhexis edge.
- Remove all but the most central iris hook.
- Turn this central iris hook upside down and use it to secure the CTS through its eyelet. Iris micrograspers can be used to make this step easier.
- The CTS is now secure and will act as a "coat hanger" to facilitate safe cataract extraction.
- Perform hydrodissection, hydrodelineation, and regular phacoemulsification and irrigation/aspiration.
- Avoid anterior chamber shallowing.
- Use additional dispersive viscoelastic as needed to tamponade any exposed anterior hyaloid.

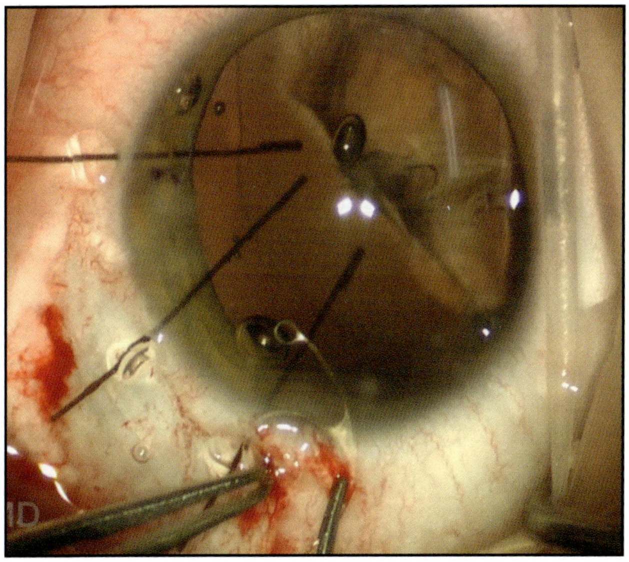

Use a curved tying forceps or Colibri forceps to insert the CTS element through the main corneal incision. Ensure that the fixation element is positioned anteriorly.

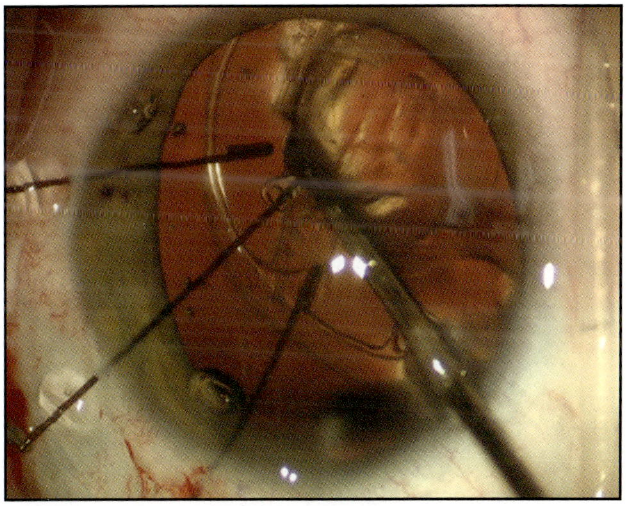

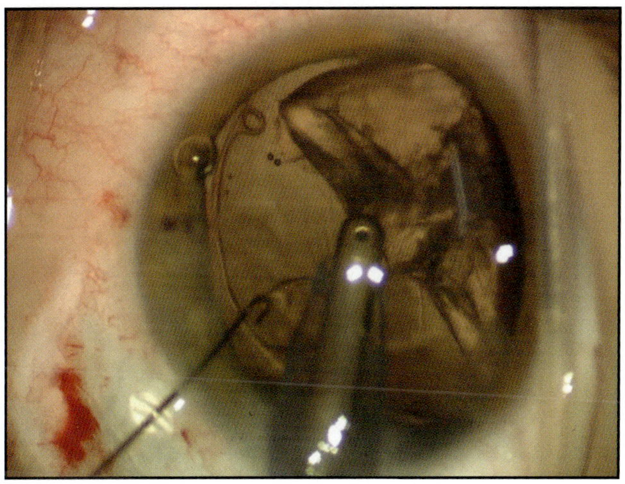

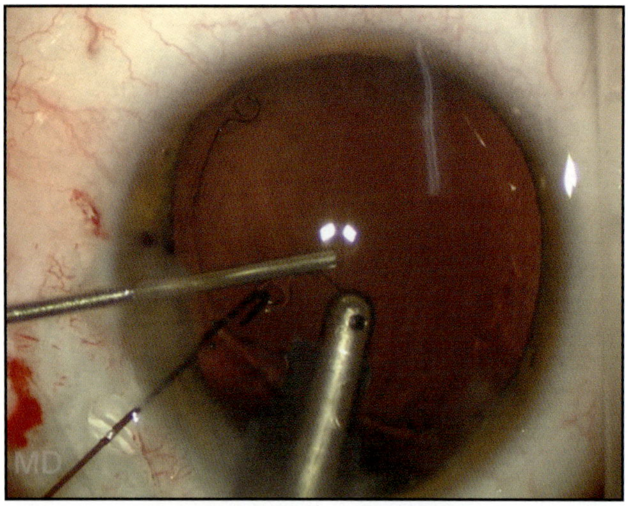

Use the nuclear disassembly that you are most comfortable with. Changing cataract surgery technique here is a mistake. Changing fluidics last minute for difficult cases can be counterproductive, although some authors advocate for low-flow "slow motion" parameters. The more familiarity, the better. Maneuvers should be limited so that remaining zonules are not damaged.

Be sure to keep the anterior chamber well pressurized during major instrument exchanges to prevent vitreous prolapse by injecting balanced salt solution (BSS) or extra OVD through the paracentesis before removing instruments.

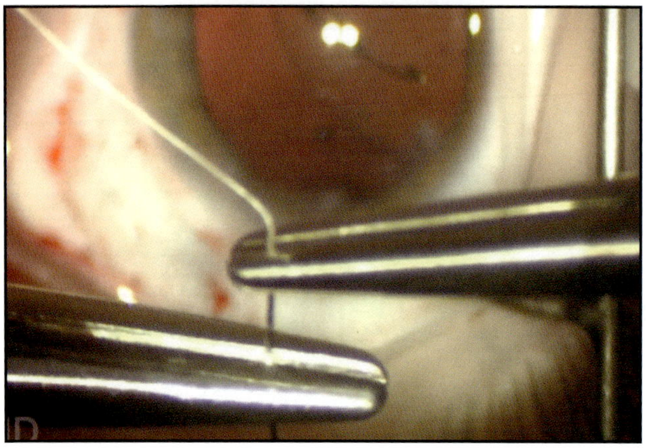

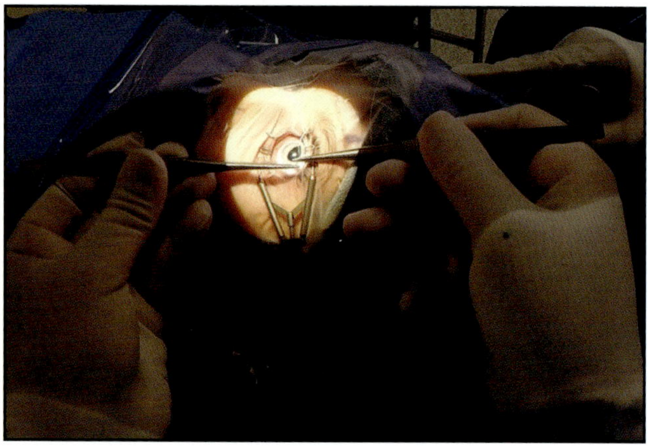

Straighten both arms of the Gore-Tex suture using a hand-over-hand technique.

Using iris micrograspers, disengage the iris hook from the CTS and bring it to the middle of the anterior chamber, oriented perpendicular to the iris plane to facilitate suture passage. Think of passing an arrow through a hoop: the straighter the line between the two, the easier the maneuver will be.

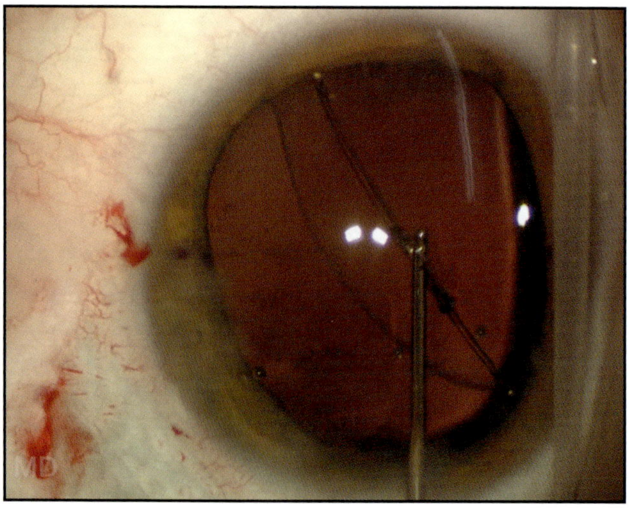

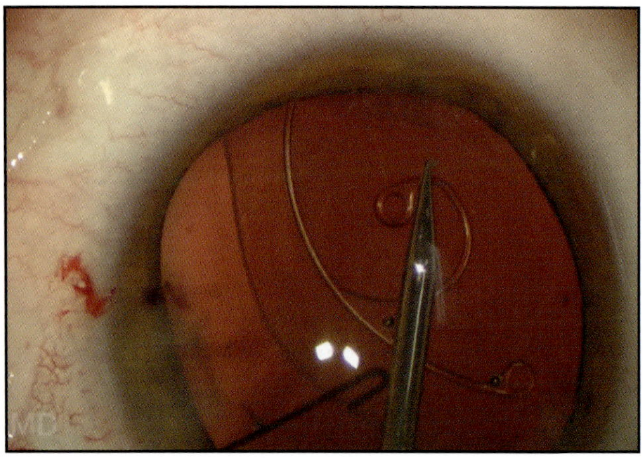

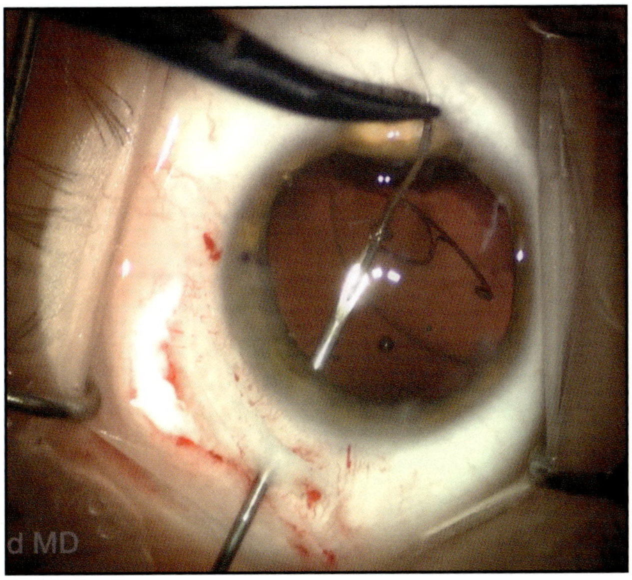

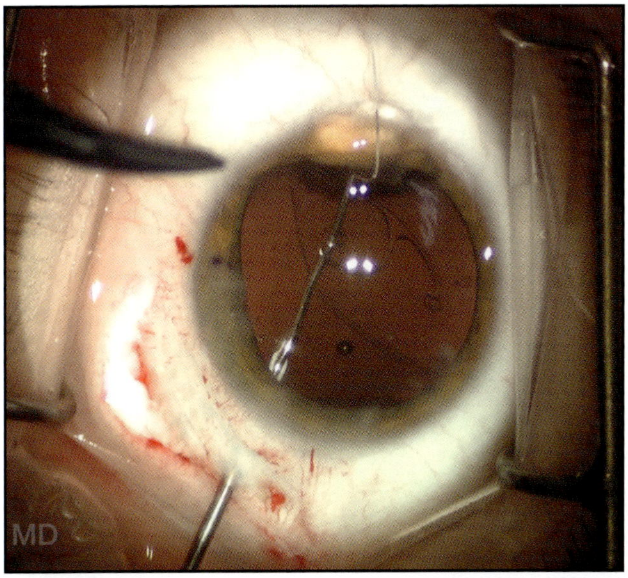

- Pass one of the straightened needles through the paracentesis incision opposite the CTS fixation site and toward the CTS fixation loop.
- To dock the suture needle, engage the 25-g hypodermic on one side of the scleral scratch incision. Enter through the sclera perpendicular to the scleral surface, then promptly turn the needle to be oriented parallel to the iris plane and head toward the Gore-Tex needle (see diagram on p 77).
- Dock the needle in the 25-g hypodermic once it has passed through the CTS fixation eyelet, and use iris micrograspers as needed to ensure that successful docking has occurred. This may require more force than anticipated in order to catch the Gore-Tex needle within the docking 25-g needle.
- Gently remove the 25-g needle from the scleral side, bringing the Gore-Tex suture along.
- Use a Sinskey hook to reposit the CTS in its correct in-the-bag position.

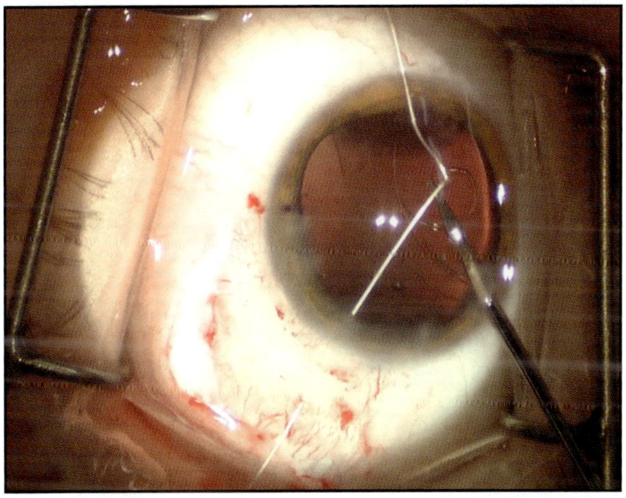

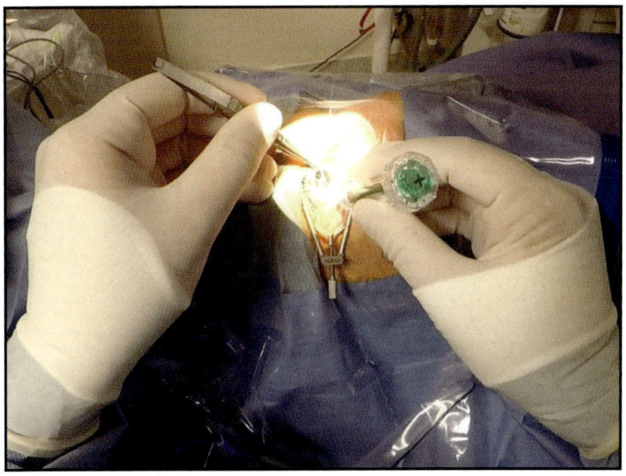

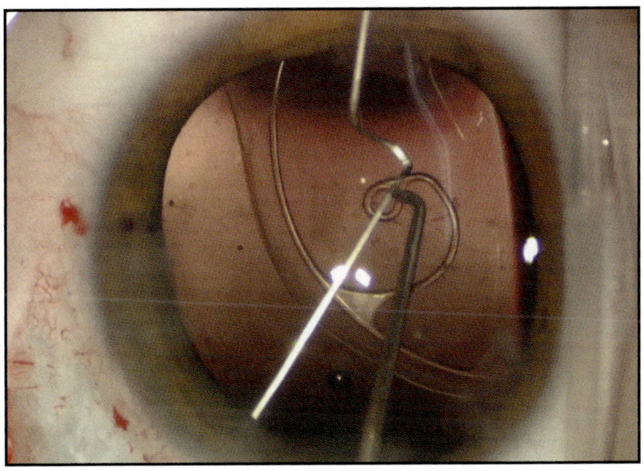

- Use the same ab interno suture passage technique described previously to pass the second arm of the Gore-Tex suture.
- Take care to ensure that no corneal fibers are trapped between the 2 suture arms.
- Enter sclera through the other end of the scleral scratch incision, about 2 mm away from the first passage.
- This time, the second Gore-Tex needle will pass anterior to the anterior capsule, requiring more anterior angulation of the 25-g needle upon entering the eye. Consider instilling some more dispersive viscoelastic to keep the peripheral capsule and anterior hyaloid away from the needle.
- Externalize the 25-g needle and cut both ends to a length that is comfortable for tying.

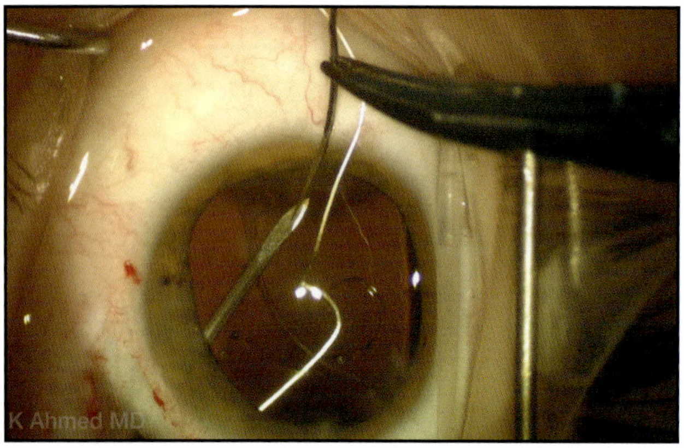

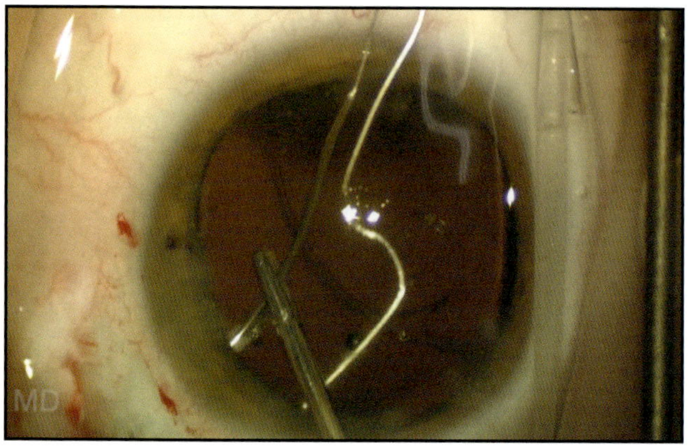

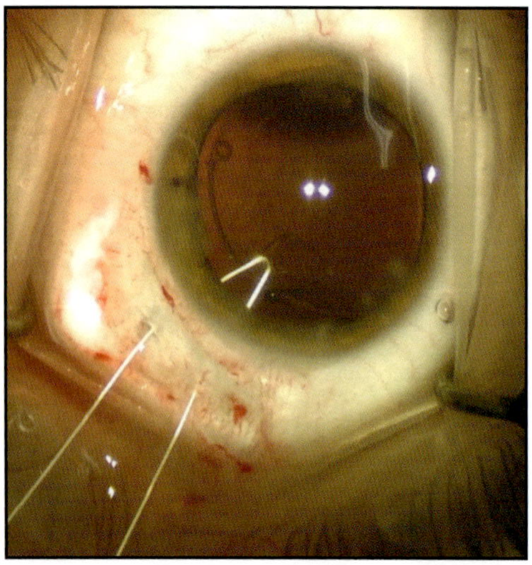

- Create a loose slip knot: Start with 2 single throws in the same direction (careful: it is NOT one double throw), then use an assistant to tighten the knot itself by pulling one of the suture ends while you grip the other suture end and the 2 sutures of the scleral side of the knot.
- Take care to avoid any movement of the CTS during this step. See additional slip knot diagrams at the end of this chapter.

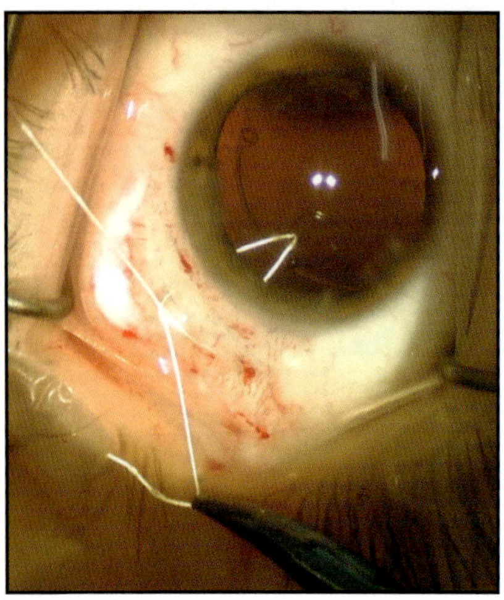

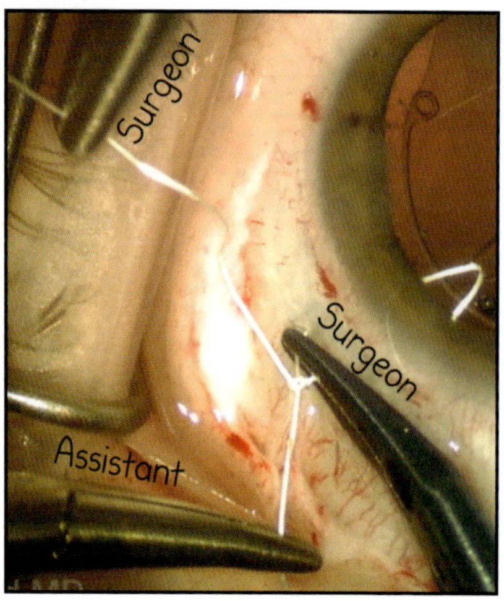

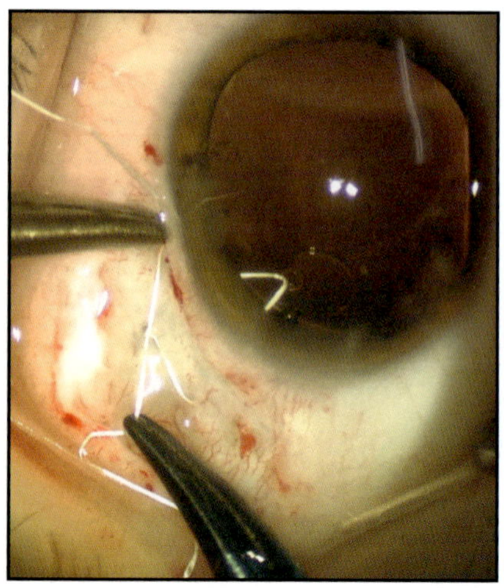

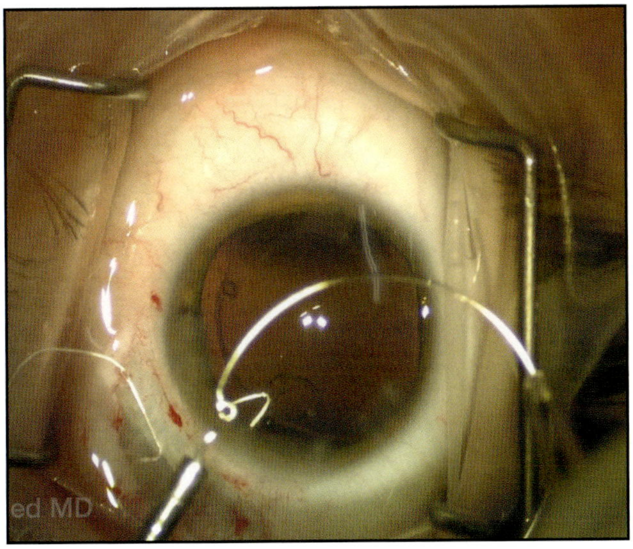

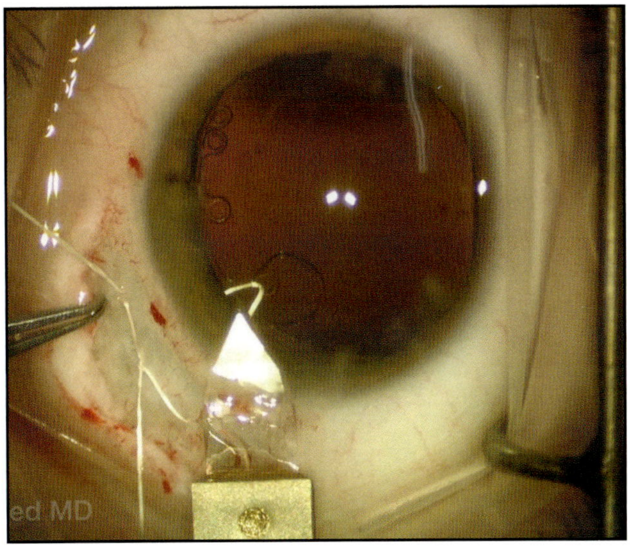

- Add additional cohesive viscoelastic in the bag. Place a CTR in the capsule, facilitated by a Kuglen hook. (Refer to Chapter 10.) CTR passage can be obstructed slightly by the CTS, but this issue is generally minimized by ensuring that the capsular bag is full of cohesive OVD. Enlarge the temporal corneal incision slightly (usually 3.2 mm) to facilitate complete insertion of the intraocular lens (IOL) injector and direct placement of the single-piece acrylic IOL in the capsular bag.
- Manually remove OVD from the capsule and anterior chamber using BSS on a blunt cannula. Take care not to remove too much OVD or decompress the anterior chamber, as shallowing can allow for vitreous prolapse.

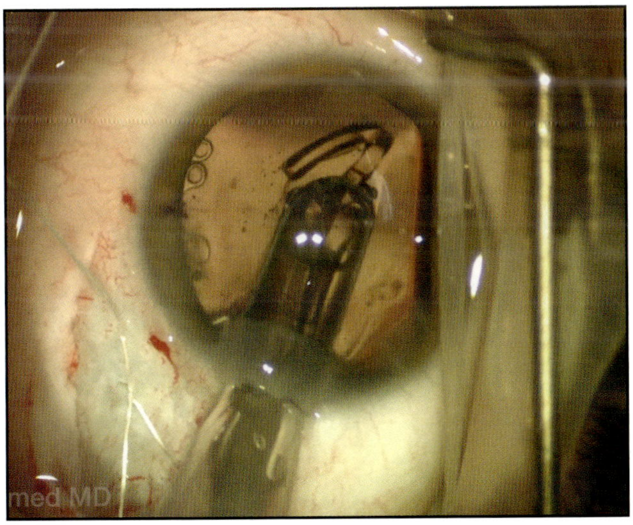

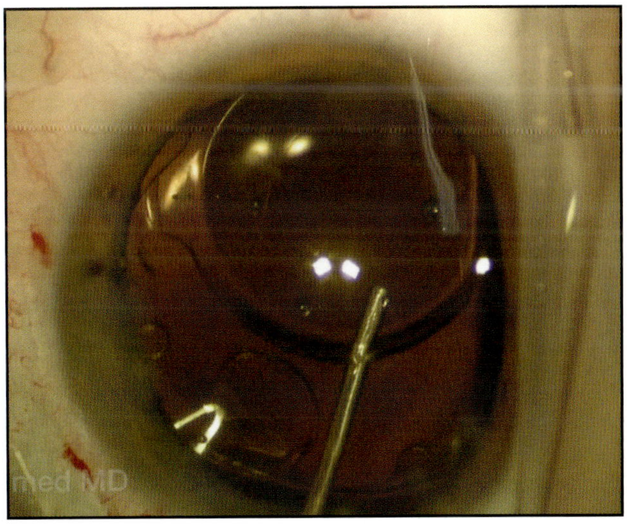

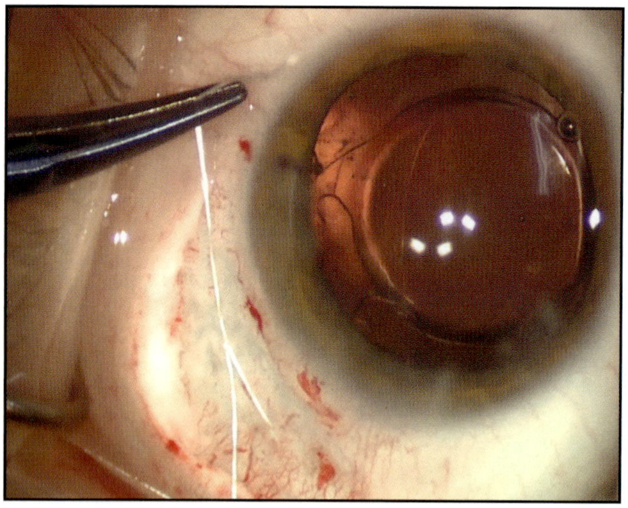

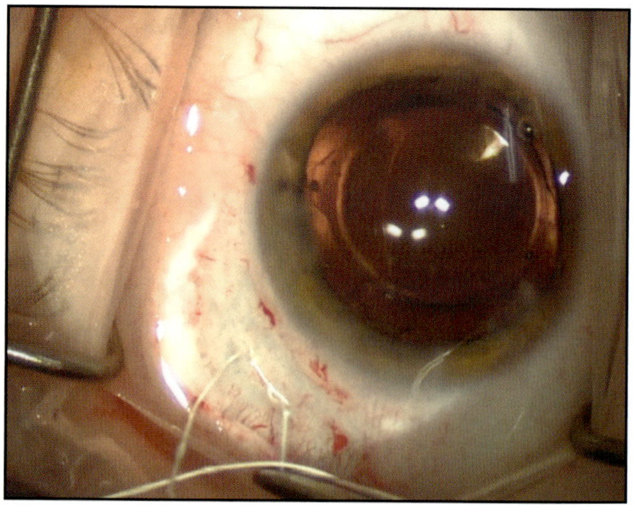

- Gently tighten the slip knot on the CTS to ensure centration of the IOL. Do not overtighten, as this can damage the capsulorrhexis.
- Once adequately tensioned, lock the suture with a reverse throw, followed by a single forward throw (see knot diagram).
- Trim the ends and bury the knot (with one arm of the needle driver, enlarge one of the sclerotomy sites and then rotate the suture so that the knot passes through the sclerotomy). Verify that the IOL is still centered and the CTS is engaged.
- Instill Miochol (acetylcholine) into the anterior chamber to confirm the pupil mioses roundly and symmetrically. Any peaking may suggest the presence of prolapsed vitreous.
- Close the conjunctival peritomy with interrupted resorbable suture such as Vicryl (Ethicon, Inc).
- Hydrate the corneal incisions and place sutures as needed to ensure a watertight closure.

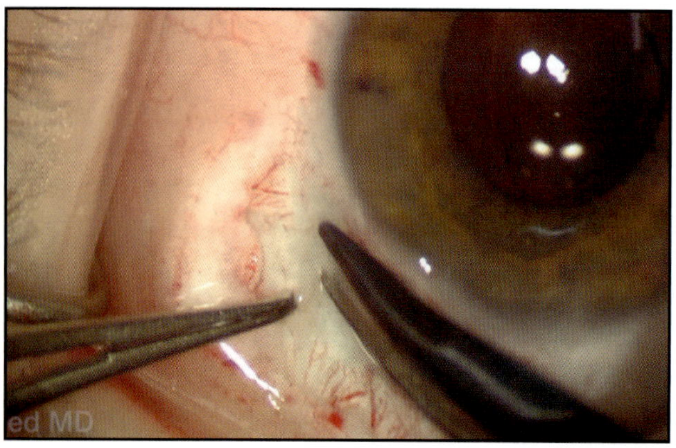

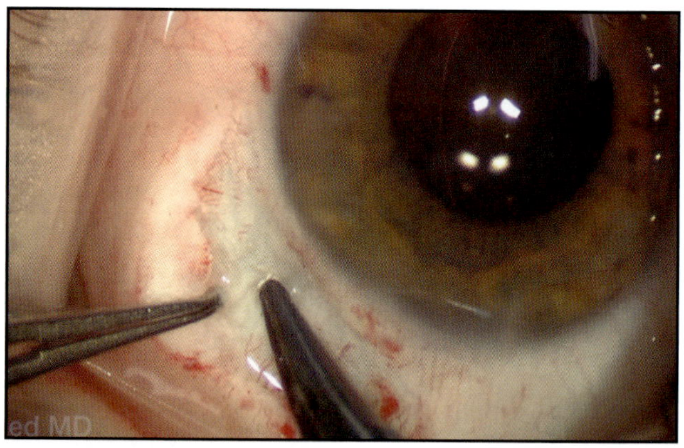

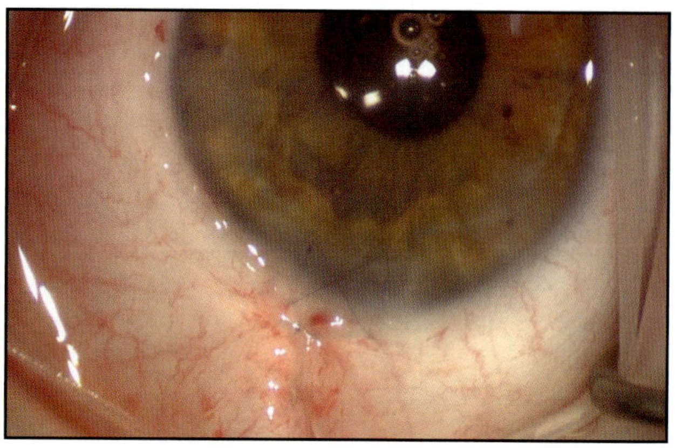

In cases of severe diffuse zonulopathy, one CTS may not be enough. A single CTS covers about 90 degrees of zonulopathy. The previously described technique is easily replicated to add a second CTS. Key points are to place both CTS elements about 180 degrees apart and to titrate suture tension using slip knots on both CTS, ensuring that the IOL is centered before the additional throws are used to lock the sutures.

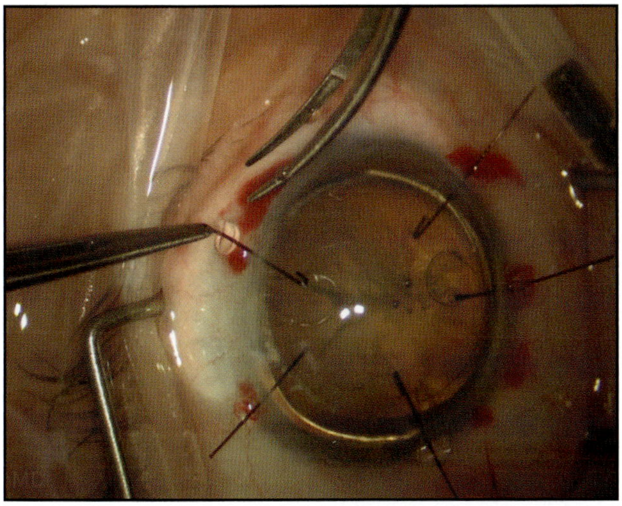

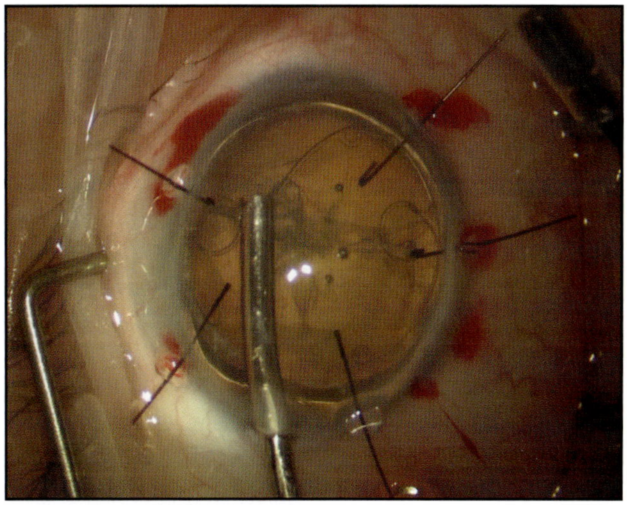

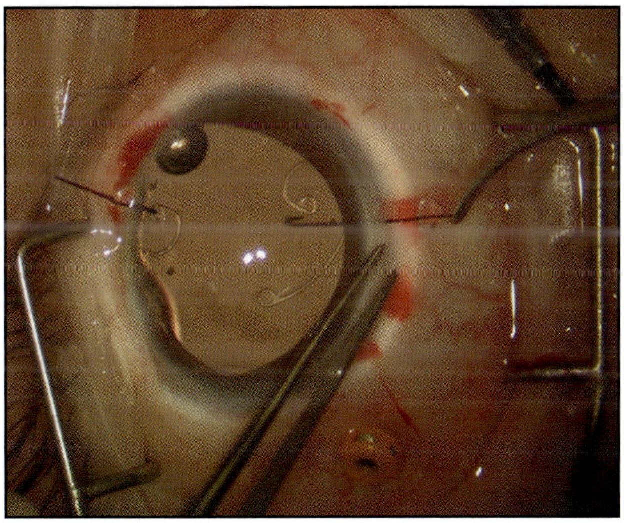

THE SLIP KNOT

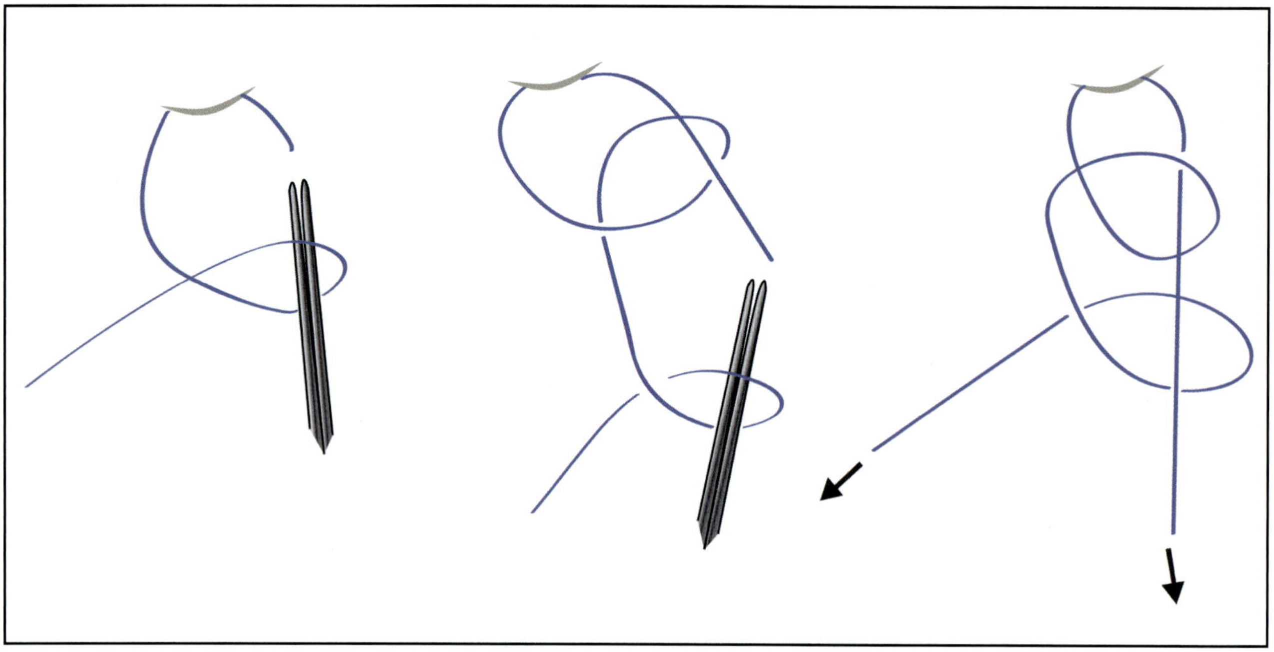

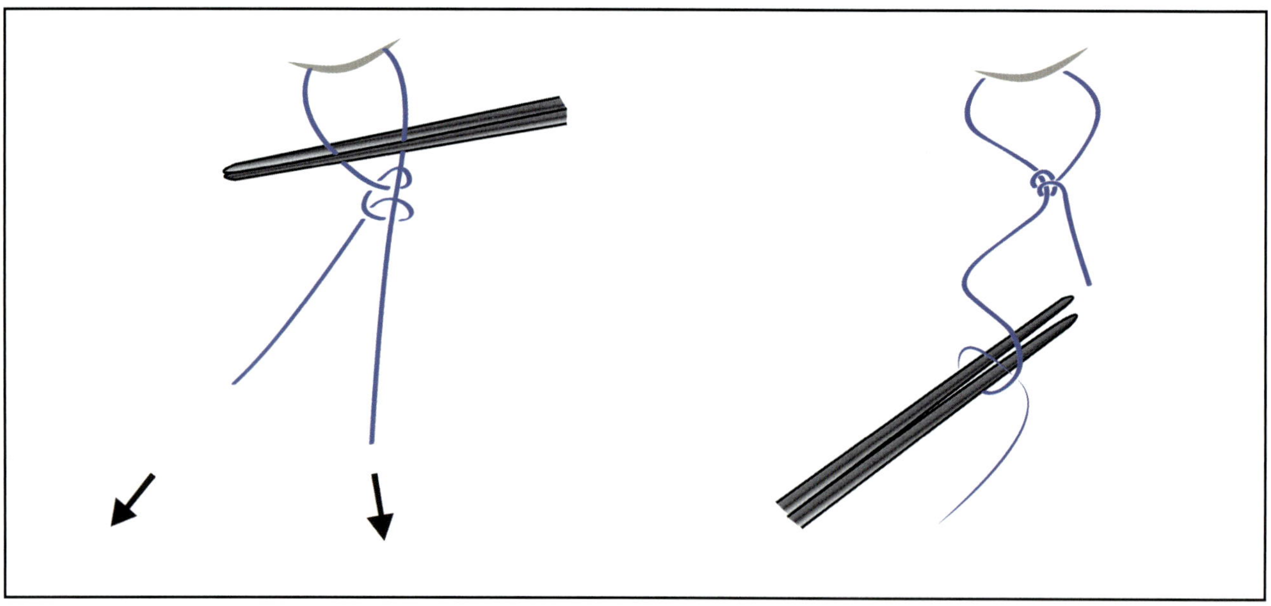

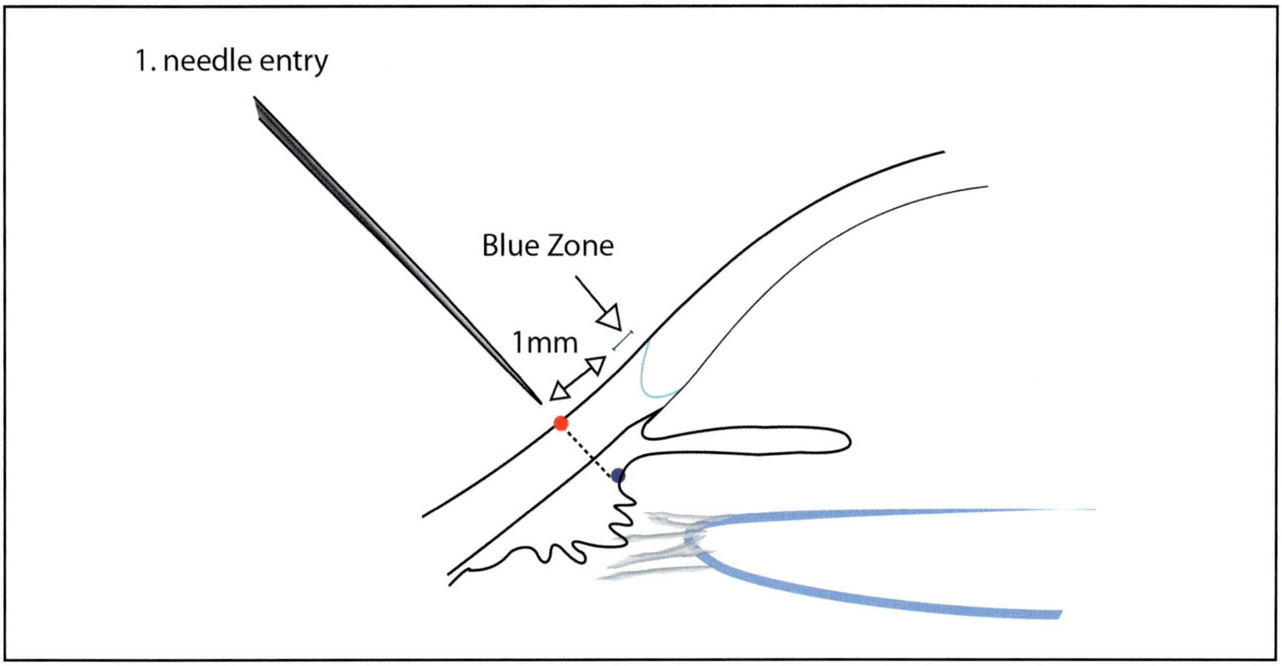

Diagram of needle entry and angle change for sulcus fixation. Needle entry should be done perpendicular to the sclera, 1 mm posterior to the end of the blue zone (corresponding to the corneal wedge). Once the needle has advanced into the scleral thickness, a 45-degree angle change should be carried out in order to enter the ciliary sulcus parallel to the iris plane (dotted arrow).

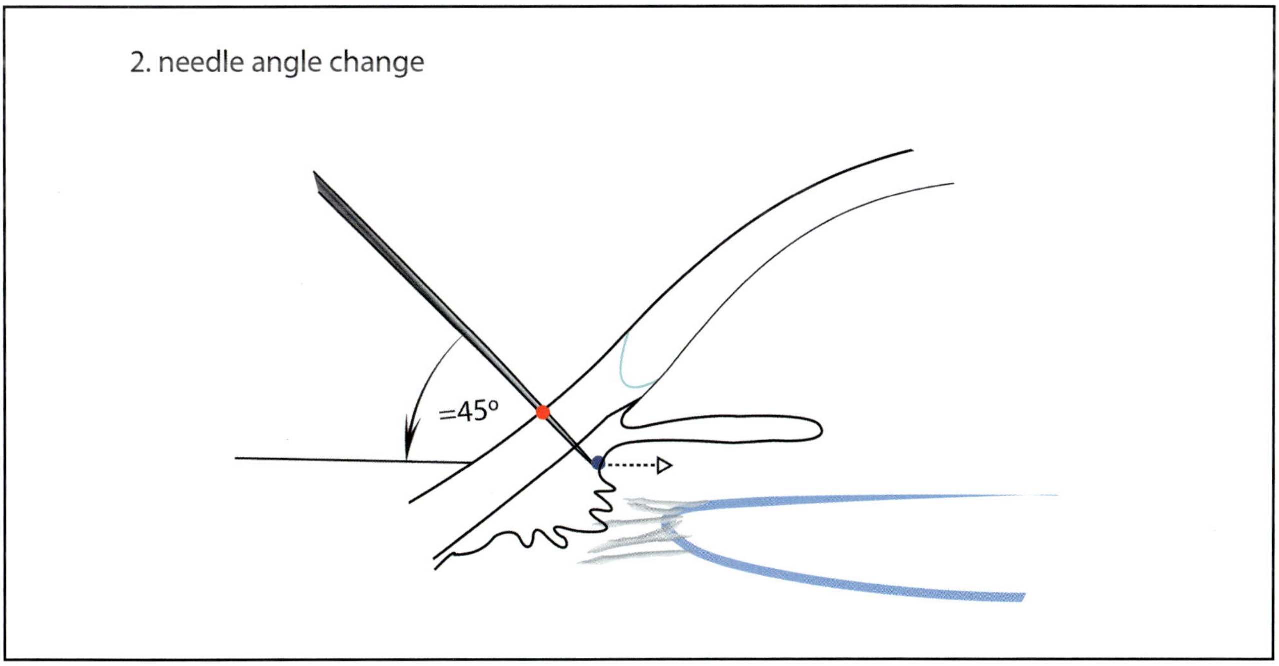

CHAPTER 12

HOW TO IMPLANT A MODIFIED CAPSULAR TENSION RING

INTRODUCTION

Modified capsular tension rings (MCTRs) can be used to support the capsular bag by fixating the device to sclera via a fixation loop that is part of the ring. This loop can be sutured to sclera while the remainder of the device is in the capsular bag.

Here, we will discuss the surgical technique and address variations of this device, including the Malyugin-Cionni ring. The Malyugin modification eliminates the shorter segment of the Cionni MCTR so that it can be injected similar to a CTR. This means it can be incorporated through a 1.8-mm incision and can even be injected after a suture has been pre-placed through the fixation loop.

KEY POINTS

- These devices cannot be used if there is any disruption of the capsule or with a discontinuous capsulorrhexis.
- If there is a posterior capsule defect, this should be converted to a small continuous curvilinear posterior capsulotomy; otherwise, the forces of these rings will extend any noncontinuous capsule defect.
- See Chapter 11 as many of the key elements come into play.
- Care must be taken not to puncture the capsular bag with the docking needle passes.

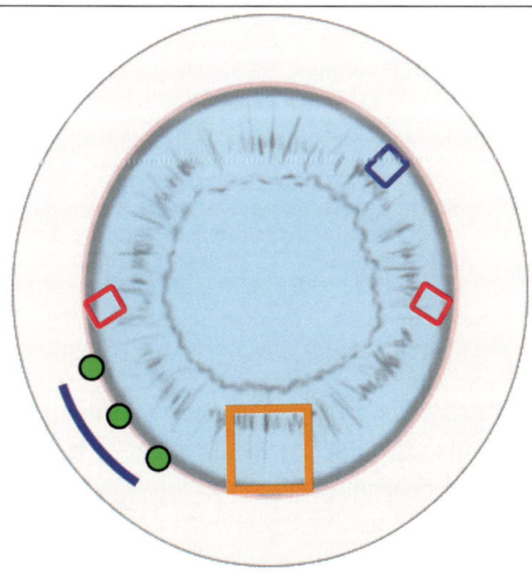

- Standard phaco + knife and fork
- Additional paracentesis approximately 180 degrees from zonular dialysis (site of capsular tension segment [CTS] fixation)
- Partial-thickness scleral scratch incision 1/4 scleral depth 1 mm posterior to the scleral spur, 3 to 4 mm in length in area of planned CTS fixation
- Iris hook incisions in area of planned CTS fixation

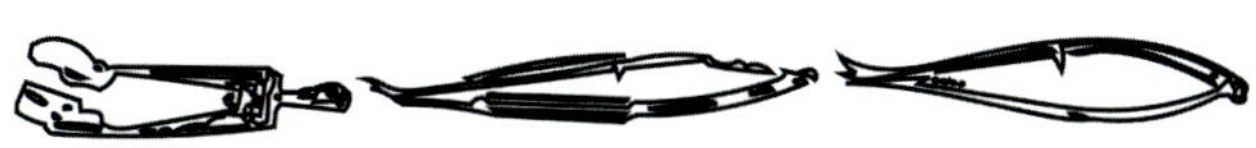

- Microsurgical Technology, Inc microforceps Gore-Tex 7-0 suture on CV-8 needle—double-armed 0.5 inch
- 25-g hypodermic needle for docking the Gore-Tex suture if using 9-0, or 27-g hypodermic needle to dock if using 10-0 Prolene (Ethicon, Inc)

Ahmed IK, Campos-Möller X, Shah M, Sheybani A. *Illustrated Advanced Anterior Segment Surgery: A Step-by-Step Guide for Challenging Cases* (pp 79-85).

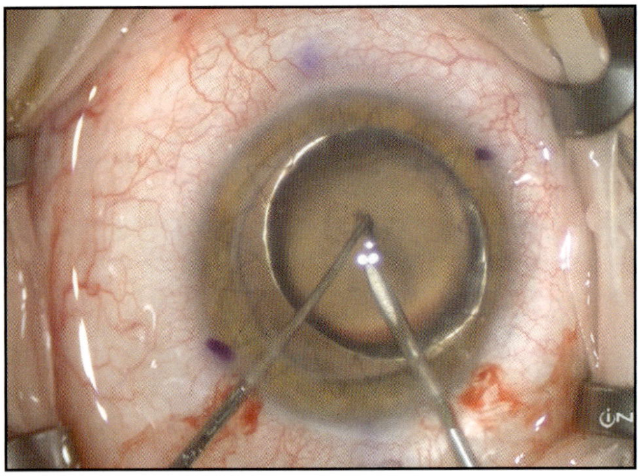

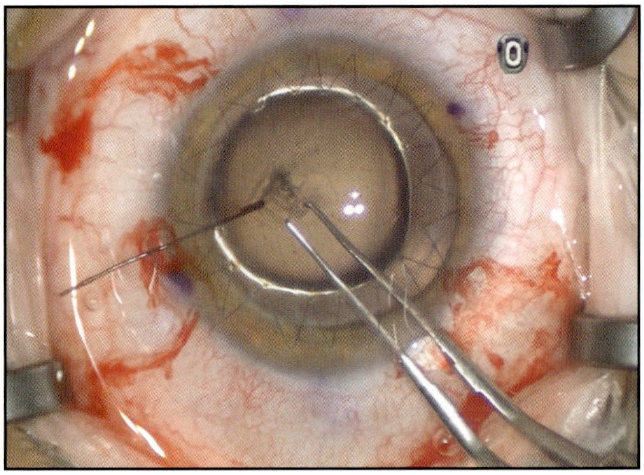

- After knife and fork paracenteses are created, a "soft shell" ophthalmic viscosurgical device (OVD) technique is used. Dispersive OVD can also be used to tamponade vitreous backward in the areas of zonular absence.
- If the zonules are diffusely weak, a Kuglen hook should be used to provide countertraction while initiating the capsule puncture. Alternatively, sharp-tipped micrograspers can be used to puncture and perform the continuous curvilinear capsulorrhexis (refer to Chapter 7).
- An iris hook is placed along the capsule to provide countertraction while the continuous curvilinear capsulorrhexis is performed. A Kuglen hook in the nondominant hand can be helpful to maintain countertraction as the rhexis is performed with the dominant hand.

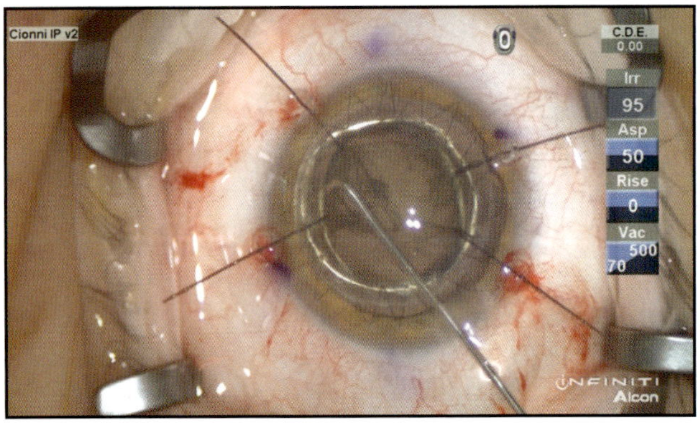

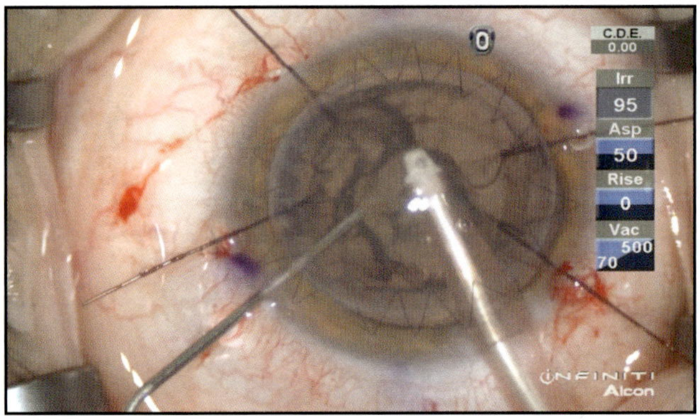

- Iris hooks do well supporting the capsule when there is low flow (unlike in phacoemulsification, where there is high flow). In this case, the lens is aspirated with the irrigation/aspiration handpiece without significant manipulation; therefore, iris hooks can be left in place. Otherwise, capsule retractors should be used if phacoemulsification is performed as iris hooks can tear the anterior capsule.
- Here, hydrodissection is performed as well as hydrodelineation. If the MCTR is placed before phacoemulsification, a cohesive viscoelastic should be used to viscodissect the cortex from the capsule to make room for the device.
- Capsule retractors can be removed to facilitate cortical cleanup.

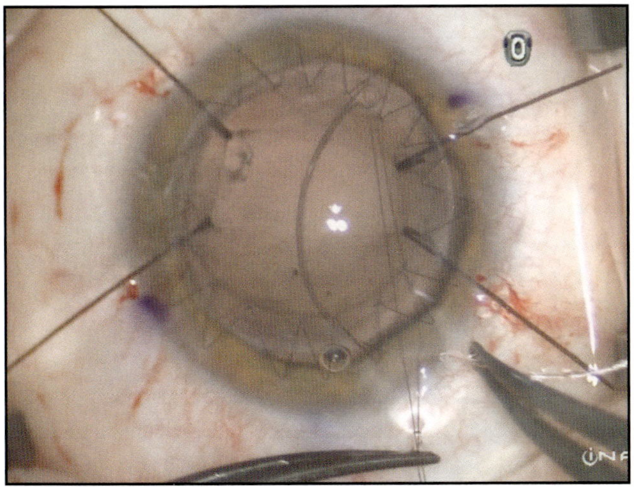

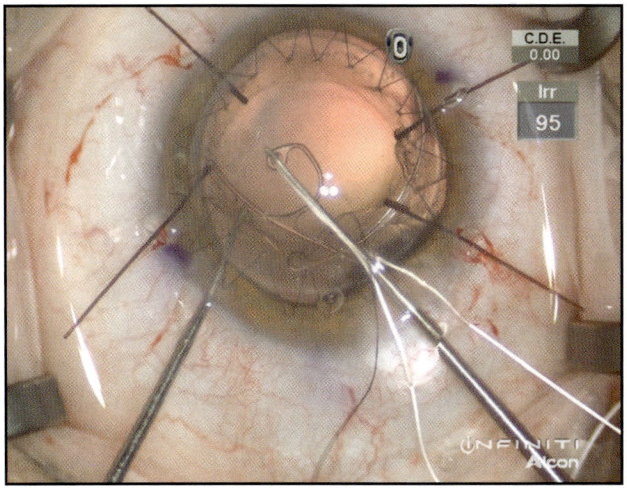

- The capsular bag is fully inflated with cohesive viscoelastic. One must ensure full expansion of the bag to minimize additional zonular trauma or capsular bag compromise. Gore-Tex suture is looped through the fixation hook prior to placement of the device, and the needles are removed. Leave the suture long enough that it remains outside the eye after insertion of the MCTR (about 4 to 6 cm). One can loop a 10-0 nylon through the leading eyelet to facilitate insertion. When the ring is fed into the capsular bag, the 10-0 nylon is pulled back through the main wound as the MCTR is fed into the eye with nontoothed forceps.
- A Sinskey hook is used through the main insion, hook down, to guide the fixation hook into the eye, rotating the MCTR to the desired quadrant.
- The hook should remain ABOVE the capsule while the rest of the MCTR is within the capsular bag. The 10-0 nylon guiding suture is cut from the proximal loop and removed.

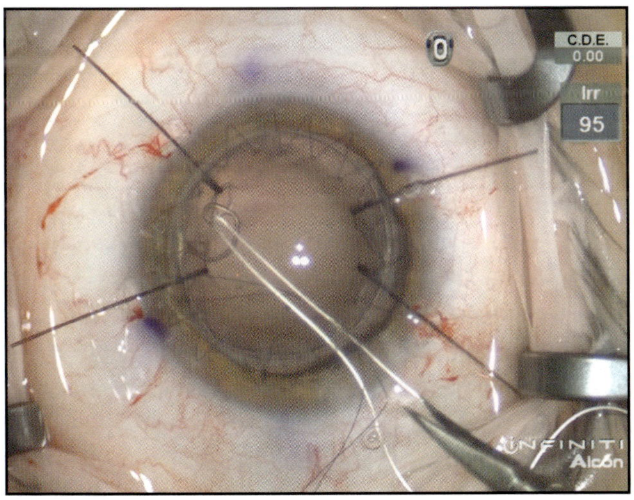

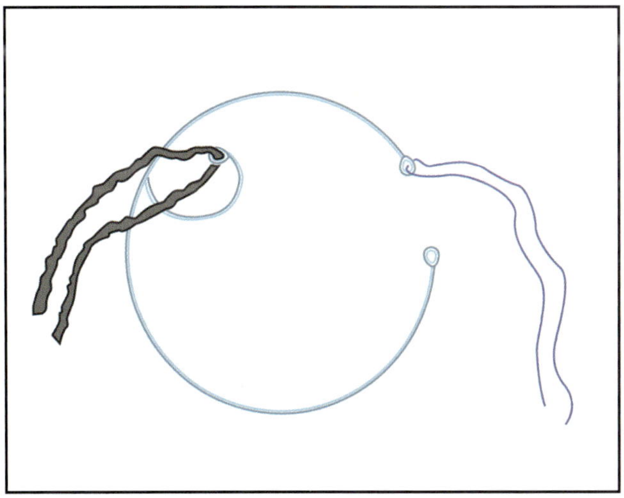

Threading an MCTR with 2 sutures: The illustration shows the proper suture configuration—nylon reign suture at the leading eyelet to facilitate passage of CTR and Gore-Tex suture at central eyelet for fixation. Avoid trapping the ring section of the CTR with the Gore-Tex suture by ensuring both suture ends are above the ring before insertion.

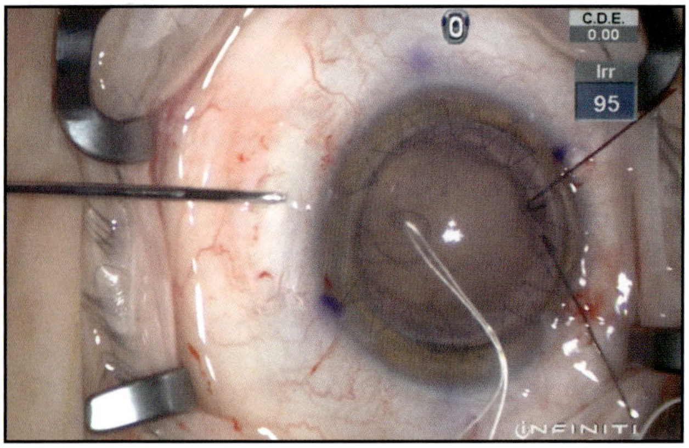

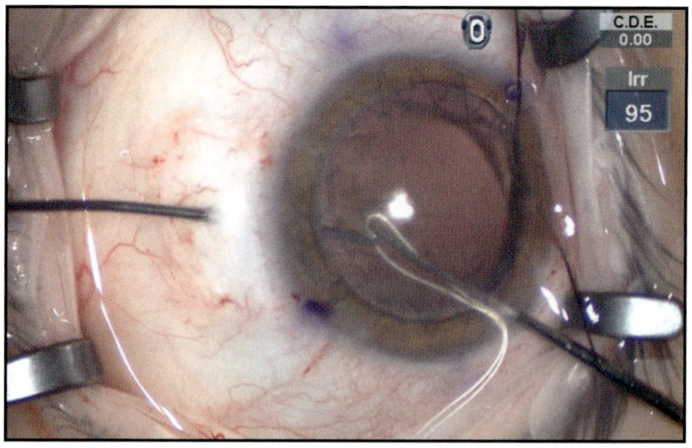

A scratch incision is made exactly as in preparation for a CTS (see Chapter 11).

The docking needle and suture passes are performed in the same fashion if the suture is not pre-placed.

If the suture is pre-placed (as in this case), micrograsping forceps are placed through the scleral incision made by the docking needle, and a loop of suture is retracted out of the eye through sclera. A Condon snare (Microsurgical Technology, Inc) can also be used to grasp this suture loop. Countertraction on the MCTR fixation loop is performed with a Kuglen hook; otherwise, the device can be drawn too far into peripheral scleral wall, disinserting the remaining opposing zonules.

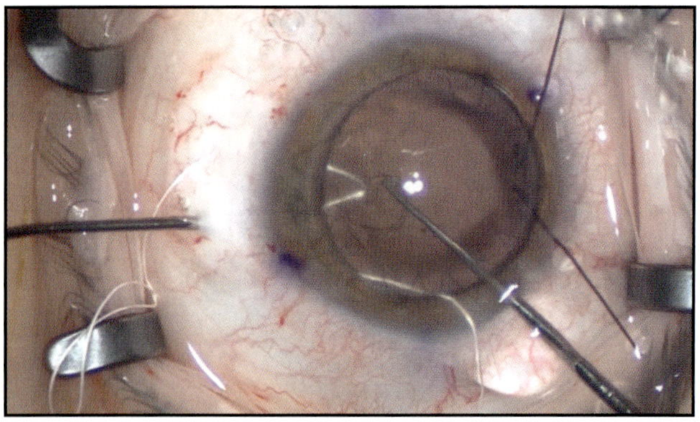

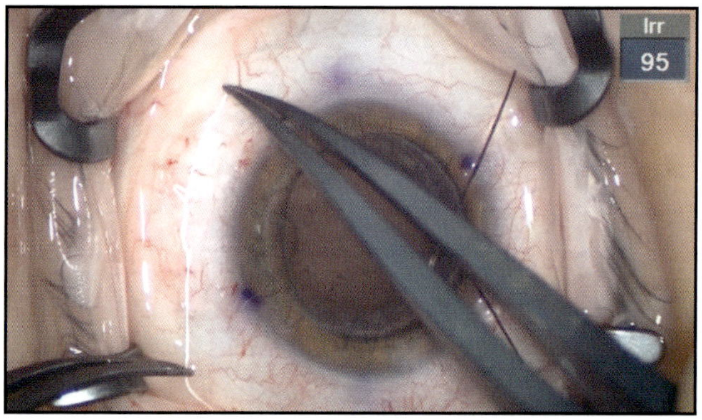

A second scleral pass is made with a needle in this case, followed by retrieval of the suture with micrograsping forceps. The suture should be grasped on the opposite side of the loop as the prior grasp.

The suture is then tied in slip knot fashion, and tension is adjusted for centration, as in Chapter 11.

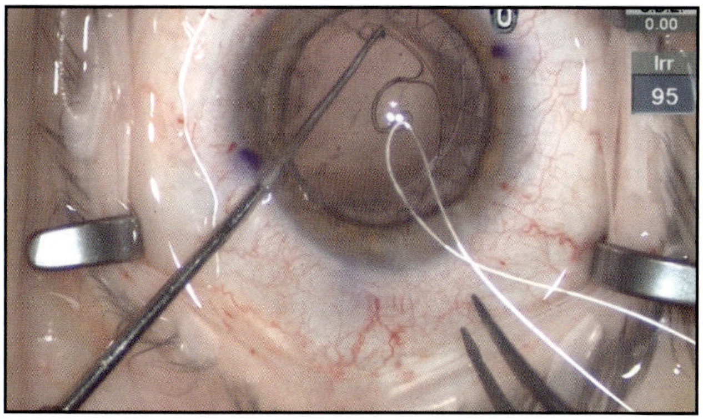

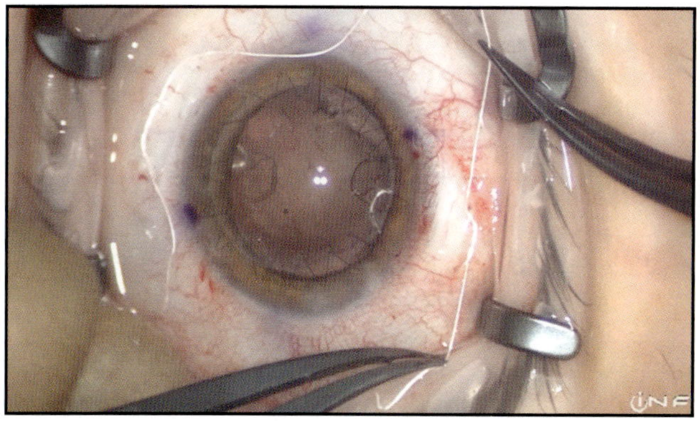

In this case with diffuse zonulopathy, a CTS is sutured 180 degrees from the sutured MCTR, in the same fashion as in Chapter 11. The intraocular lens (IOL) can now be injected INTO the capsular bag. Avoid wound-assisted injections. Manipulation of the IOL as it unfolds should be swift; the more it unfolds and the more pressure required to place the IOL into the bag, the higher the chance of iatrogenic zonular damage.

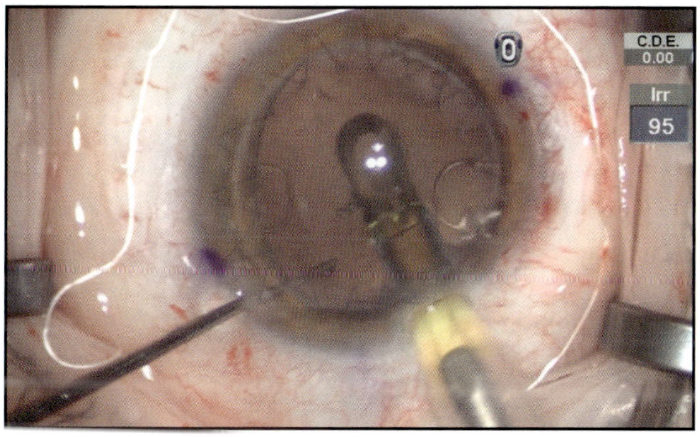

Centration of the IOL can be achieved by selectively tightening the slip knots on each side. Remember to not overtighten! Slip knots are hard to loosen, so it is better to go back and forth between opposite sides than to overtighten one of them and have a decentered IOL bag complex.

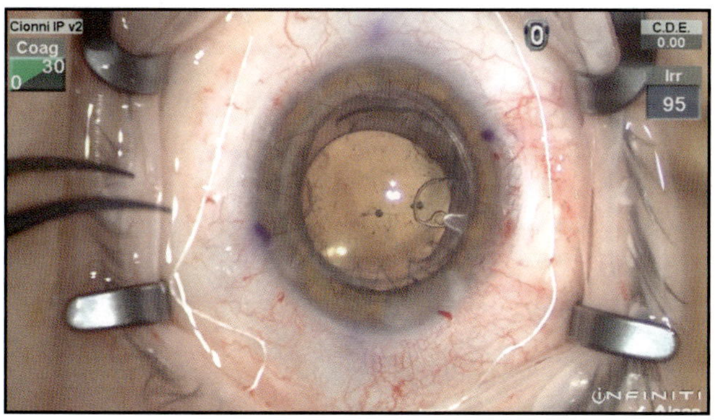

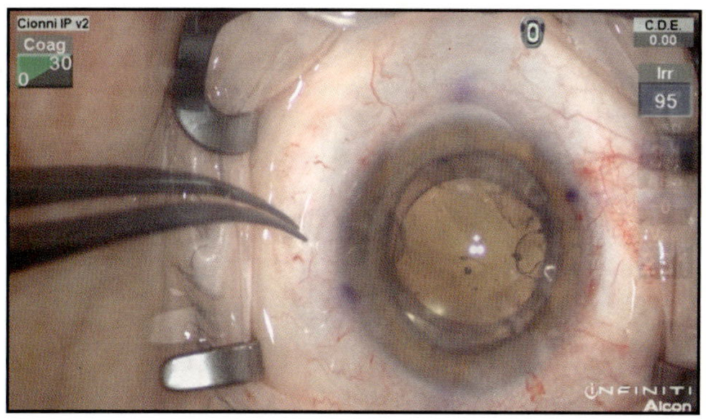

HOW TO IMPLANT THE MALYUGIN-CIONNI MCTR

This device can be injected even when pre-placed sutures are used. Here, we describe insertion of the device.

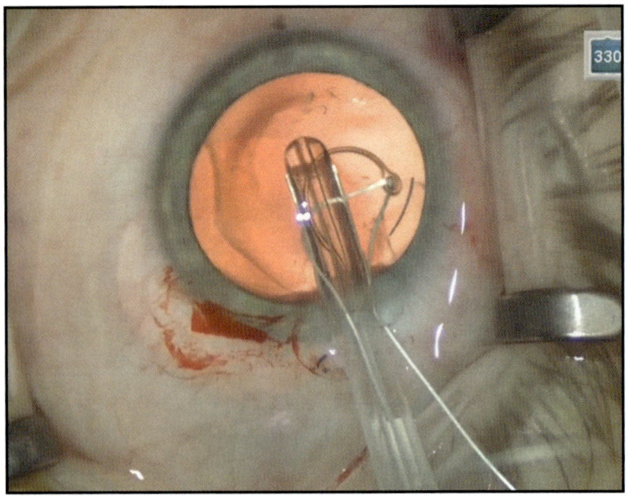

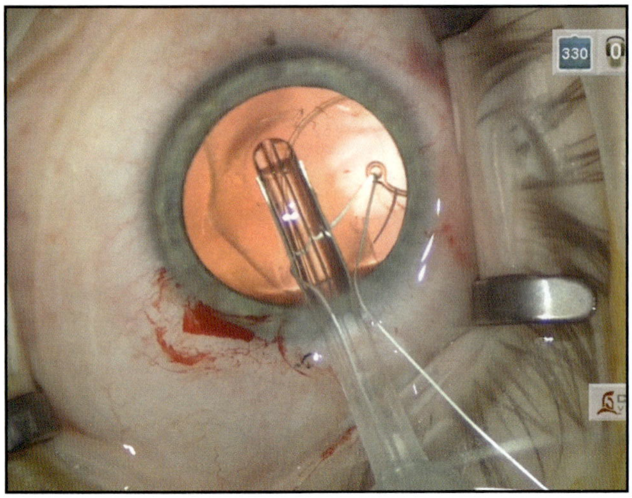

- Loop the Gore-Tex suture through the device. Have the needles cut off the suture (as previously described in this chapter).
- The device can be loaded into an injector in a similar fashion to a CTR. In this case, the leading edge is the side with the pre-placed suture through the fixation loop. The suture remains OUTSIDE the injector after the device is drawn in.
- As the device is injected, make sure undue tension is not occurring on the pre-placed sutures. Sometimes, a Sinskey hook is used to guide the device and rotate it to position.
- The device is secured as the CTS and MCTR are performed (described previously).

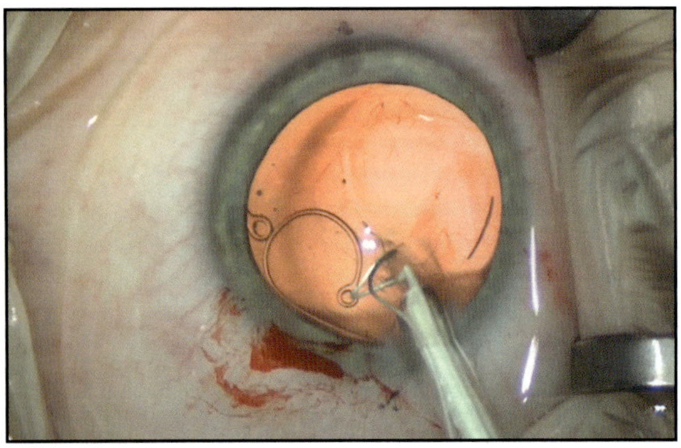

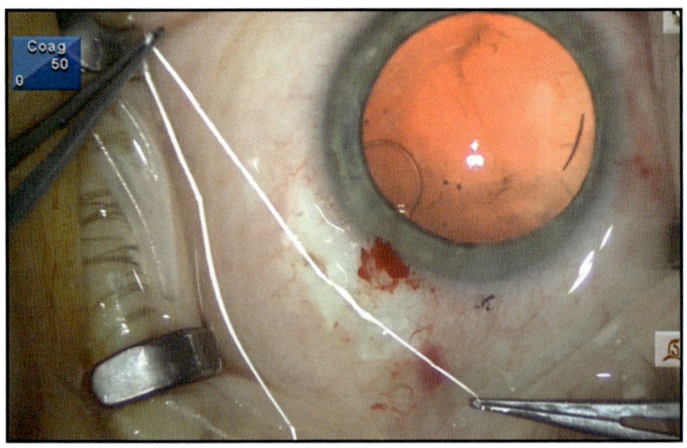

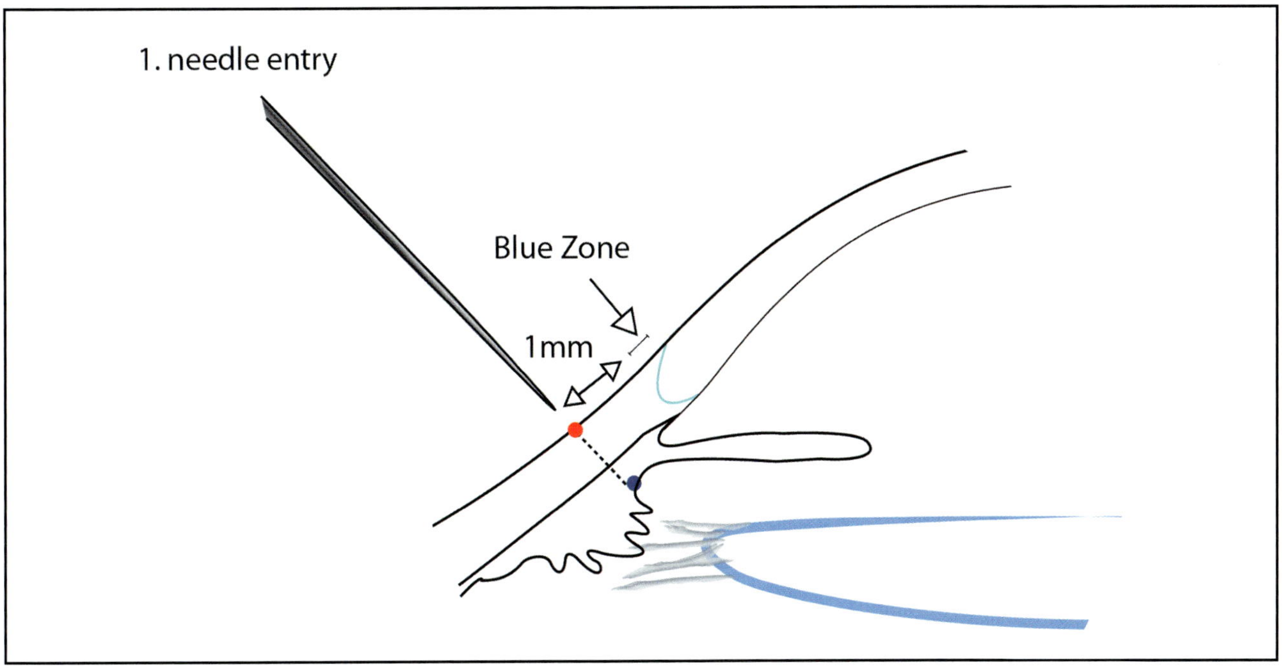

Diagram of needle entry and angle change for sulcus fixation. Needle entry should be done perpendicular to the sclera, 1 mm posterior to the end of the blue zone (corresponding to the corneal wedge). Once the needle has advanced into the scleral thickness, a 45-degree angle change should be carried out in order to enter the ciliary sulcus parallel to the iris plane (dotted arrow).

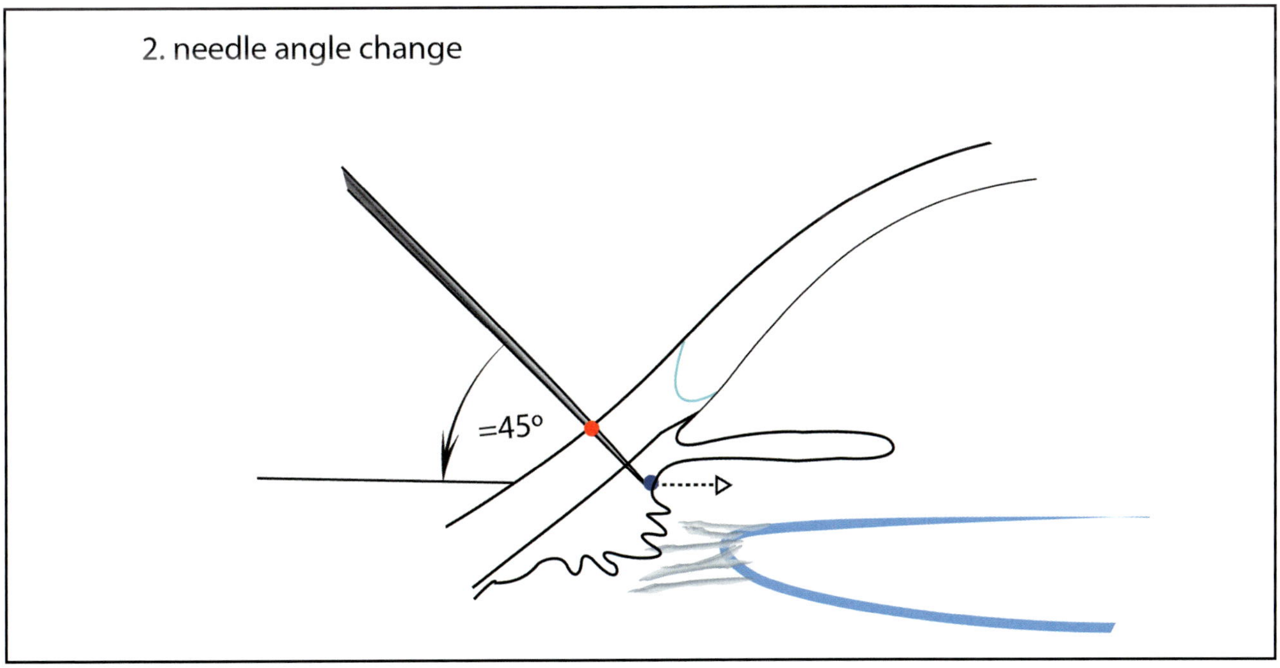

SPECIAL THANKS TO DR. ROBERT CIONNI FOR PROVIDING SURGICAL PHOTOS IN THIS CHAPTER.

CHAPTER 13

VITRECTOMY PEARLS

INTRODUCTION

When facing complex anterior segment challenges, facility and comfort in managing the anterior vitreous is essential. The basics of vitrectomy for the anterior segment surgeon follow some common principles—management of fluidics, maintenance of chamber pressurization, understanding cut rates, and control of aspiration. In a variation from our standard chapter structure, we offer you some pearls on approaching the vitreous.

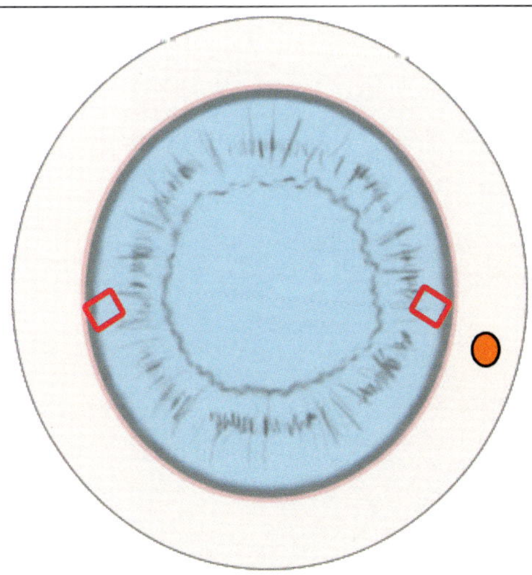

- Paracentesis sized to the diameter of the vitrectomy unit being used. A pars plana entry may also be used.

KEY POINTS

- Be comfortable performing vitrectomy through either an anterior approach (limbal/corneal incisions) or the pars plana.
- There are specific indications for choosing one approach over the other, but for most situations, an anterior approach is typically adequate.
- Dilute preservative-free triamcinolone is very helpful in staining vitreous to improve visualization. It has an added benefit of providing some anti-inflammatory coverage in the postoperative period.
- Know your machine (settings, foot pedal controls, etc). You should be able to switch between settings with ease.
- Always keep the anterior chamber well formed and prevent any sudden decompression. Use balanced salt solution (BSS) or ophthalmic viscosurgical device (OVD) freely to maintain anterior chamber (AC) formed when exchanging instruments.
- Keep incisions tight and suture all large wounds when not in use.
- Using continuous irrigation during phacoemulsification will make vitreous management potentially more difficult as irrigation should be turned off when viscoelastics are placed; otherwise, the viscoelastic and vitreous may be forced out of the eye. We prefer having complete control over irrigation/aspiration.

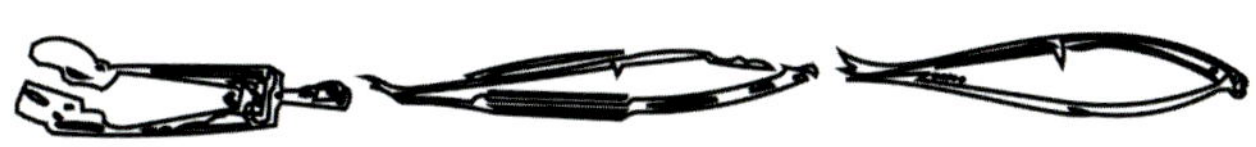

- Vitrectomy kit

Ahmed IK, Campos-Möller X, Shah M, Sheybani A. *Illustrated Advanced Anterior Segment Surgery: A Step-by-Step Guide for Challenging Cases* (pp 87-92).

Vitrectomy Unit Settings

Cut rate:

- High cut rates are ideal for segmenting vitreous strands without generating excessive traction. Cut rates above 2500 cuts per minute are desirable, whenever available. Lower cut rates, in combination with high aspiration flow/vacuum, allow for removal of larger particles such as nuclear fragments, cortical material, and capsule.

Cut on/off:

- When cut is off, only flow is activated when the foot switch is activated. Some phacoemulsification platforms do not have an on/off function. Instead, the foot switch can be programmed to activate either "vacuum before cut" (vacuum on position 2 and cut on position 3), or "cut before vacuum" (cut on position 2 and vacuum on position 3). These settings are generally termed "IA/cut" or "cut/IA."

Vacuum/flow:

- In general, moderate vacuums are preferred to reduce traction. Flow should be high enough to draw cut vitreous into the shaft, but not so high that it generates traction.

Irrigation:

- The purpose of irrigation in vitrectomy is solely to maintain the eye formed. High irrigation pressures should be avoided because this causes unnecessary turbulence.

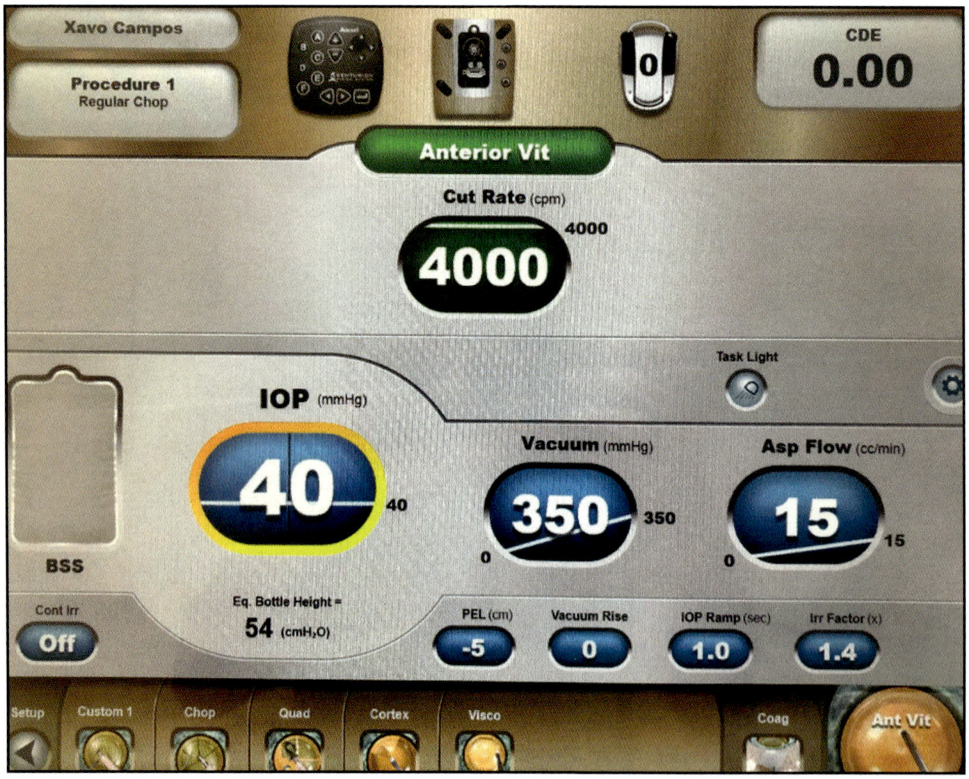

- Several techniques and devices are available to access the pars plana, but perhaps the easiest method is through the use of a valved 23-g trochar, as this does not require a conjunctival peritomy and usually does not require sutures for closure.
- Subconjunctival lidocaine can be instilled into the area of pars plana entry.
- Use the caliper end of the trochar inserter to measure 3.5 mm posterior to the limbus for aphakic or pseudophakic patients, or 4 mm for phakic patients.

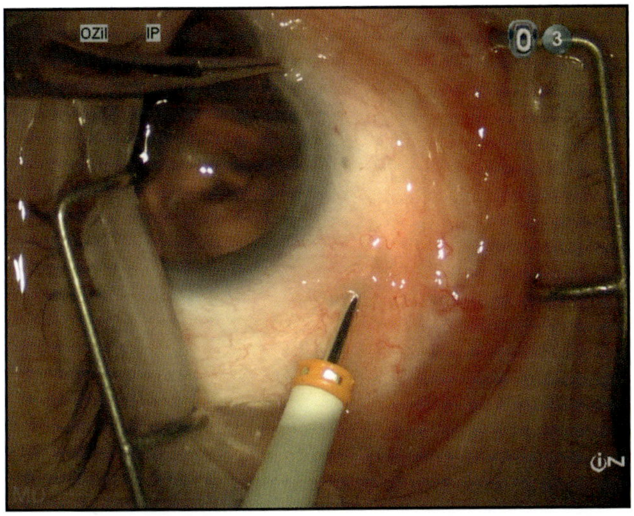

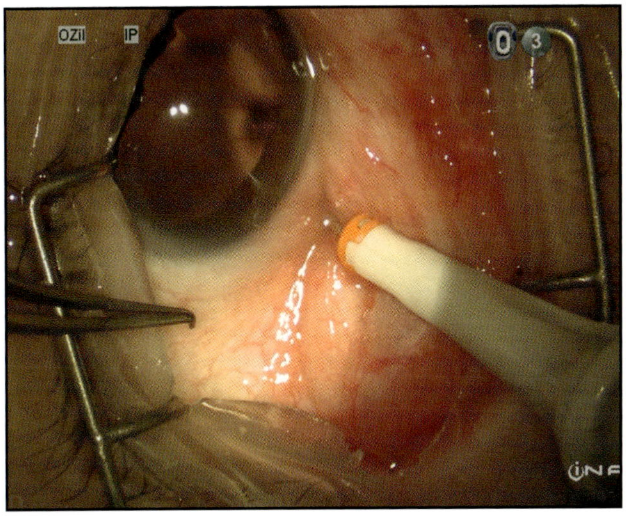

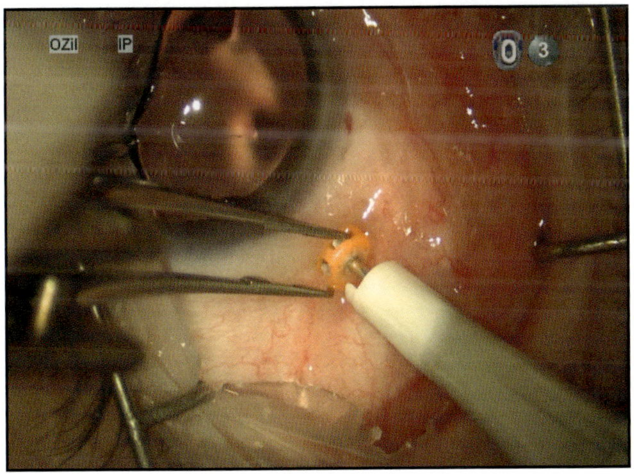

- Grasp the conjunctiva and episclera with Colibri forceps to ensure you have control of the globe.
- Use the microvitreoretinal blade end of the trochar inserter to first enter conjunctiva, tunnel under conjunctiva, and then engage sclera in a bevelled, tunneled fashion.
- Once through sclera, turn the trochar such that the blade end is facing the optic nerve (think posterior, not central).
- Use the Colibri forceps to grasp the top of the trochar, and remove the inserter while maintaining pressure on the globe to keep the trochar opposed to the sclera.
- This entry port can be used to remove vitreous at various points throughout the case, and the trochar can remain in place until it is time to close.

Removal

- Begin to remove the trochar while keeping the cutter in the eye.
- Once the trochar is removed, let go of it and place a Weck-Cel spear (Beaver-Visitec International) near the scleral insertion site to distract the conjunctiva over the sclerotomy and facilitate closure of the self-sealing scleral tunnel.
- Remove the cutter from the eye while in foot position 2 (cutting only, no aspiration).
- Ensure no vitreous has come forward or become incarcerated in the sclerotomy.

How and When to Use the Vitrectomy Handpiece

- Vitreous must not be aspirated without being cut—this creates traction, which can result in retinal tears or a retinal detachment.
- Utilize a high cut rate when managing vitreous alone. Consider reducing the cut rate when trying to cut and aspirate more solid structures, such as residual cortical material or dropped nuclear fragments (a lower cut rate can allow more vacuum to build during occlusion and allow more time for these pieces to be aspirated). Note that this will generate more traction on any vitreous that has not been previously cut.
- Do not cut when managing residual cortex or other material around tissue that needs to be preserved, such as the capsule or iris. However, be sure to adequately and thoroughly remove vitreous at a high cut rate before switching to aspiration.
- When aspirating cortex or lens fragments alone, be sure to obtain occlusion. Failure to do so can draw more vitreous forward and generate traction on the retina.
- When removing vitreous, remember that the vitrectomy unit aspirates and, thus, can draw vitreous toward it wherever it is. Because the goal of a vitrectomy is to keep vitreous back, keep the vitrectomy unit posterior to the posterior capsular plane.
- Be mindful of the direction of the aspiration port and cutter, and do not get too close to the iris or capsule!

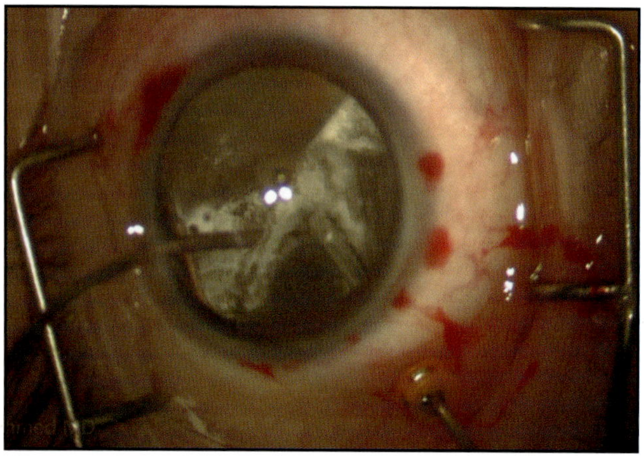

Triamcinolone used to visualize the vitreous gel. Notice the irrigation handpiece is directed posteriorly, toward the vitrector shaft. In this case, irrigation flow is preventing aspiration of the dislocated lens.

How to Use the Irrigation Handpiece

- Consider dry vitrectomy (no irrigation) when excess turbulence in the eye would be problematic. In such a situation, consider maintaining some AC pressurization with BSS on a cannula in your nondominant hand.
- When performing vitrectomy with irrigation, orientation of irrigation is important. Aim the irrigation cannula posteriorly, toward the cutting end of the vitrector.
- You can use the irrigation cannula as an extra manipulator in the eye to ensnare vitreous or help feed lens or cortical remnants into the vitrector.
- Whenever removing the irrigation unit from the eye, be sure to maintain AC pressurization with OVD or BSS prior to removal. Sweep the vitreous away from wounds with the irrigation cannula or the cutter as you cut the strand.

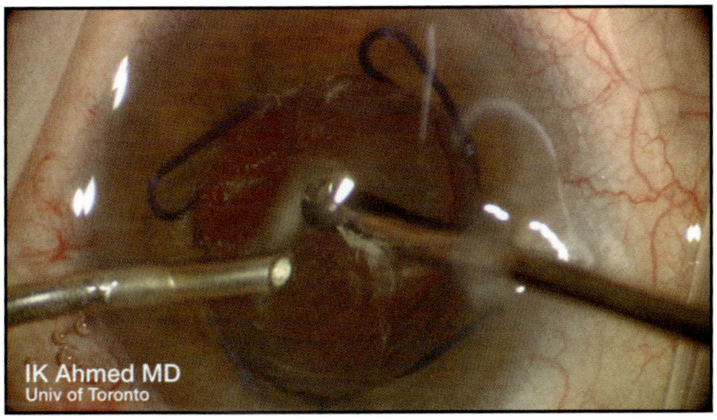

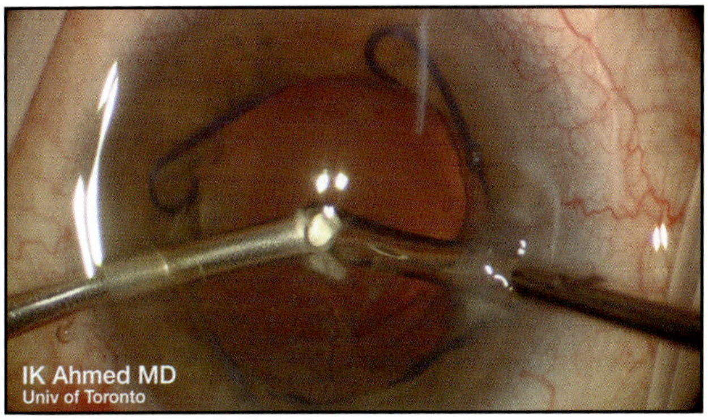

Anterior vitrectomy approach with triamcinolone stain of the vitreous. The vitrector shaft is posterior to the irrigation. In this case, a high cut rate with moderate vacuum is used to clear out vitreous (cut/IA mode).

Once vitreous has been cleared from the AC, higher vacuum with no cut can be used to clean up cortex from the capsular bag (IA/cut mode). Changing hands and using multiple incisions can facilitate reaching fragments throughout the entire AC.

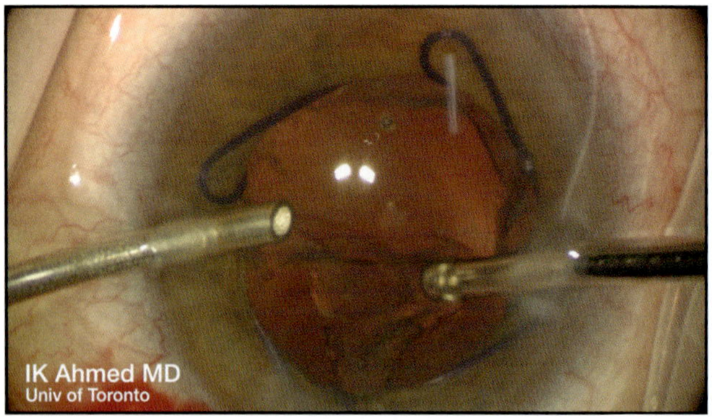

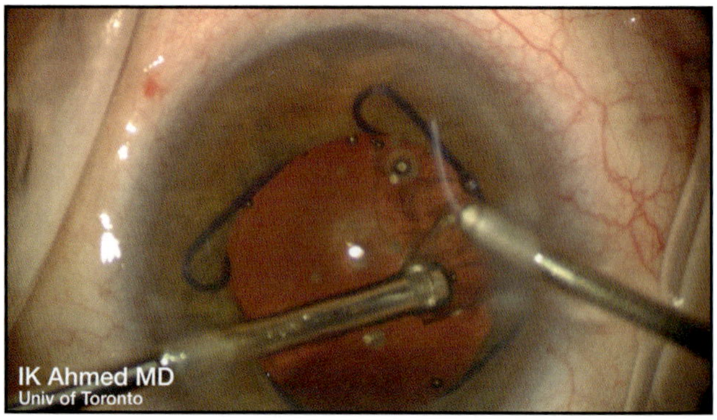

Keeping the AC formed is essential. Whenever removing instruments from the eye, BSS and/or dispersive OVD should be used to prevent anterior vitreous prolapse.

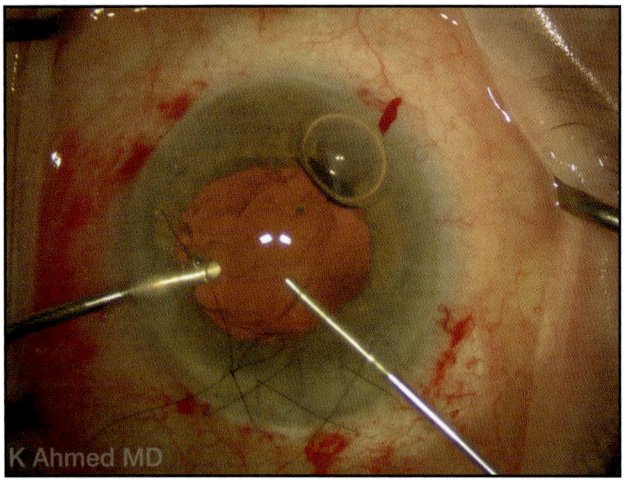

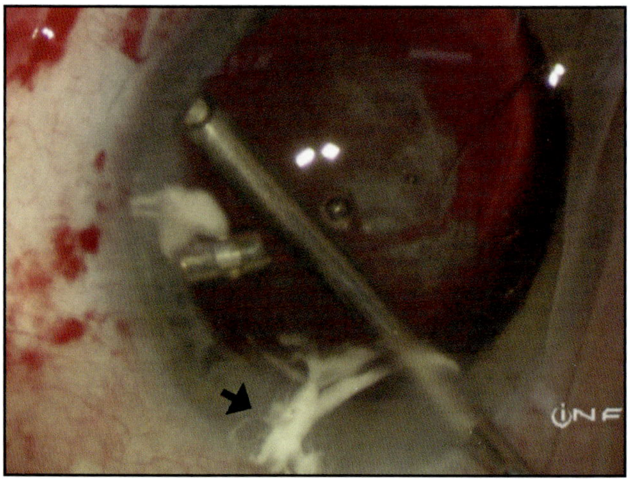

Larger wounds (like the main incision) should be sutured. Vitreous follows the path of least resistance, and larger wounds will have recurrent vitreous prolapse through them, as shown to the right (arrow).

CHAPTER 14

HOW TO OPTIC CAPTURE AN INTRAOCULAR LENS

INTRODUCTION

Intraocular lens (IOL) optic capture can be used to ensure stabilization and adequate centration of a sulcus-placed lens. In essence, the IOL is wedged in the rhexis with the haptics in a different plane than the optic. Optic capture can be utilized in the setting of a posterior capsule rent with adequate anterior capsular support in which a 3-piece IOL can be placed in the sulcus and the optic in the capsular plane and away from the iris.

KEY POINTS

- This technique requires adequate capsulorrhexis size and shape. Ideally, the opening should be slightly smaller than the optic, and round, continuous, and curvilinear.
- Capsule runouts or rents will radialize if trying to optic capture an IOL in those situations, worsening the problem.
- Do not perform optic capture for weak zonules. The manipulation required can potentially make zonulopathy worse.
- Optic capture can be performed with 3-piece IOLs.
- For single-piece IOLs, reverse optic capture should be used, as single-piece acrylic haptics should not be placed in the ciliary sulcus.

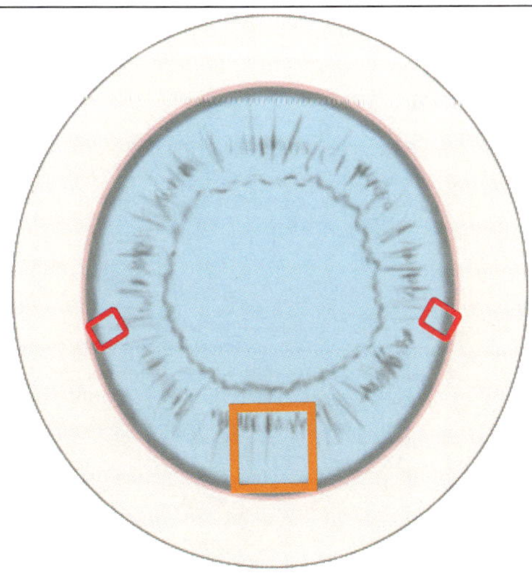

- Standard phaco with knife and fork

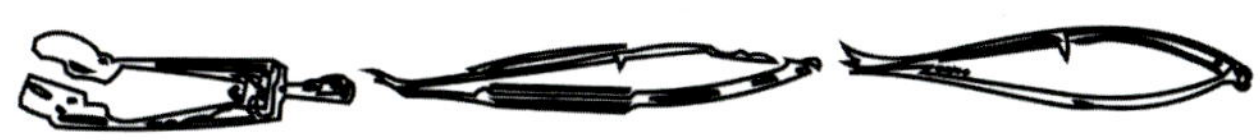

- Angled Kuglen hook
- Angled Sinskey hook
- 23-g Microsurgical Technology, Inc micrograspers
- Miochol (acetylcholine)

Ahmed IK, Campos-Möller X, Shah M, Sheybani A. *Illustrated Advanced Anterior Segment Surgery: A Step-by-Step Guide for Challenging Cases* (pp 93-97).

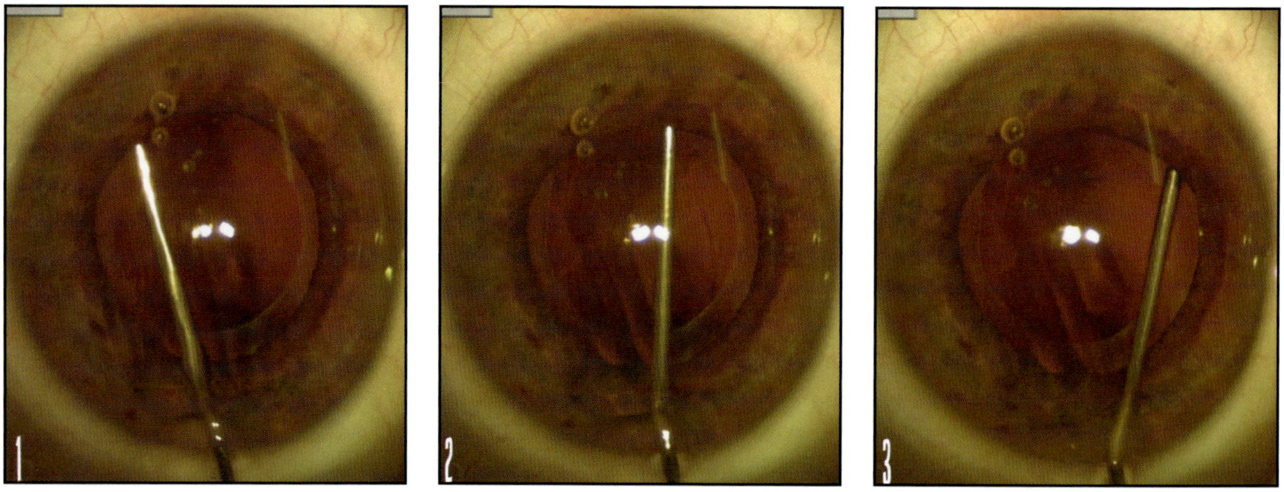

Inject cohesive ophthalmic viscosurgical device under the nasal iris to separate it from the anterior capsule leaflet, creating space for the leading IOL haptic. This step is important to prevent implantation of the leading haptic in the capsular bag.

Implant the IOL completely into the sulcus space to facilitate optic capture. Begin injection of the IOL such that the leading haptic emerges from the injector parallel to the iris plane and slides into the sulcus space without going under the anterior capsule leaflet. This will require a clockwise rotation of the injector as the leading haptic emerges. As the IOL continues to be injected and the optic presents, there will be a tendency for the IOL to flip upside down—begin to rotate the injector counterclockwise to prevent this. If using a screw-type injector, inject slowly and take your time. The trailing haptic can be left outside the eye and rotated into the sulcus using a Kuglen or Sinskey hook, engaging at the optic haptic junction. After successful implantation of the IOL into the sulcus, optic capture through the anterior capsulotomy can be achieved. See Magic Hands below each image; notice the position of the injector's "wing" to understand this rotation.

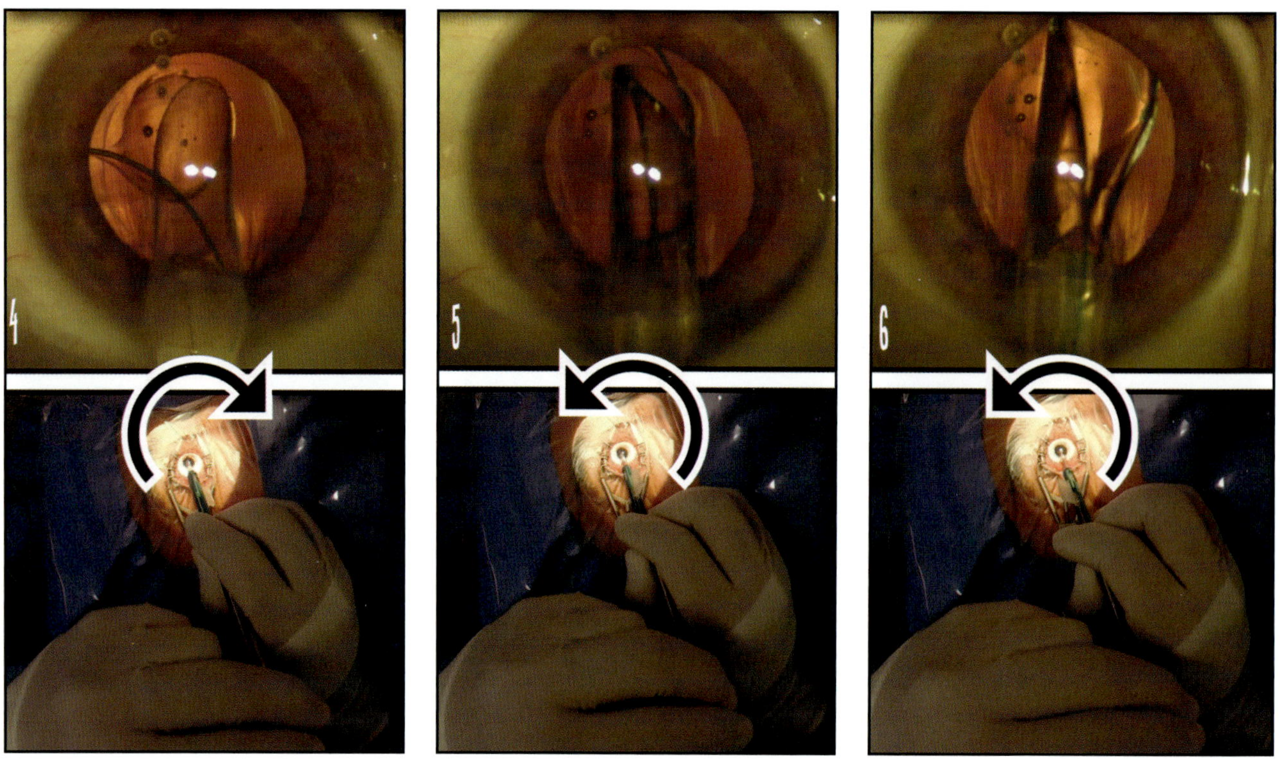

Guide the trailing haptic into the sulcus space by rotating the IOL with a Kuglen hook from the optic-haptic junction.

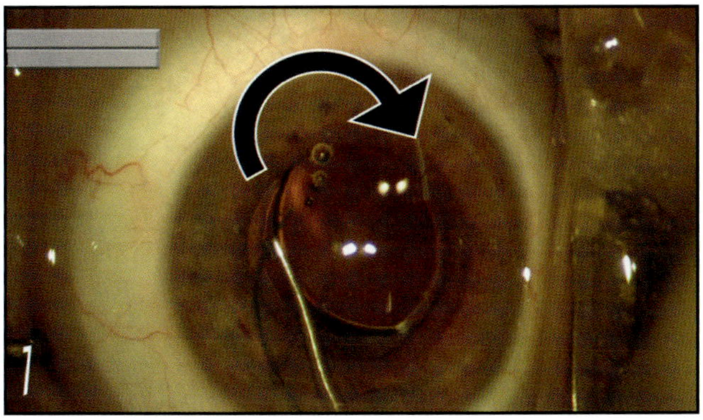

Use a Sinskey hook to gently push one edge of the optic behind the rhexis. The haptics must remain anterior to the capsular plane.

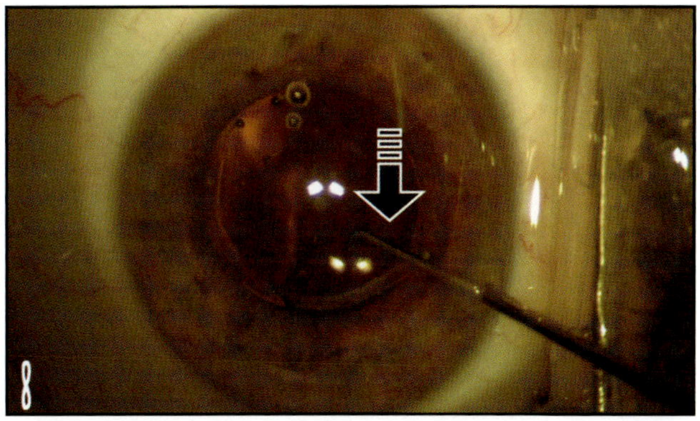

Slide one side of the optic under the rhexis and displace the IOL further under the rhexis leaflet so that the optic edge 180 degrees apart can be placed beneath the opposite rhexis edge. It is important to exert pressure with the Sinskey hook at 90 degrees from the haptic-optic junction to ensure adequate capture. A Kuglen hook can also be used in the nondominant hand to stretch the rhexis while the dominant hand uses a Sinskey hook to slide the remaining optic under the rhexis. A properly sized rhexis makes this step easier—it should be large enough for the IOL to pass, but small enough to support the entire optic of the IOL. Usually 5 to 5.5 mm is ideal.

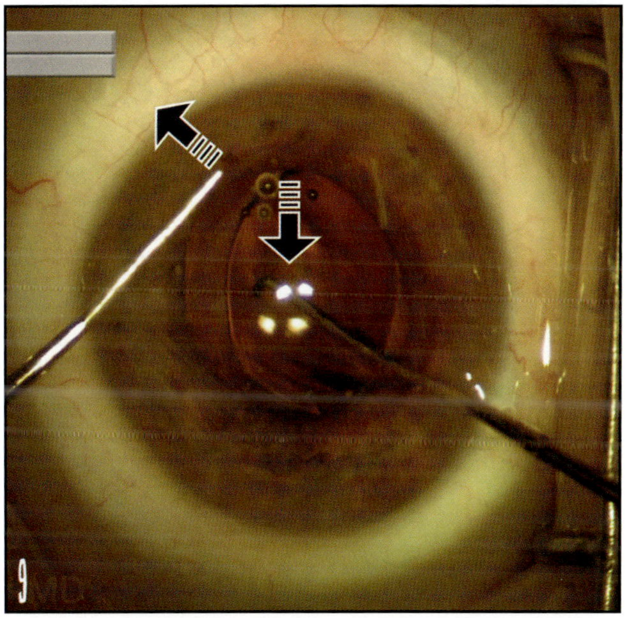

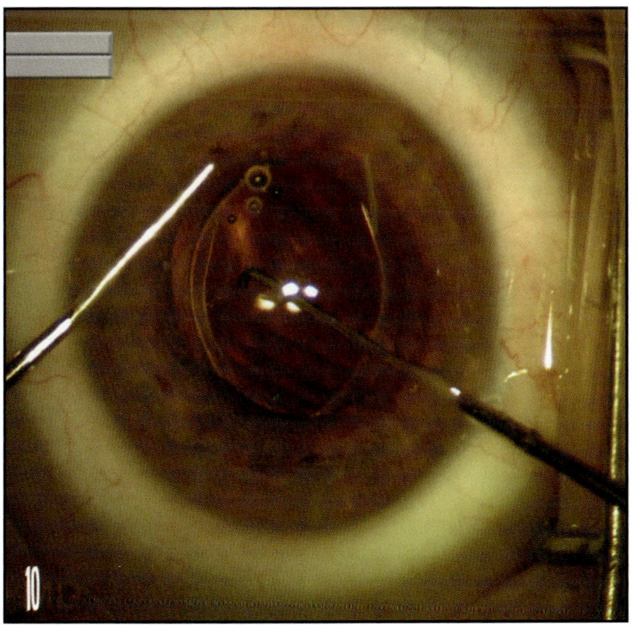

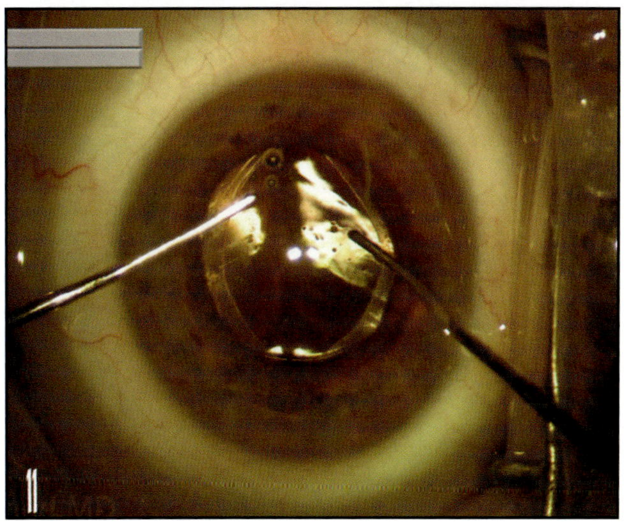

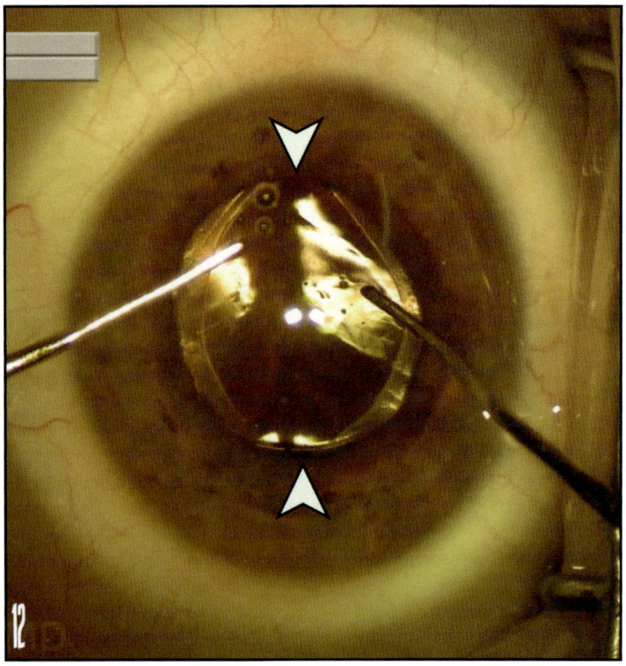

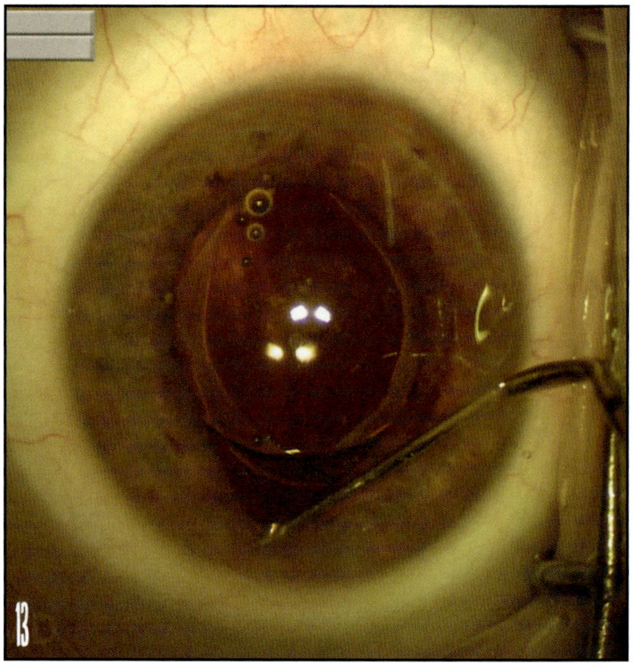

The capsulorrhexis should now be ovalized instead of round, with its largest diameter corresponding to the optic-haptic junctions (arrows, 12) and a rectification of the capsulorrhexis curvature.

If there is a rounded portion, recheck that the IOL is truly optic captured. This can be done by using a Kuglen hook to retract the iris at all 4 quadrants (13, 14) and ensuring that the rhexis edge is covering the IOL optic (except at the optic-haptic junction, where it will go under the haptic). At the end of the case, an intracameral miotic agent can be used.

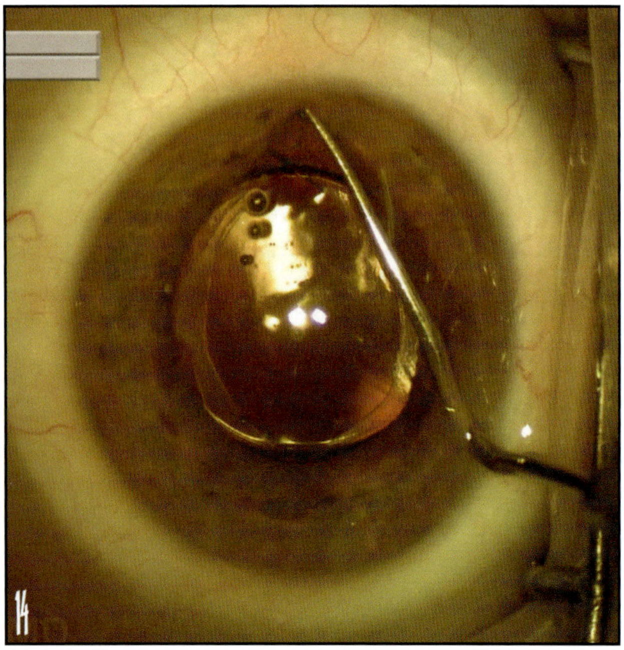

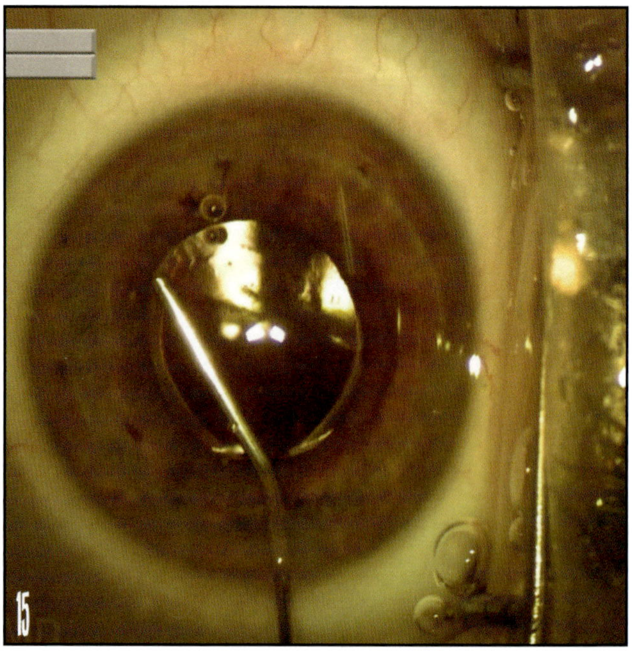

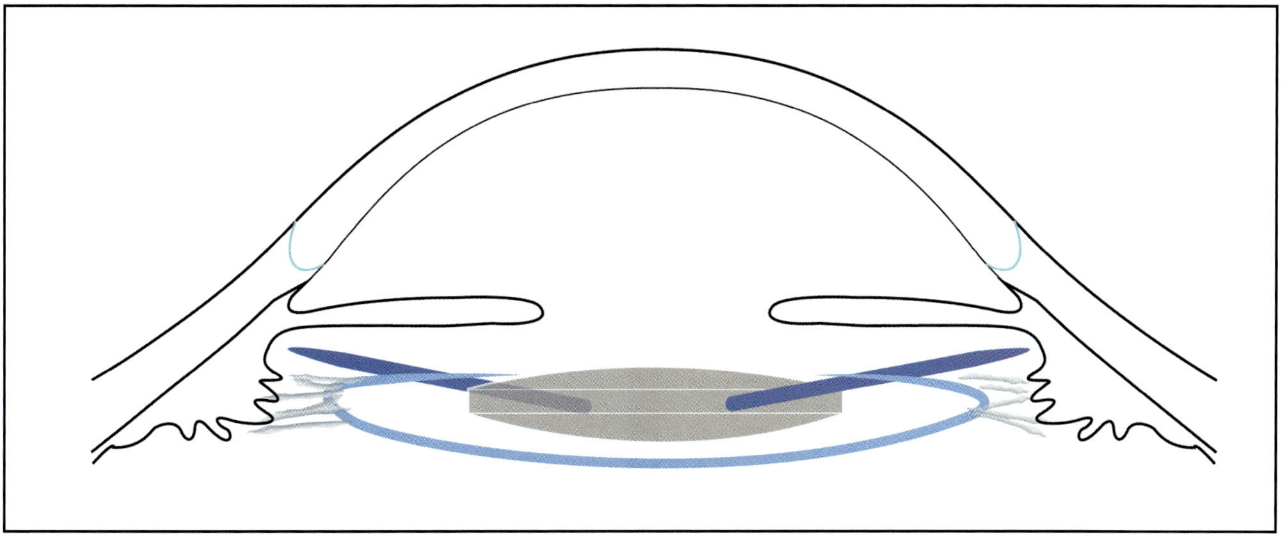

CHAPTER 15

HOW TO POSTERIOR OPTIC CAPTURE

INTRODUCTION

Posterior optic capture involves placing the optic of the intraocular lens (IOL) behind the posterior capsule, after performing a posterior capsulorrhexis. It is beneficial to perform a posterior optic capture in several instances. If the anterior capsulorrhexis is discontinuous, a sulcus lens can still be placed and optic captured through the posterior capsule. In cases where toric IOL rotational stability is in question, posterior optic capture can be performed to hold the IOL in position. Also, in pediatric cataracts, one can perform a posterior capsulorrhexis without the need for a vitrectomy and posterior optic capture the IOL through the posterior rhexis to barricade vitreous and ensure IOL stability.

KEY POINTS

- The posterior rhexis should be adequately sized—roughly around 4.5 mm in order to be able to optic capture the IOL.
- When performing a posterior rhexis, a 27-g hypodermic needle is placed on the end of a viscoelastic cannula in order to immediately inject a dispersive viscoelastic once the posterior capsule is incised so that vitreous is barricaded.
- Make sure the viscoelastic is primed to the end of the needle so that air does not obstruct your view. Air in the posterior segment is trickier to remove as aspiration can draw vitreous anteriorly.
- If there is a posterior capsule opening, incorporating this into a continuous curvilinear rhexis is optimal; otherwise, posterior capsule runouts can occur.

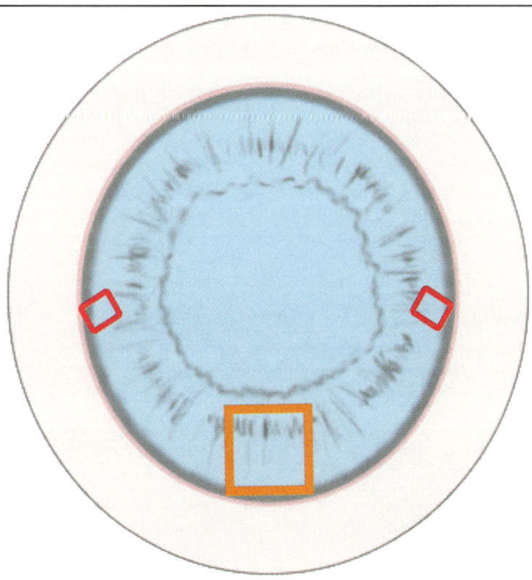

- Standard phaco with knife and fork

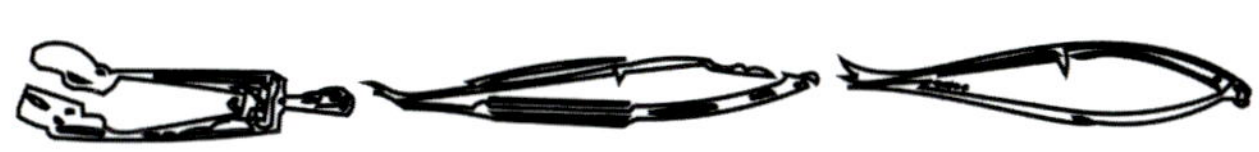

- Microsurgical Technology, Inc microforceps
- 27-g hypodermic needle
- Sinskey and angled Kuglen hooks

Ahmed IK, Campos-Möller X, Shah M, Sheybani A. *Illustrated Advanced Anterior Segment Surgery: A Step-by-Step Guide for Challenging Cases* (pp 99-105).

Once the cataract or IOL is removed, steps must be taken to ensure the posterior rhexis is centered. Cohesive ophthalmic viscosurgical device is used to lightly stretch the bag. Avoid overfilling as this will displace the posterior capsule so far back that it will be hard to reach for posterior curvilinear capsulorrhexis. A 27-g hypodermic needle is used to penetrate the posterior capsule just off-center, creating a small opening. Dispersive viscoelastic is injected through the opening gently, just after puncturing. Overfilling can cause the posterior rhexis to bow too far anteriorly, causing a runout.

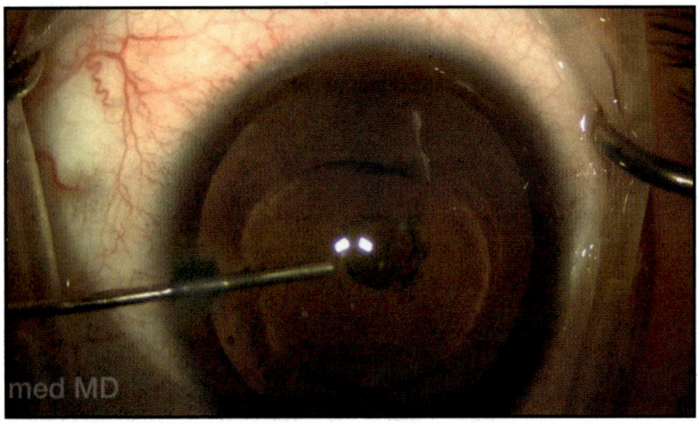

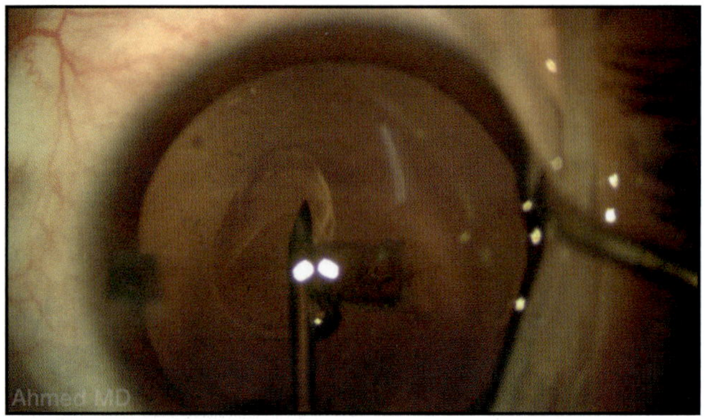

Microsurgical Technology, Inc microforceps are used to create a continuous curvilinear capsulorrhexis. Be wary of the fact that the vector forces for posterior capsulorrhexis are different than for anterior capsulorrhexis. The posterior zonules tend to provide less traction than the anterior zonules. Dispersive viscoelastic is used to ensure vitreous is barricaded. The bag is filled with cohesive viscoelastic in order to create space IN THE BAG for IOL implantation. Previously overfilling behind the posterior capsule will make this step suboptimal.

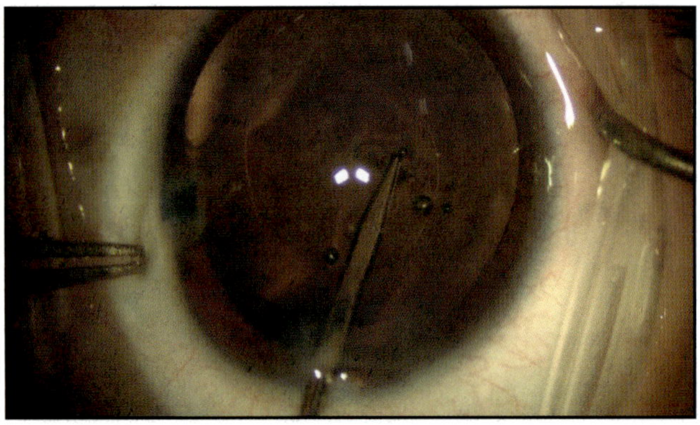

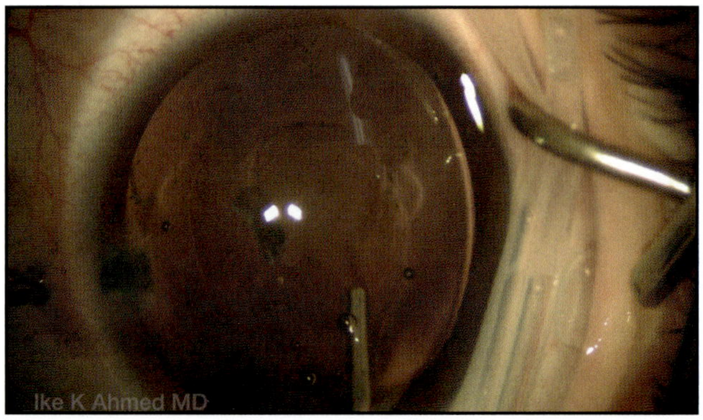

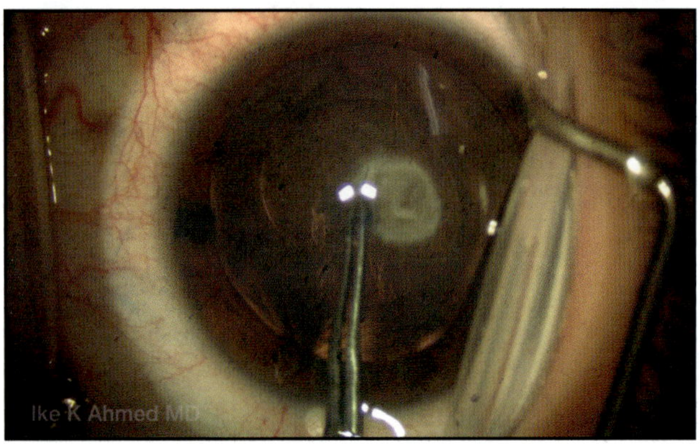

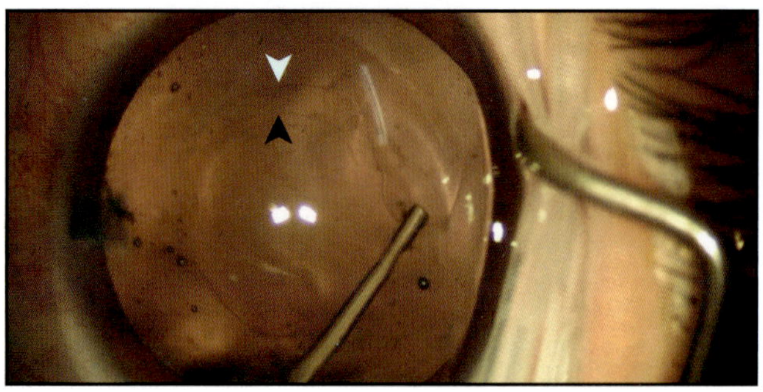

White arrow: Anterior capsulorrhexis edge
Black arrow: Posterior capsulorrhexis edge

- The tip of the injector cartridge is placed in the anterior chamber, positioning the IOL in the bag, behind the anterior capsule and in front of the posterior capsule. Have a second instrument ready in order to position the IOL in the bag before the IOL completely unfolds.
- In the case of a toric IOL, position the IOL first before performing posterior optic capture.
- Closing the large main incision, even with a temporary tie, can prevent chamber shallowing and vitreous prolapse and is recommended.

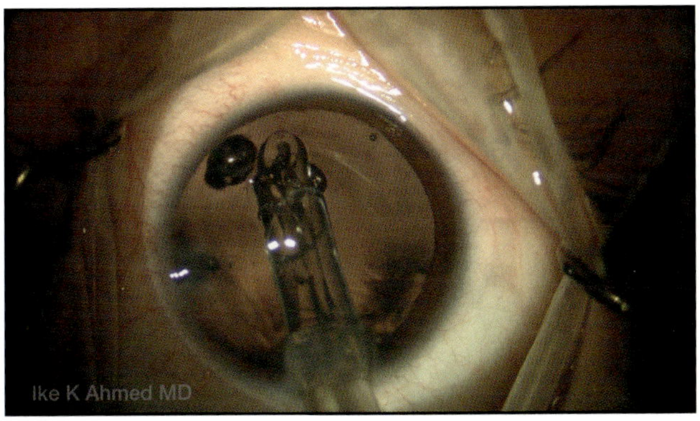

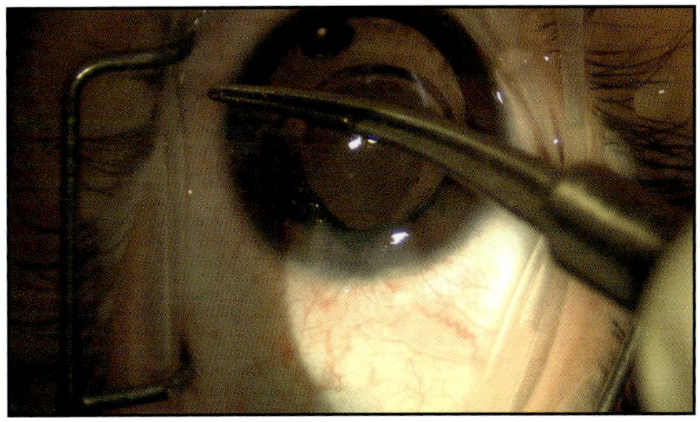

- The IOL optic is pushed behind the posterior rhexis with a blunt cannula or Sinskey hook. This is repeated for the opposite side of the optic in a similar fashion to a traditional optic capture maneuver (see Chapter 14).
- Viscoelastic is manually removed with caution using balanced salt solution on a blunt cannula to prevent chamber shallowing and vitreous prolapse.
- The patient is placed on ocular pressure-lowering agents for at least the first several days because not all viscoelastic can be removed.

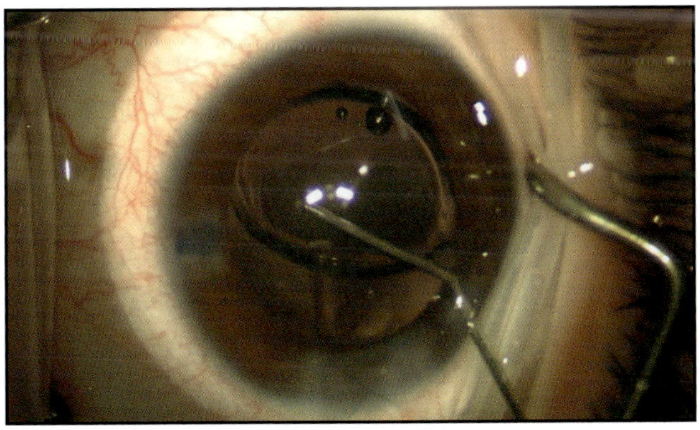

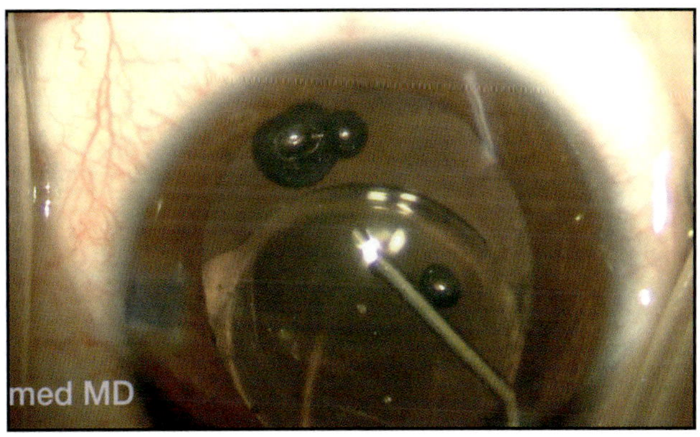

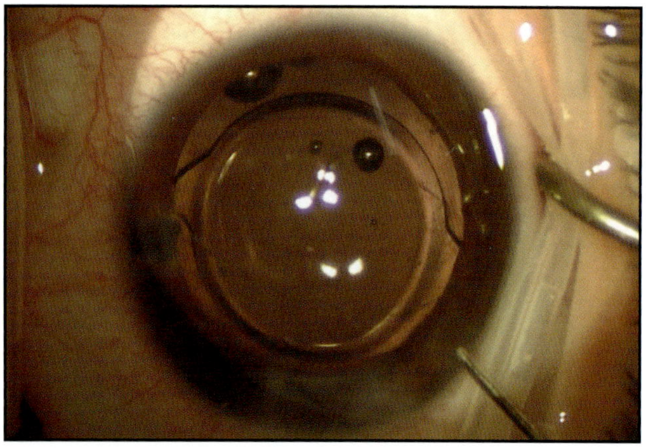

When the optic is adequately captured behind the posterior capsule, the capsulorrhexis takes on an ovalized shape, peaked at the optic-haptic junctions.

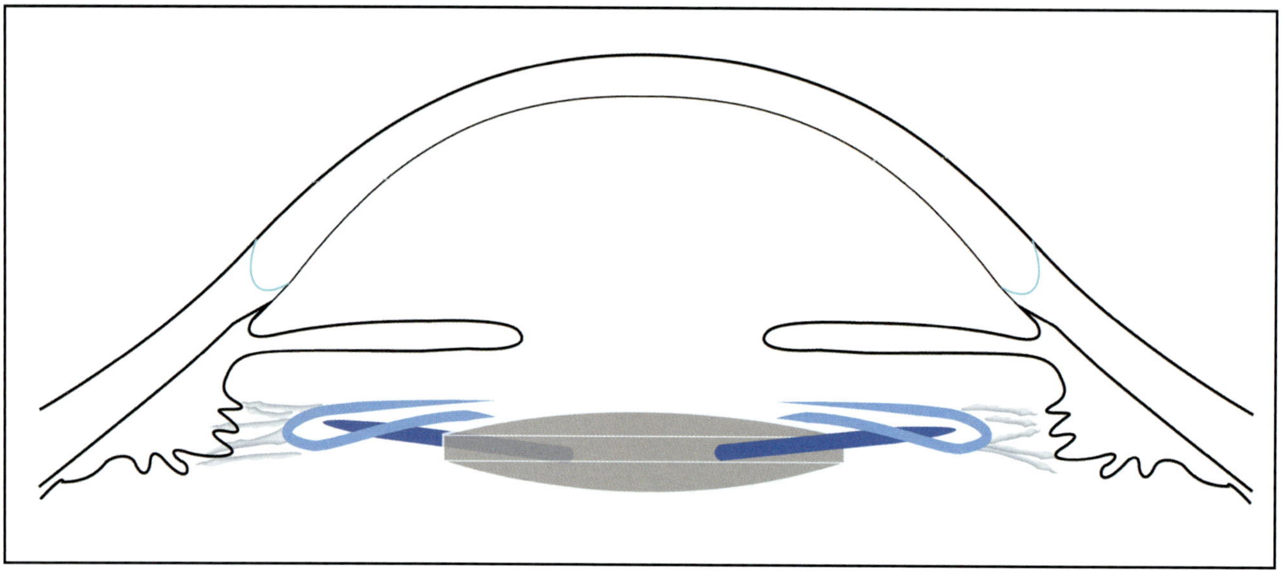

Posterior optic capture: Notice the IOL haptics are in the bag, while the optic is captured behind the posterior capsulorrhexis.

HOW TO DOUBLE OPTIC CAPTURE

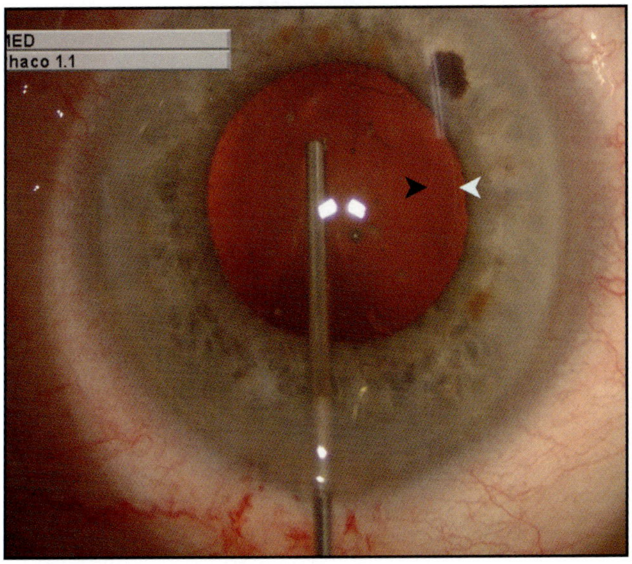

How to Perform Double Optic Capture

In the setting of an intact peripheral capsule and adequate capsulotomy size, ideally less than 6 mm, a double optic capture technique can be utilized. This is often used in the setting of an IOL exchange in which the anterior and posterior capsules are fused. If a posterior capsulotomy has not already been performed, one can be fashioned intraoperatively. Refer to earlier in this chapter to review how to perform a primary posterior capsulorrhexis. It is important to make sure that this capsulorrhexis is also less than 5.5 mm. The anterior hyaloid face is tamponaded with dispersive viscoelastic, and the sulcus space is inflated with a cohesive viscoelastic, thus facilitating sulcus placement of a 3-piece IOL. Using a Sinskey and a Kuglen hook, the 2 edges of the optic that are 90 degrees away from the haptic-optic junction are "dunked" under the fused anterior and posterior capsules, one at a time. In doing so, the optic will now be posterior to the posterior capsule, while the haptics will remain anterior to the anterior capsule in the sulcus space. Thus, a double optic capture has been performed. The IOL optic is secured and stable, minimizing pseudophacodonesis. The "sulcus-friendly" haptics are also stable. The posterior vault of the 3-piece IOL facilitates this configuration readily.

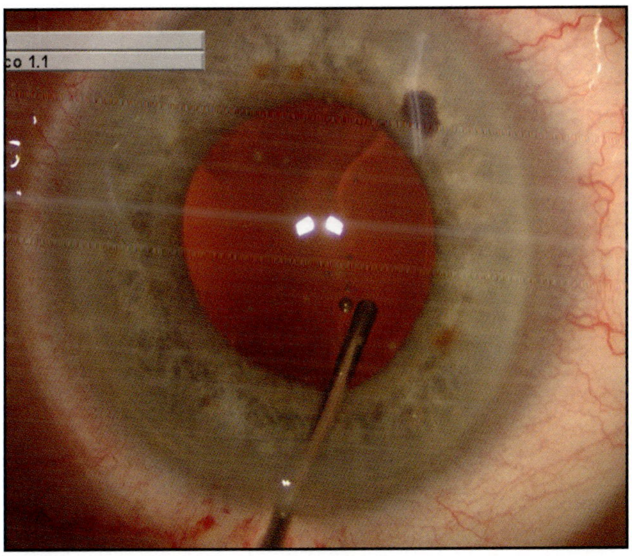

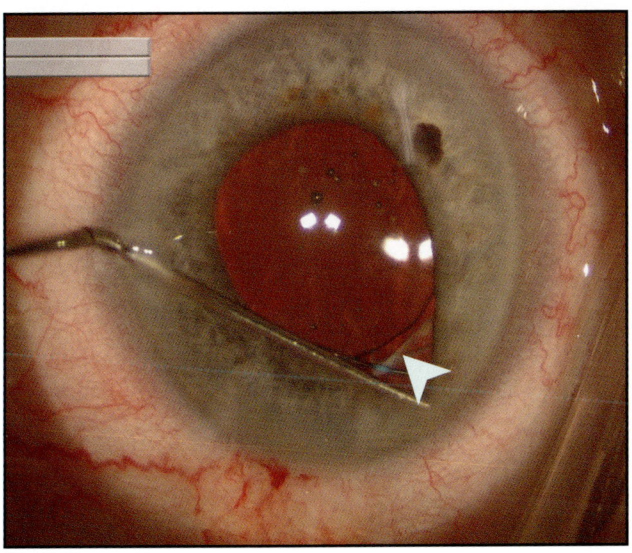

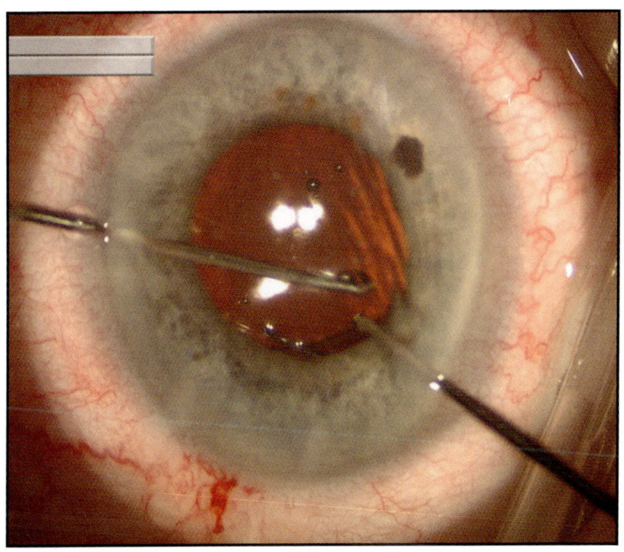

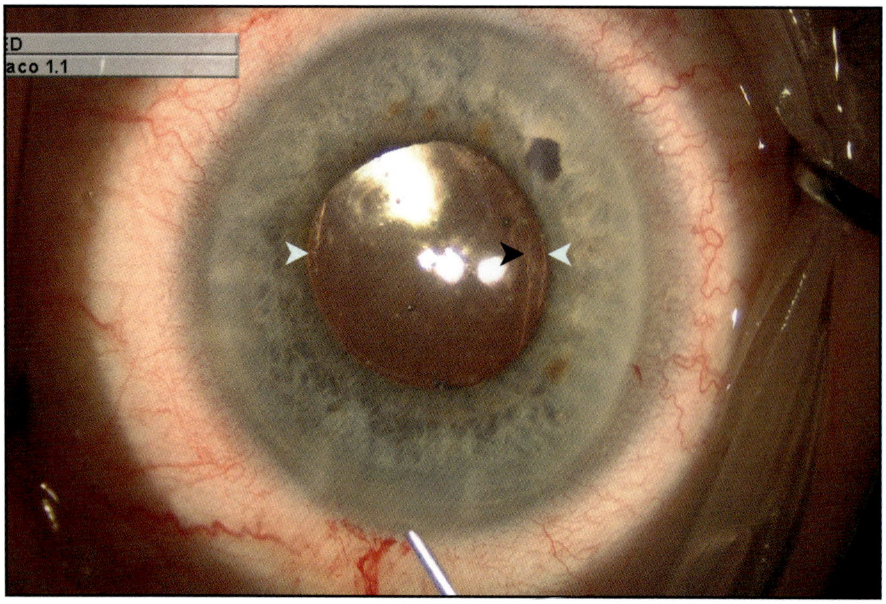

Make sure the IOL optic is posterior to both the anterior and posterior capsules. This can be evidenced by ovalization and rectification of the curve of the capsulorrhexis. White arrows mark the anterior rhexis edge and the black arrow marks the posterior rhexis edge.

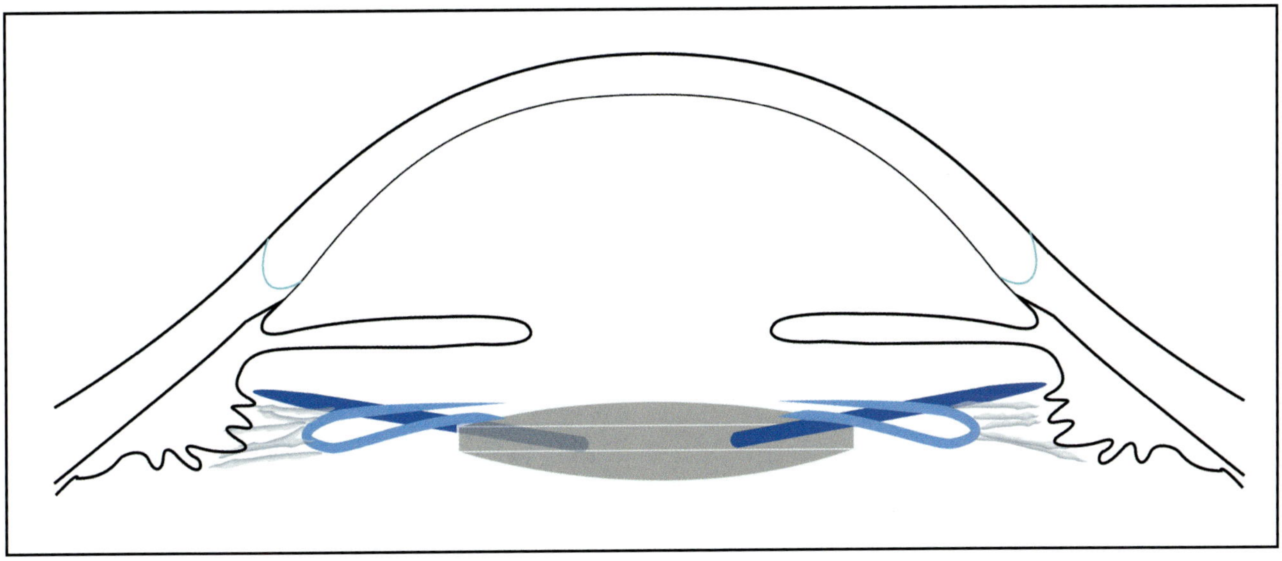

Double optic capture: Notice how the IOL haptics are in the ciliary sulcus, whereas the optic is captured behind both anterior and posterior capsulorrhexes.

CHAPTER 16

HOW TO REVERSE OPTIC CAPTURE A SINGLE-PIECE INTRAOCULAR LENS

INTRODUCTION

Reverse optic capture is a technique in which the optic of an intraocular lens (IOL) is captured anterior to the capsulorrhexis, while the haptics remain in the capsular bag. This technique can be used to reposition a dislocated IOL when the capsular bag is centered but with posterior capsule disruption. It can also be used to treat negative dysphotopsia and to prevent toric IOL rotation in large eyes.

KEY POINTS

- The capsulorrhexis must be small enough to support the optic of the IOL; otherwise, the optic will fall back into the bag. This is especially true for single-piece acrylic lenses.
- This technique can be performed with acrylic 1- or 3-piece IOLs.
- In order to perform this in some situations with either poly(methyl methacrylate) lenses or when the rhexis is too small, relaxing incisions can be made on the rhexis with microscissors. In order to increase the effective opening, care must be taken as a small phimotic rhexis can sometimes radialize when there is significant force; therefore, multiple relaxing incisions in an equatorial fashion might be necessary.

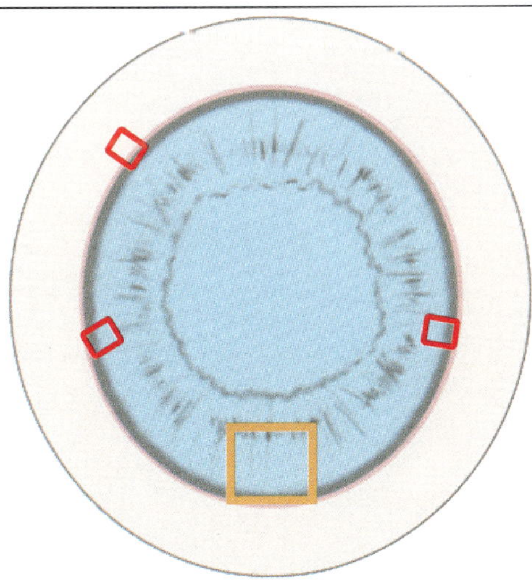

- Standard knife and fork configuration with an extra paracentesis if necessary

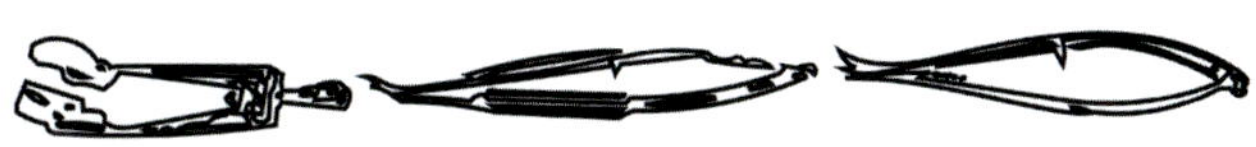

- Angled Kuglen hook
- Angled Sinskey hook
- Cohesive and dispersive ophthalmic viscosurgical device (OVD)
- Microsurgical Technology, Inc micrograspers

Ahmed IK, Campos-Möller X, Shah M, Sheybani A. *Illustrated Advanced Anterior Segment Surgery: A Step-by-Step Guide for Challenging Cases* (pp 107-112).

Micrograspers are used to separate the rhexis from the optic. A Sinskey hook is inserted in this space. The Sinskey hook can be used to mechanically separate the capsule from the optic by pressing on the optic under the capsule leaflet. Gently lifting on the micrograsper can hold the space open for placement of a cohesive OVD cannula. The OVD can be used to viscodissect around the optic edge and haptics, thus freeing the IOL. See Chapter 24 for more details.

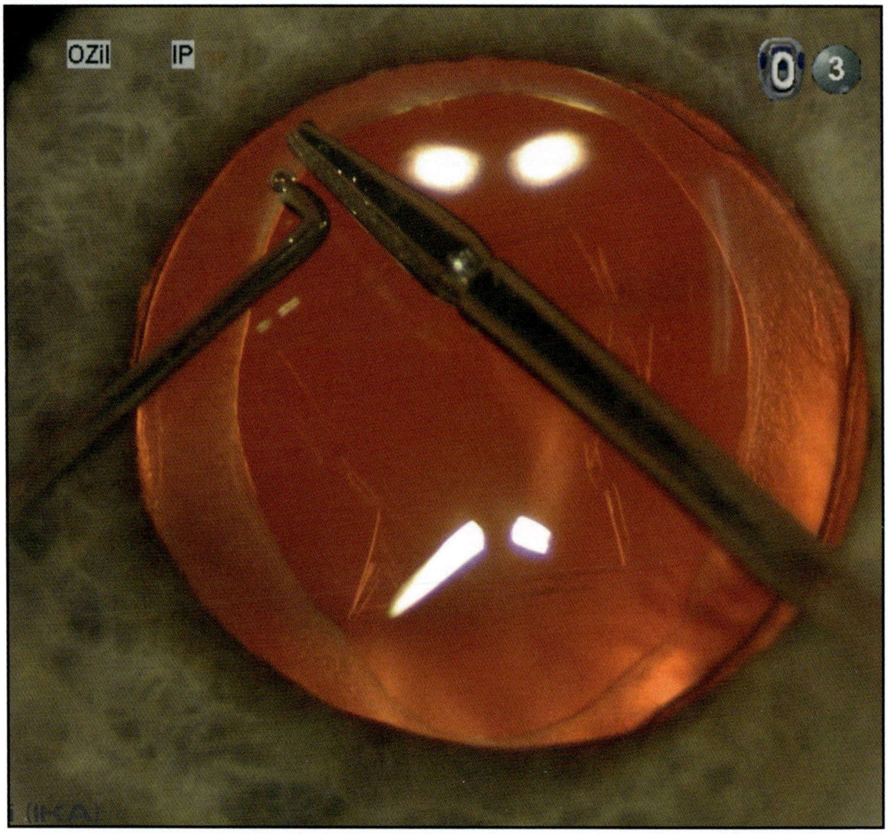

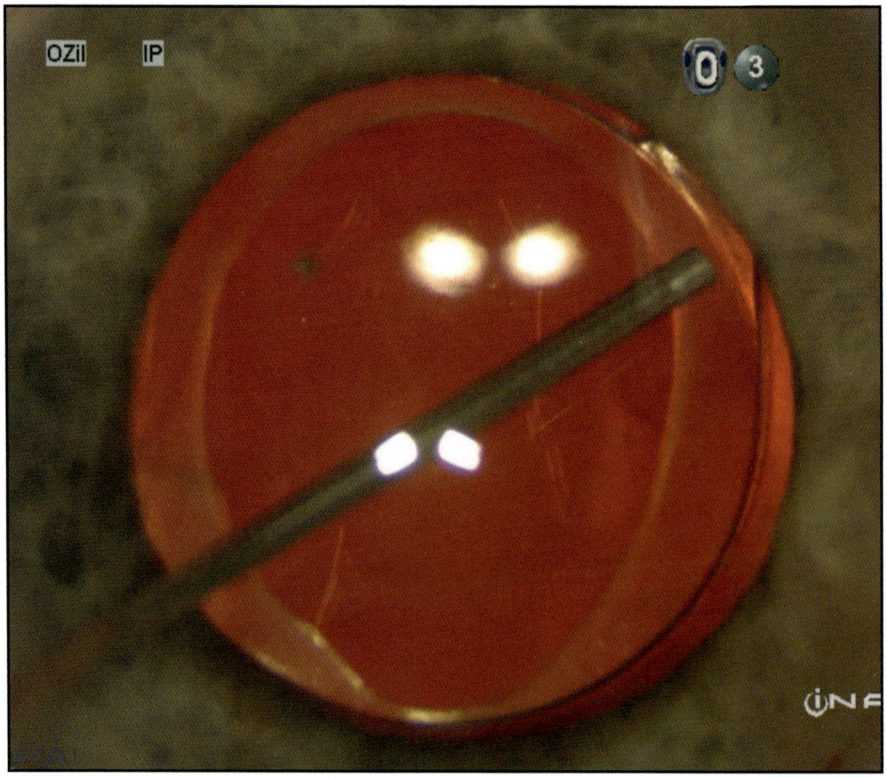

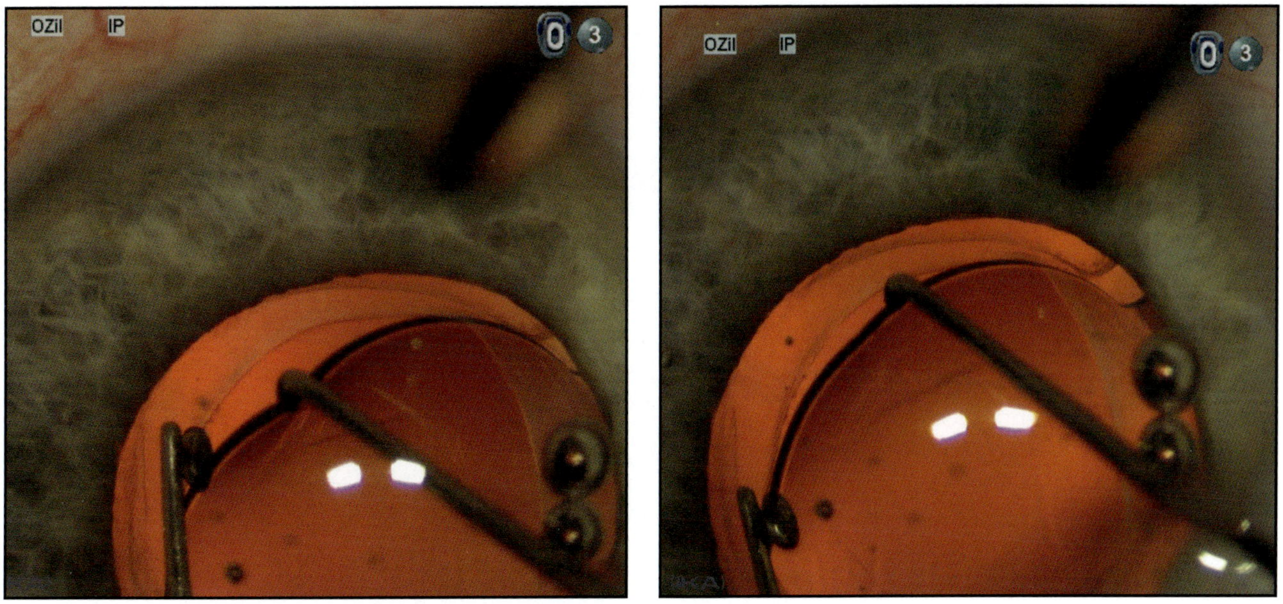

The optic must be placed anterior to the capsule except at the optic-haptic junction. Images above show a bimanual maneuver, where the Sinskey hook holds the edge of the IOL at one point while the Kuglen hook sweeps the periphery of the optic, releasing it from adhesions and bringing it forward. Once the edge is free, the 2 hooks can be used in a "chopstick" fashion to displace half of the optic above the capsulorrhexis leaflet. This is repeated on the opposite side of the optic.

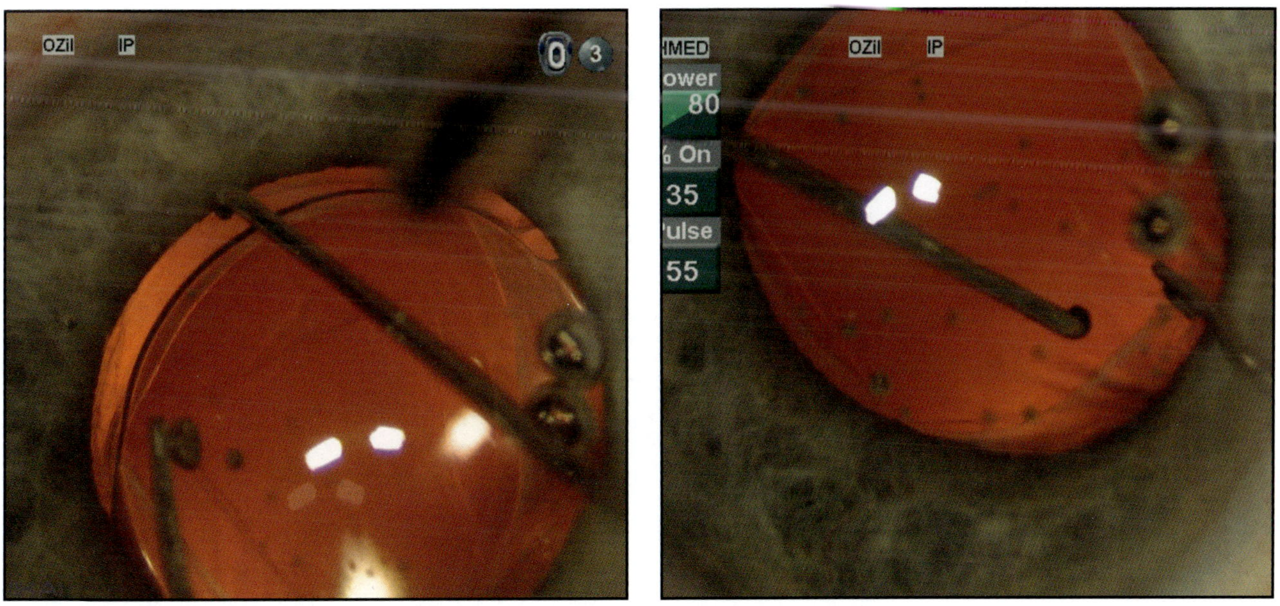

The Kuglen hook can also be used to retract the anterior capsule, creating space for the optic to pass, while the Sinskey wraps around the optic to lift it anteriorly. In some cases, the IOL must be rotated to maximize the overlap of the optic with the capsule. This can be done in the bag when the posterior capsule is intact, but it is safer to bring the entire IOL into the sulcus for rotation when the posterior capsule is compromised. Once in the right orientation, the haptics can be tucked in place with the use of a Sinskey hook and a micrograsper.

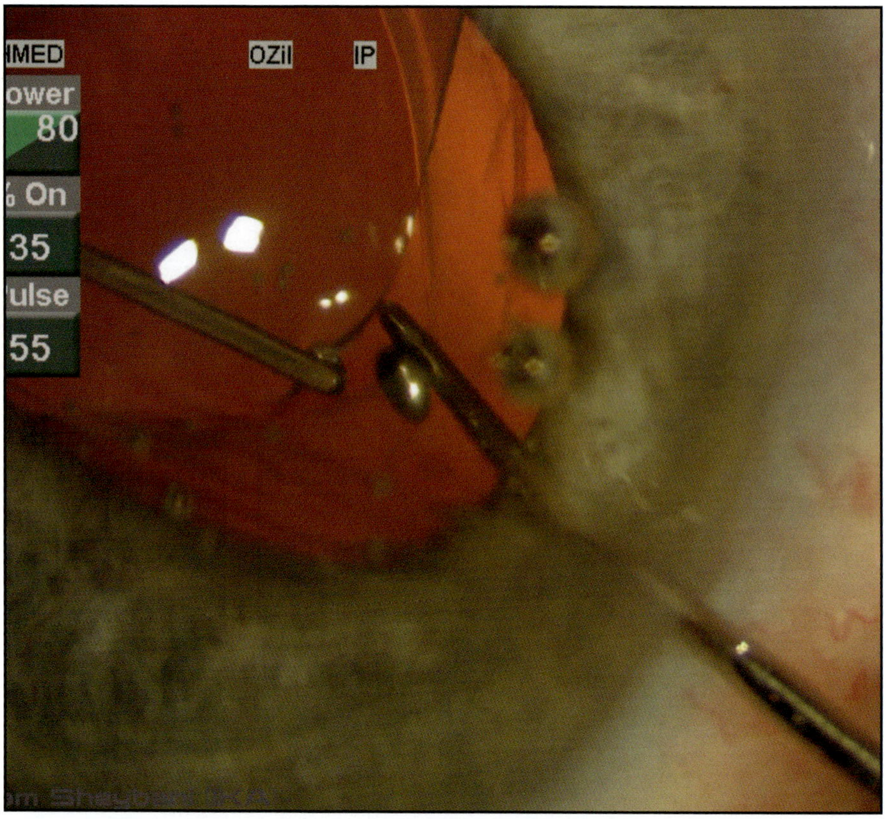

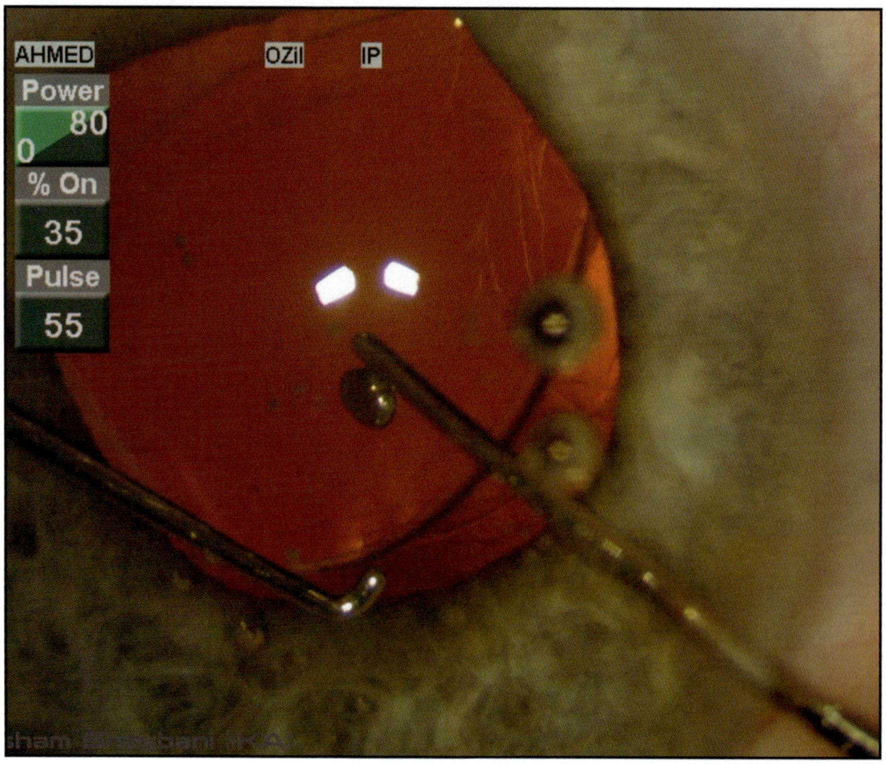

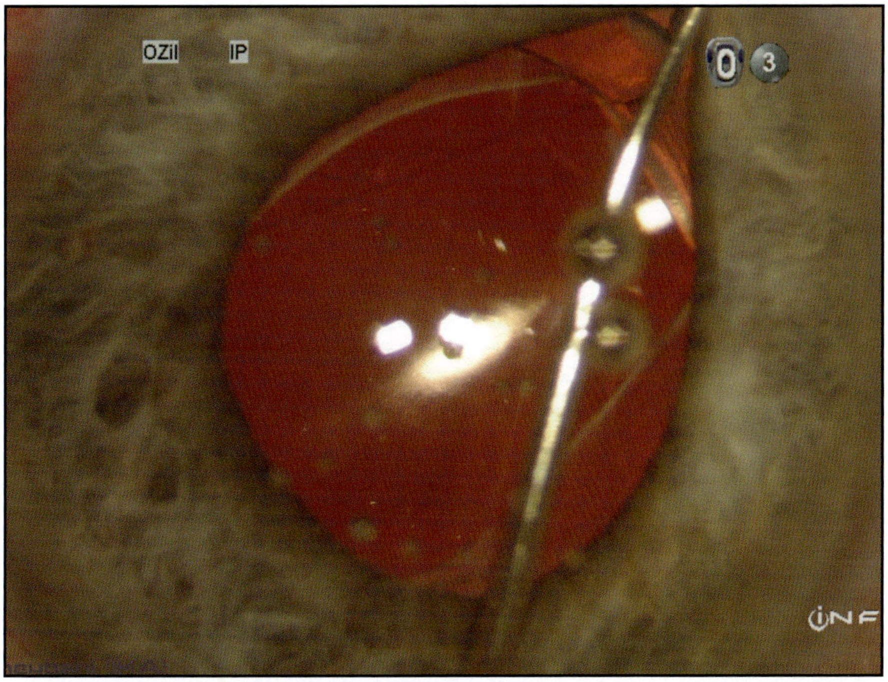

At the end of the repositioning, verify that the haptics are still in the bag by using a Kuglen to displace the pupil peripherally. The capsulorrhexis should now be ovalized with the peaks right at the optic-haptic junctions. There should be a bridge of rhexis edge above the haptic, and the rest of the optic should be above the rhexis edge.

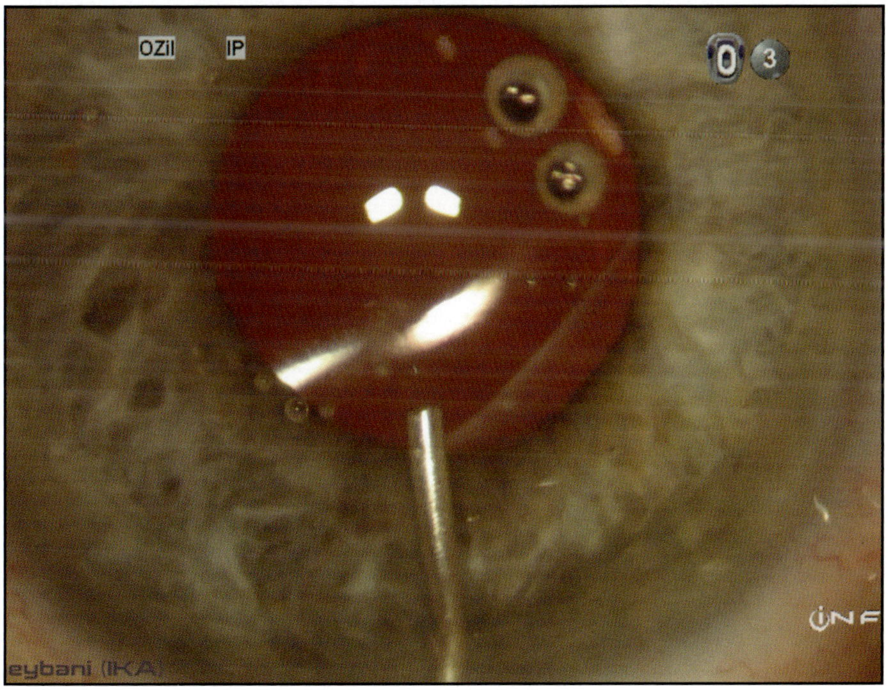

OVD is removed manually with a 27-g cannula.

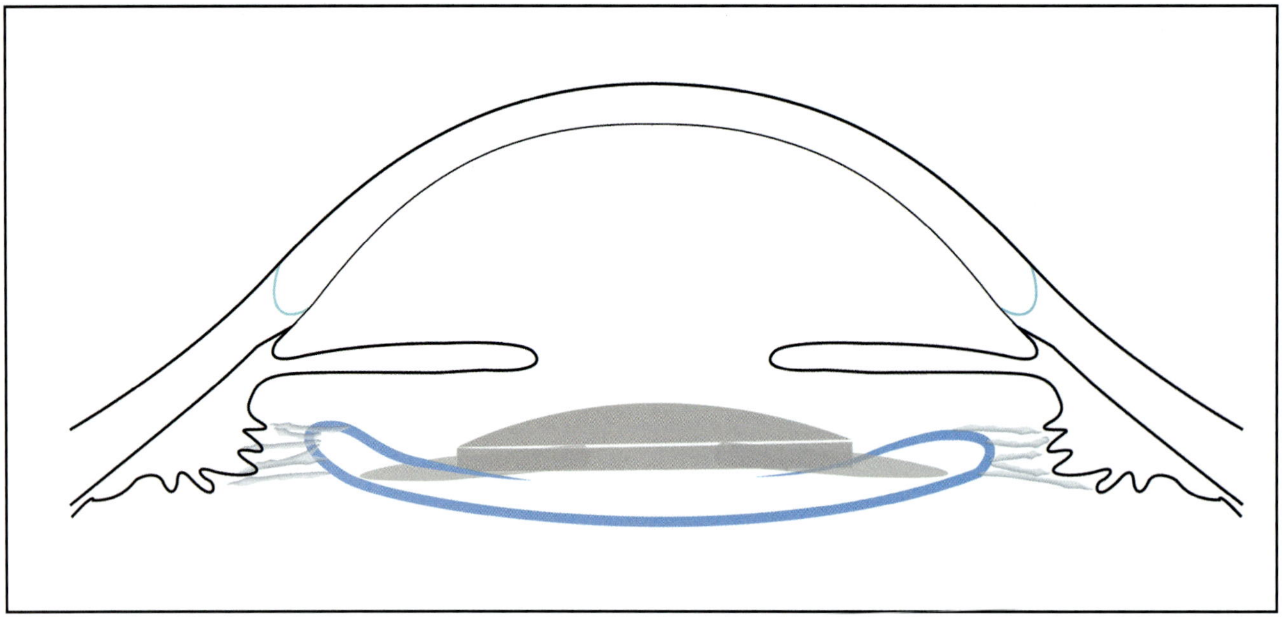

Reverse optic capture: Notice how the IOL haptics are in the bag, whereas the IOL optic is captured anterior to the capsulorrhexis.

CHAPTER 17

HOW TO INSERT AN ANGLE-SUPPORTED ANTERIOR CHAMBER INTRAOCULAR LENS

INTRODUCTION

Angle-supported anterior chamber intraocular lenses (ACIOLs) are single-piece poly(methyl methacrylate) IOLs that can be implanted in the absence of capsule support. They do not require intraocular suturing and are technically easier to place than iris claw IOLs. Another advantage of ACIOLs is their wide availability throughout the world.

KEY POINTS

- It is very important to size ACIOLs correctly; usually 0.5 mm longer than the measured white-to-white distance and must be placed in the same orientation measured.
- A peripheral iridectomy or iridotomy is required to prevent pupil block.
- Correct orientation is key. The haptics take 2 turns off of the optic.
- The lens vault should be anterior. The initial curve of the haptic from the optic is in a backward "S" when placed correctly. Improper orientation can increase the risk of iris chafing.
- Clear corneal wound construction can limit iris prolapse and avoid disrupting conjunctiva that could be used for future glaucoma surgery.
- We avoid using a lens glide unless there is very poor iris support. A lens glide can gape the wound, allowing for chamber shallowing and vitreous prolapse.
- Do not "push" the IOL once most of the optic is in. This can force the IOL behind the pupil. Instead "pull" the IOL into the angle from a side port using a Sinskey or Kuglen hook.
- Oversizing can peak the pupil.
- Undersizing can allow the IOL to rotate, causing iris chafing.
- Pupil suturing should be performed when the pupil is larger than the IOL's optic zone to prevent monocular diplopia.
- Overly mydriatic pupils sometimes do not offer enough support and, rarely, dislocation through the pupil can occur.

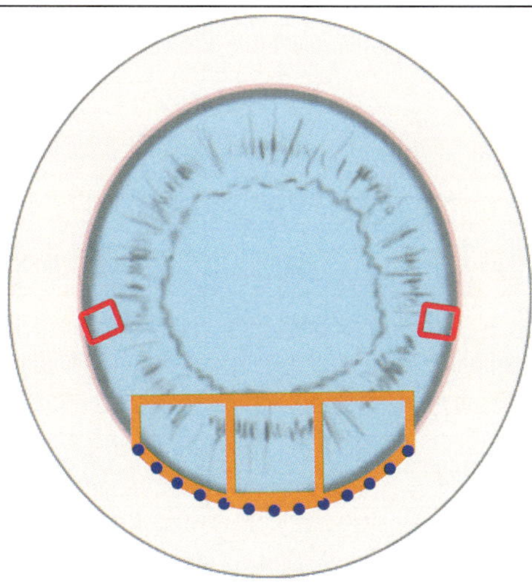

- Limbal 300-μm groove
- Bevelled, 3-step, and triplanar 6-mm corneal
- Knife and fork paracentesis

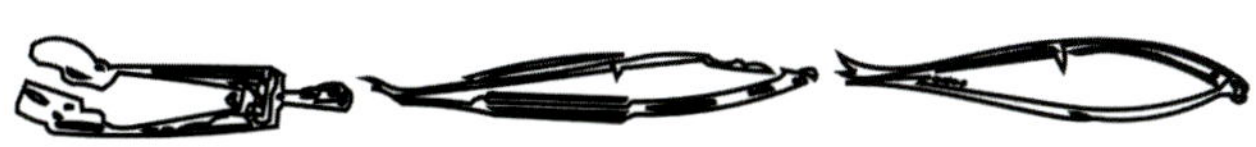

- 1.2-mm side port and 3-mm keratome
- Vitrector for peripheral iridectomy
- Microsurgical Technology, Inc micrograspers and microscissors
- Cohesive and dispersive ophthalmic viscosurgical device
- Miochol (acetylcholine)

Ahmed IK, Campos-Möller X, Shah M, Sheybani A. *Illustrated Advanced Anterior Segment Surgery: A Step-by-Step Guide for Challenging Cases* (pp 113-117).

- White-to-white distance is measured with a caliper, and the lens is sized 0.5 mm larger than the largest measured white-to-white. Sometimes, measuring multiple meridians will help determine the best orientation to limit under- or oversizing of the IOL.
- Miochol is injected or swept into the anterior chamber (AC) to constrict the pupil.
- If vitreous prolapse through the pupil is suspected, triamcinolone acetonide can be used to stain the vitreous gel and aid in its visualization. A limited anterior vitrectomy may be performed if necessary.

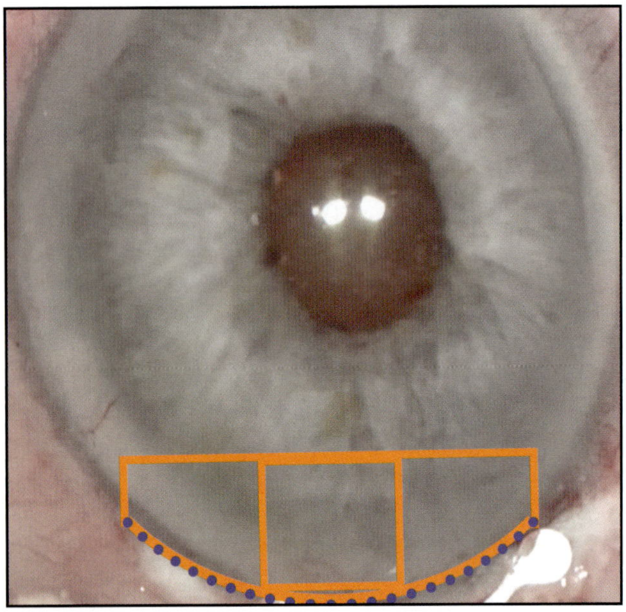

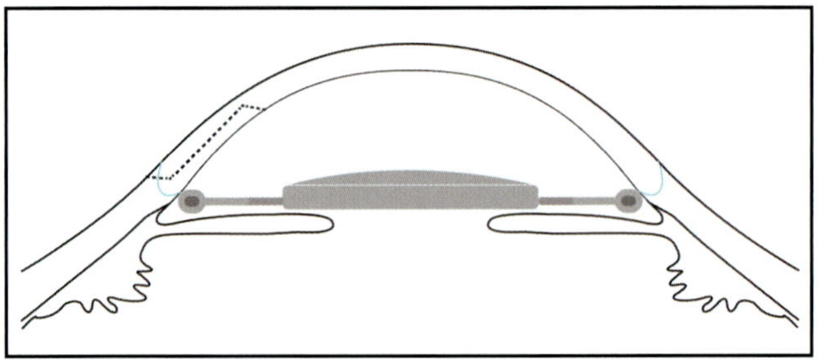

Create the corneal incision by first creating a 6-mm limbal groove, 300 μm in depth. Enter this groove with the keratome in order to create a triplanar corneal incision. Going well into clear cornea creates a step that will make IOL implantation easier by preventing prolapse of the trailing haptic.

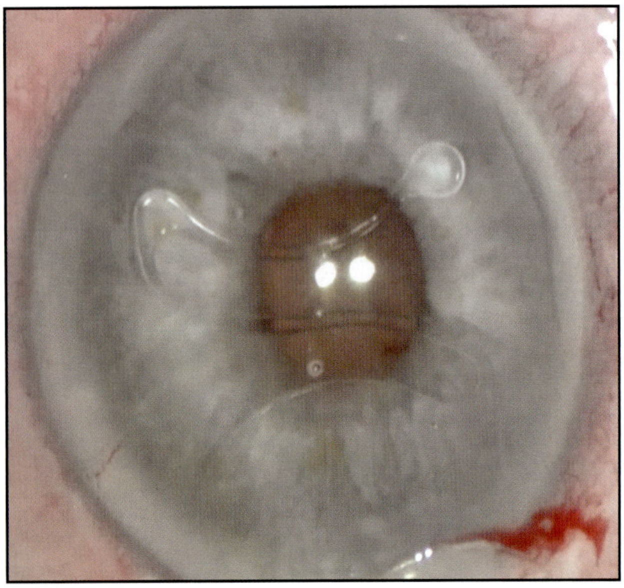

The IOL is inserted through the clear corneal incision, initially controlled by curved tying forceps. Pay attention to orientation as it is not advisable to rotate the IOL inside the AC for risk of iris or angle structure trauma.

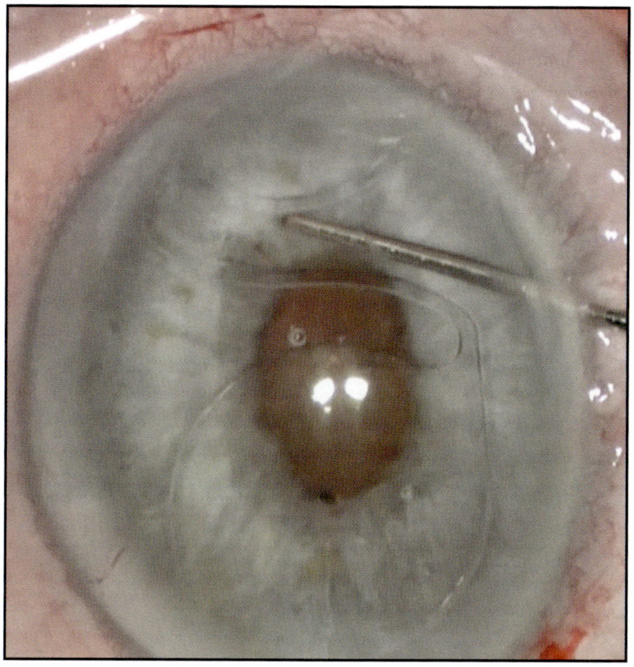

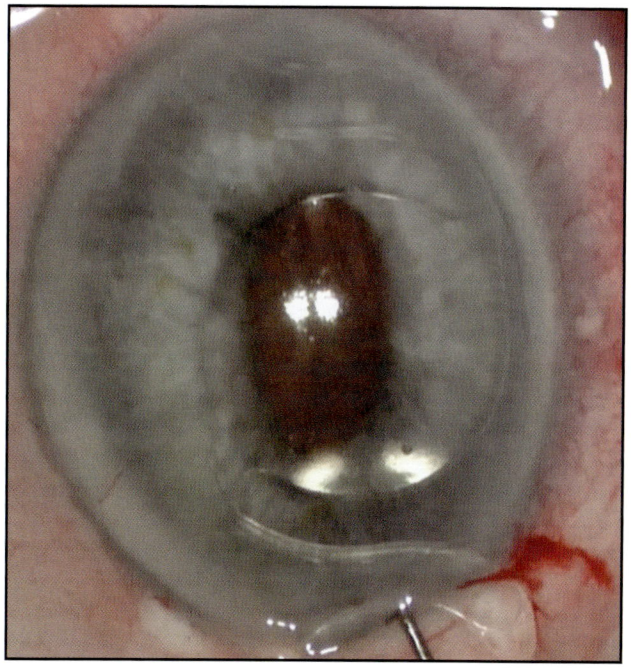

- Once most of the IOL optic is in the AC, a Sinskey hook is used through a paracentesis to pull the IOL the rest of the way into the angle.
- Use a Sinskey or Kuglen hook to push the trailing haptic into the AC, just below the lip of the corneal wound.
- If necessary, IOL rotation can be performed by pulling the distal haptic toward the pupil to release it from the angle while rotating and pushing the proximal haptic in a similar fashion (either simultaneously or in sequence) with small rotation maneuvers until the IOL is in the desired orientation. Avoid excessive rotation.

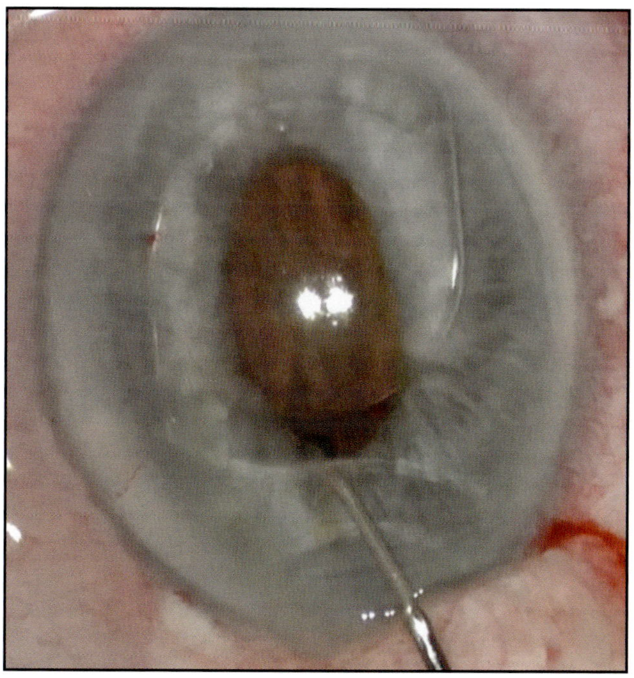

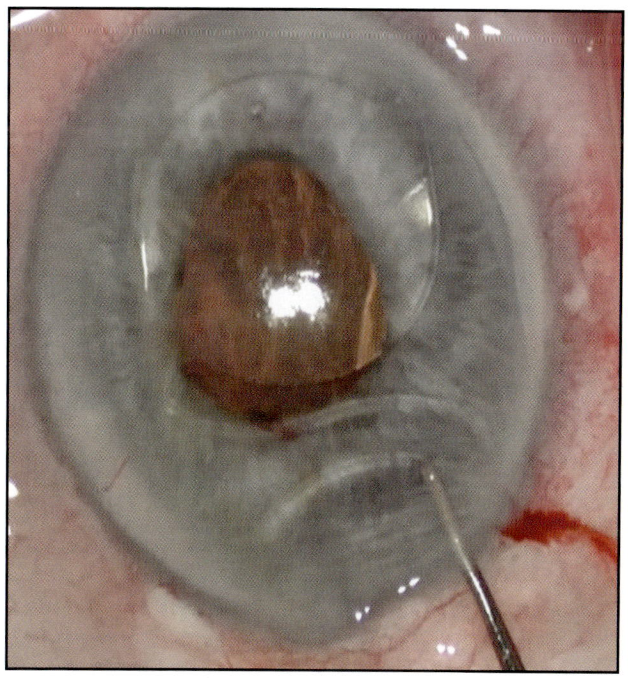

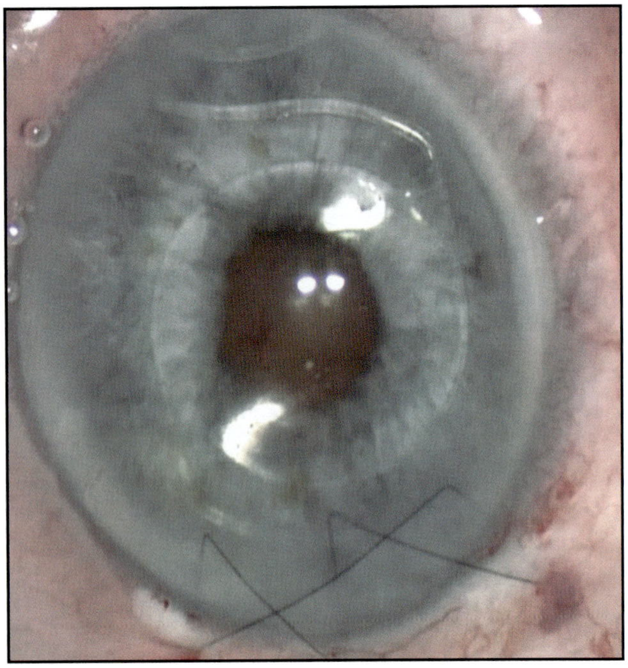

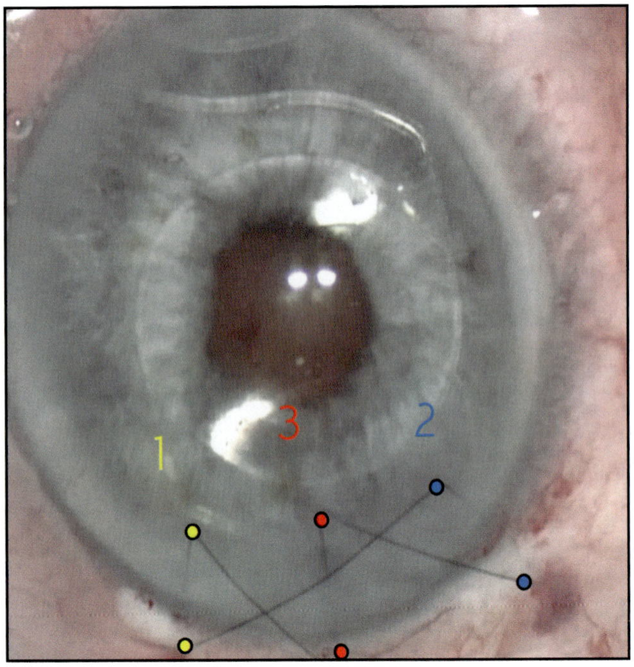

- The corneal incision can be sutured with either a continuous suture or interrupted sutures. The sequence of suture passes is explained on the top right image. See also Chapter 18 for Artisan implantation for more on this suture technique.
- A peripheral iridectomy should be performed to prevent pupil block. Our preferred technique is with the aid of a vitrector, on IA/cut setting.
- Remove viscoelastic manually, but prevent chamber shallowing. Oral or topical intraocular pressure–lowering agents can be utilized as needed in the postoperative period.

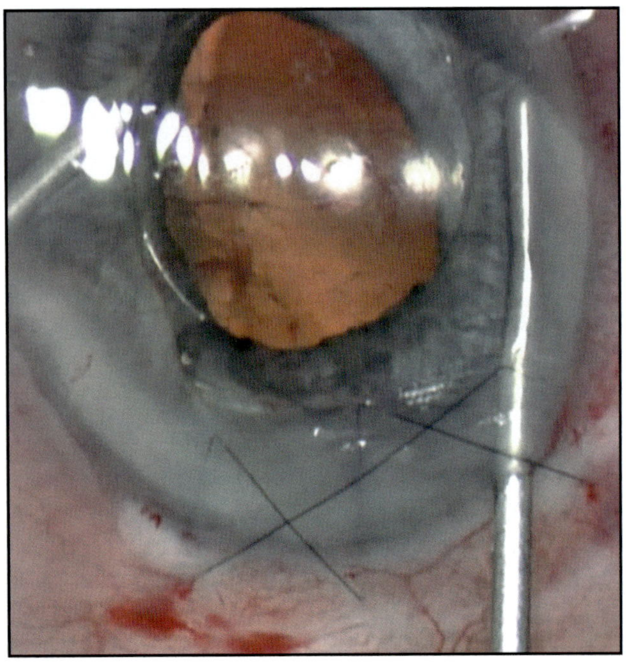

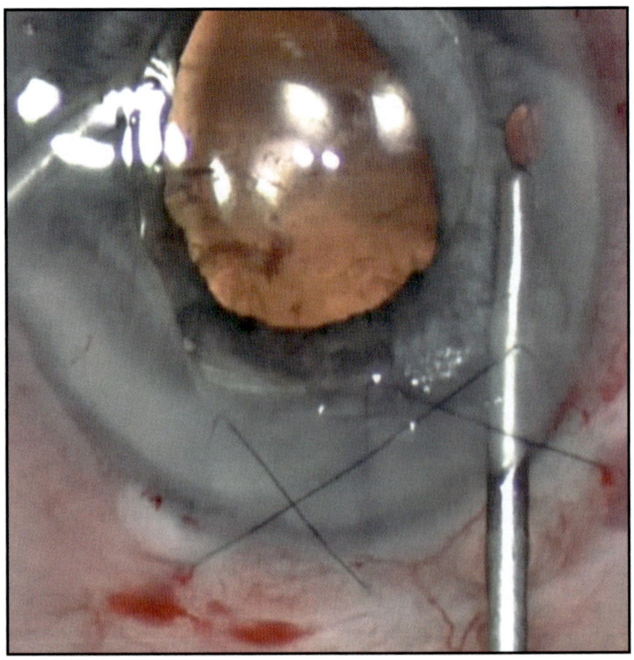

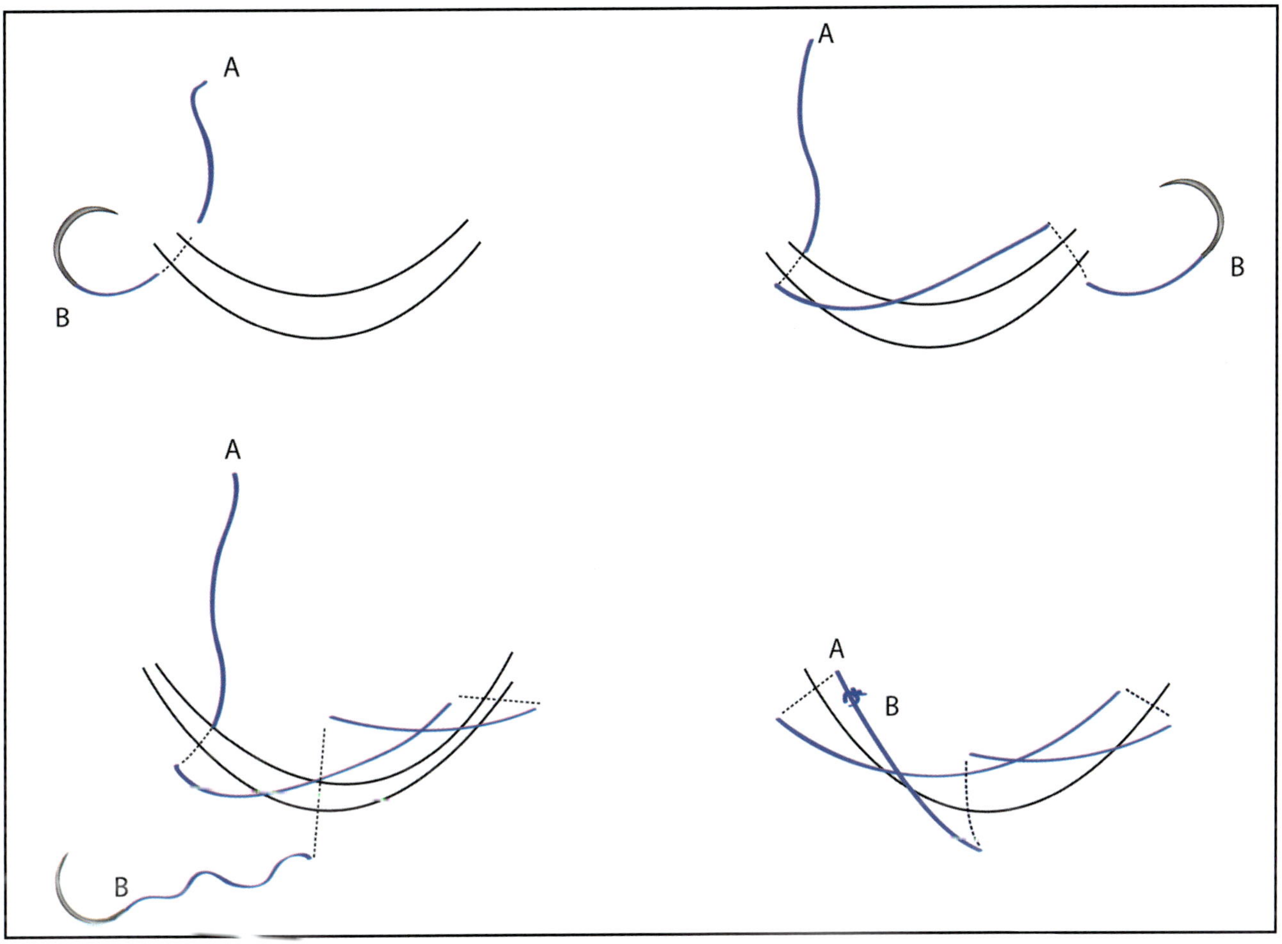

Corneal XX suture: The first needle pass is at one end of the incision. The second pass is at the opposite end, and the third pass is in the center of the incision. The trailing end A can then be sutured to the needle end B. Burying the knot is easier if using a bimanual technique, where one tyer pushes the suture and the other pulls in the same direction.

CHAPTER 18

HOW TO IMPLANT AN IRIS CLAW ARTISAN INTRAOCULAR LENS

INTRODUCTION

Iris claw lenses have potential advantages when compared to angle-supported anterior chamber intraocular lenses (ACIOLs) in that they are in contact with angle structures and do not have to be sized as meticulously. They simply need to be sized for an adult vs pediatric-sized anterior chamber. As they are enclavated to the iris, they cannot rotate, but there does remain a small risk of de-enclavation and resultant dislocation. Depending on anterior chamber anatomy and concern for endothelial cell loss, these versatile IOLs can be affixed to the anterior or posterior side of the iris.

KEY POINTS

- Preoperative endothelial cell count is crucial. If there is a chance of endothelial failure, we recommend posterior fixation of this lens or planning a posterior to iris IOL.
- A careful vitrectomy and any iris work should be done prior to ACIOL insertion.
- Pay attention to orientation as the IOL has an anterior vault.
- Pull the IOL into the eye instead of trying to push it in. This avoids wound gape, iris prolapse, hypotony, vitreous presentation, and the IOL getting pushed behind the iris.
- A peripheral iridectomy should be made peripherally out of the way of the IOL. Avoid excessively large sizes or dysphotopsias can occur. Make sure it is free of vitreous posteriorly (vitreous can block the peripheral iridotomy and pupil block can still occur).
- Use intraocular pressure medication and/or possibly oral acetazolamide postoperatively for 2 to 3 days, as all the viscoelastic may not have been evacuated.

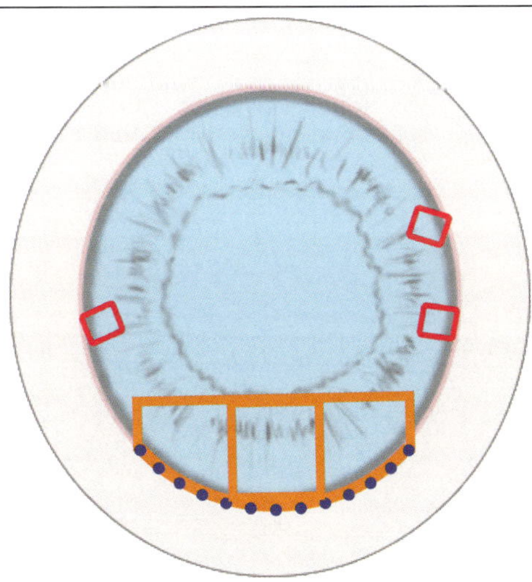

- Limbal 300-μm groove
- Bevelled, 3-step and triplanar 6-mm corneal incision
- Knife and fork paracentesis
- Additional paracentesis for nasal haptic enclavation angled toward nasal peripheral iris

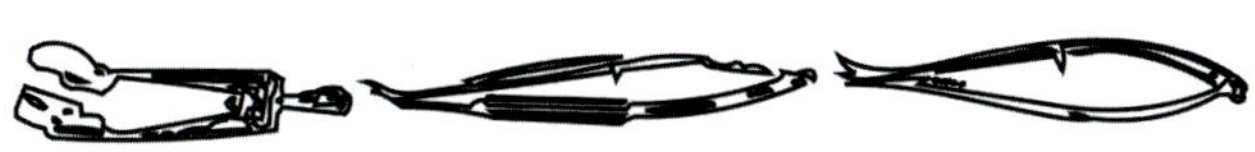

- Side port blade and main keratone
- Microsurgical Technology, Inc microtyers
- Microsurgical Technology, Inc microforceps
- 10-0 nylon suture for closure
- Preservative-free triamcinolone for vitrectomy
- Miochol (acetylcholine)

Ahmed IK, Campos-Möller X, Shah M, Sheybani A. *Illustrated Advanced Anterior Segment Surgery: A Step-by-Step Guide for Challenging Cases* (pp 119-126).

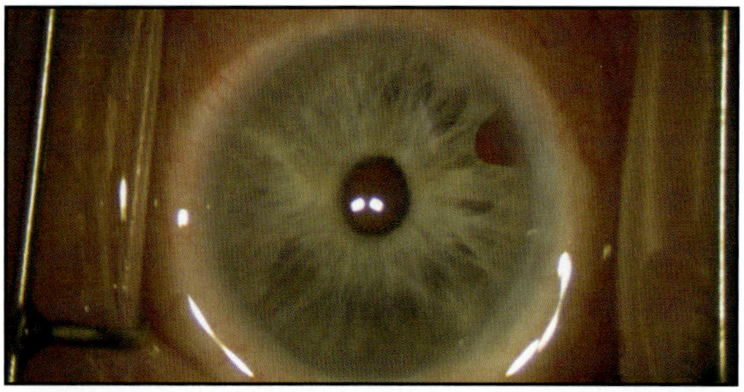

In this chapter, we are implanting an iris-claw Artisan ACIOL in a patient with traumatic aphakia. Notice that an iridectomy had been previously created.

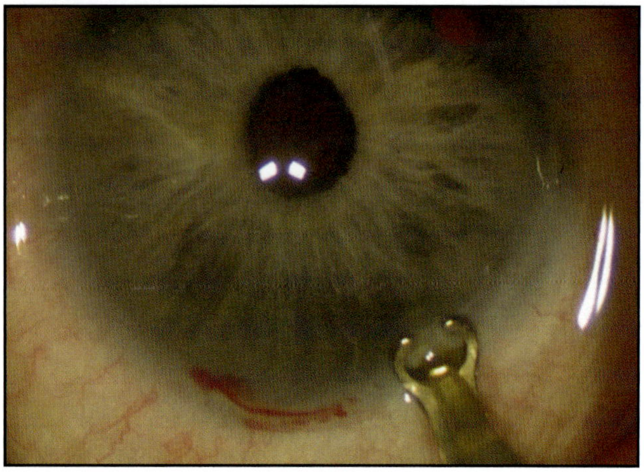

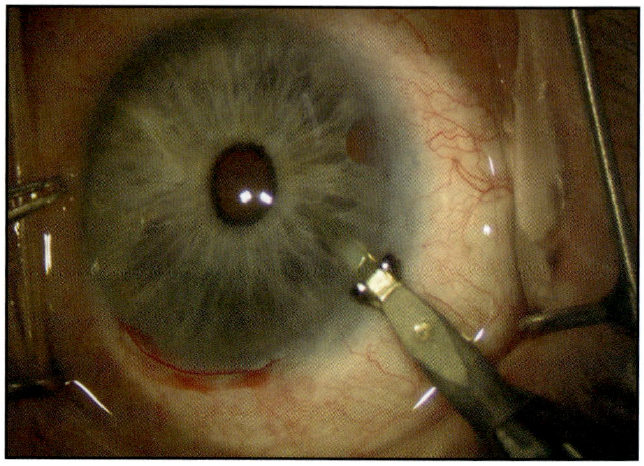

A 6-mm limbal groove is created at 300-μm of depth to achieve a 3-step incision. Do not enter the anterior chamber at this incision yet. Side ports are created first (see incision template).

Dispersive ophthalmic viscosurgical device (OVD) is used to protect the corneal endothelium and cohesive OVD to create space in the anterior chamber. A small amount of additional dispersive OVD can be used through the pupil to create a tamponade, preventing vitreous prolapse.

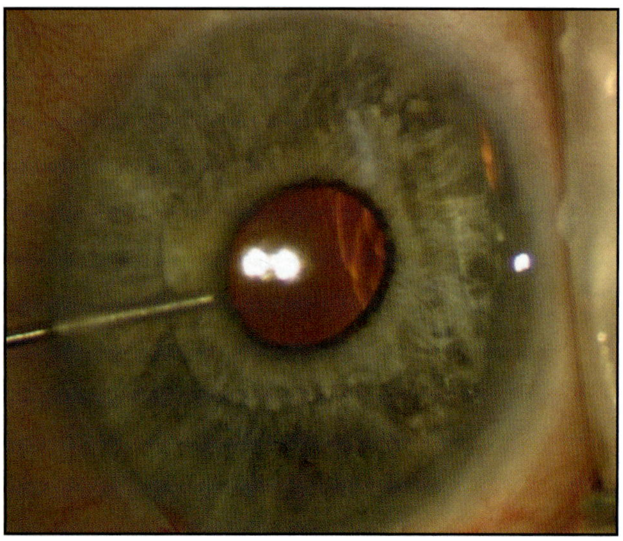

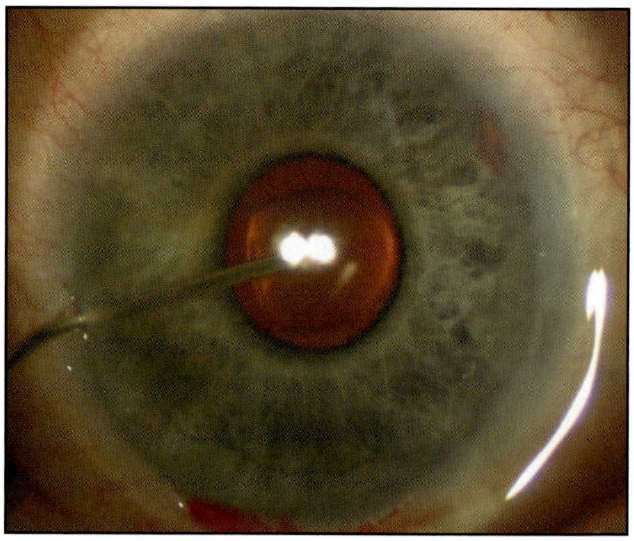

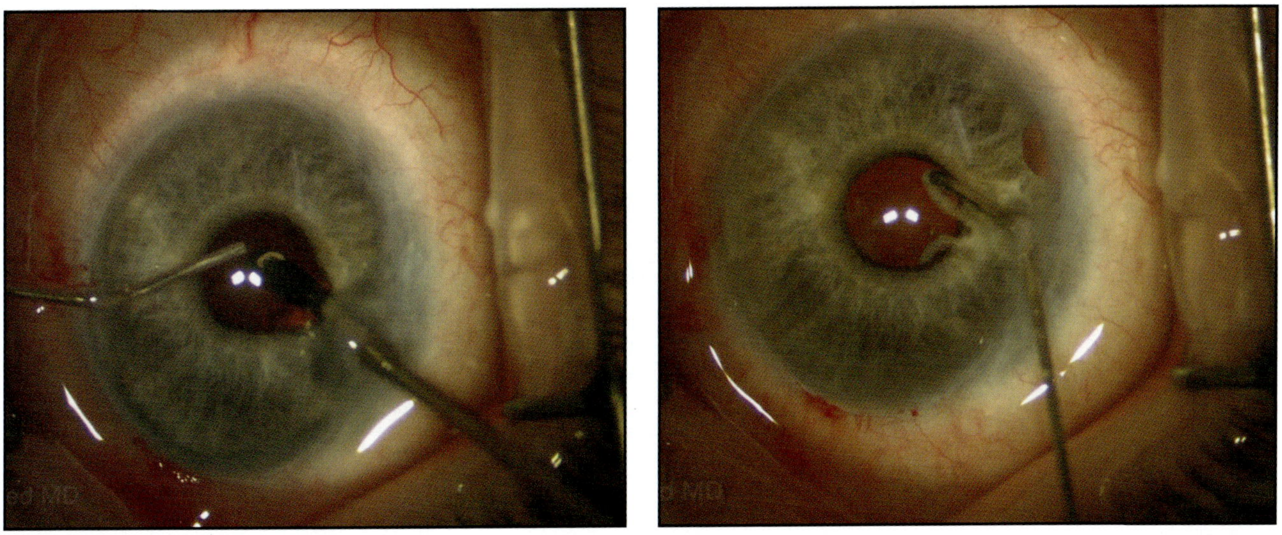

Anterior vitrectomy may be necessary. Diluted triamcinolone acetonide (Kenalog) can be very useful for staining vitreous, thus aiding its visualization. High cut rate with low, linear aspiration are our preferred settings. Vitreous that is in the anterior chamber and in the way of surgery should be removed exclusively. Avoid extensive vitrectomies and causing secondary hypotony.

Creating an incision with a 3 plane architecture ensures adequate wound healing and minimizes astigmatism. Enter the anterior chamber with a 2.75- to 3-mm keratome at the center of the previously created limbal groove (blue dotted line) and then cut sideways to the left and right.

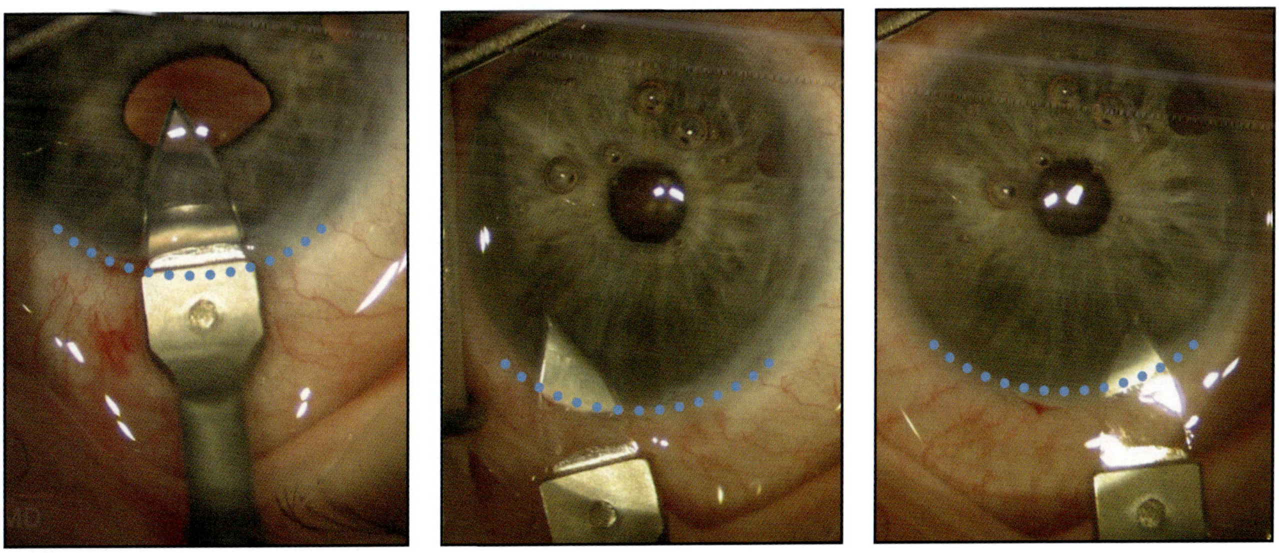

Insert the lens into the anterior chamber by holding the optic with a tyer (1). Do not lift the anterior lip of the wound to avoid anterior chamber shallowing. The IOL can then be centered on the pupil with a Sinskey hook (2).

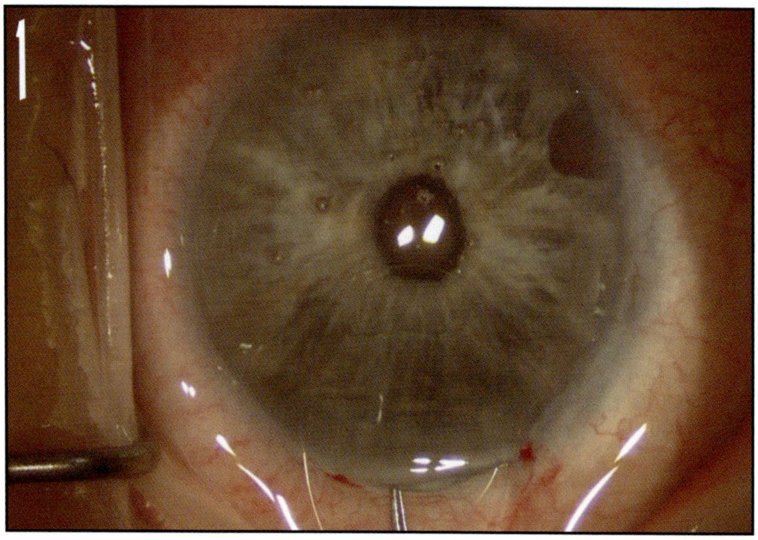

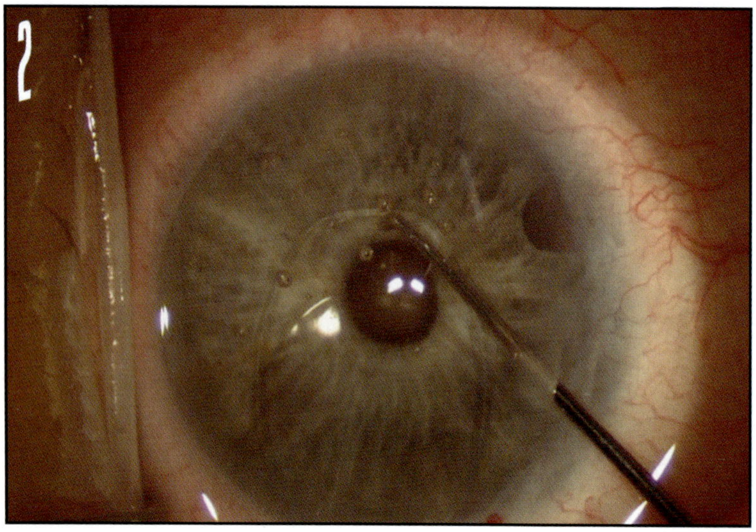

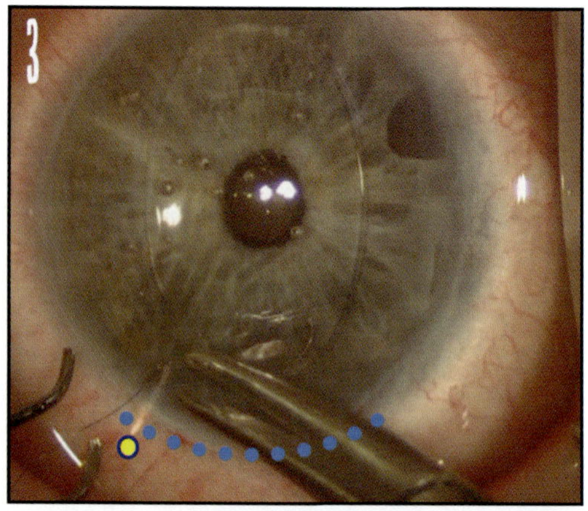

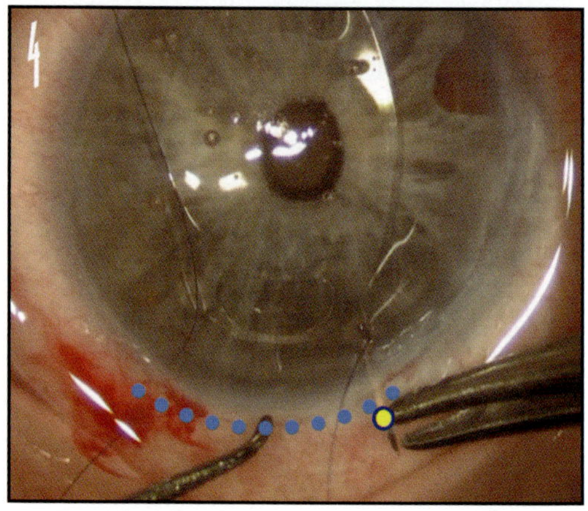

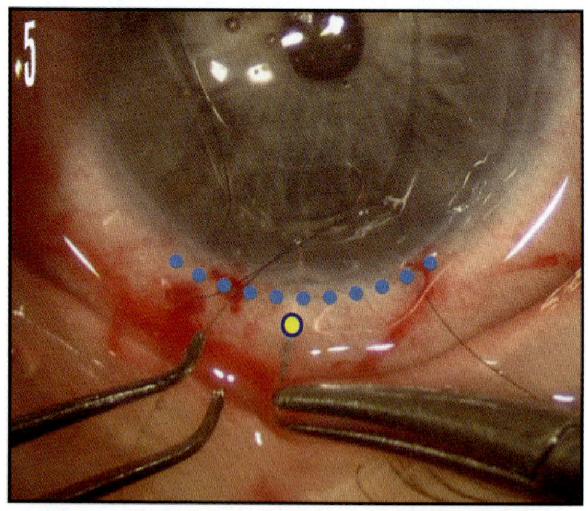

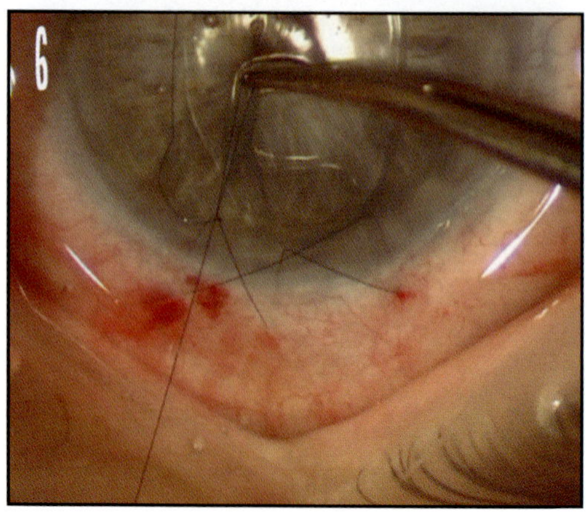

Images 3 through 6 illustrate our preferred "XX" continuous anastigmatic suture technique to close large incisions. The blue dotted line shows the extent of the incision, and the yellow dots indicate where the needle passes are made. At this point, a temporary knot can be created to secure the wound. We will later titrate suture tension and create a permanent knot.

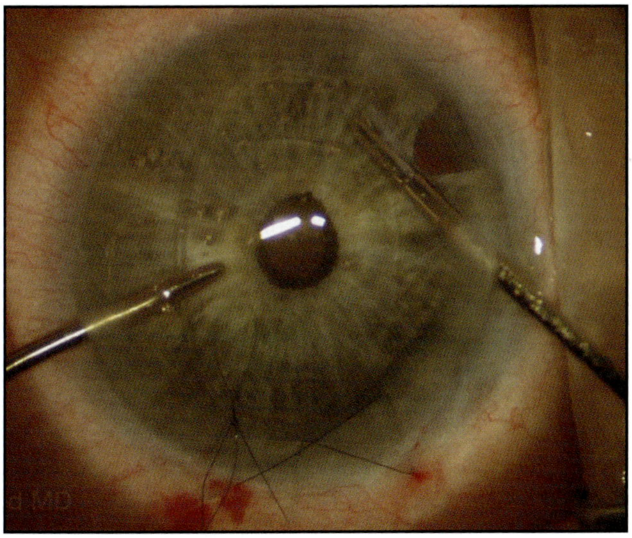

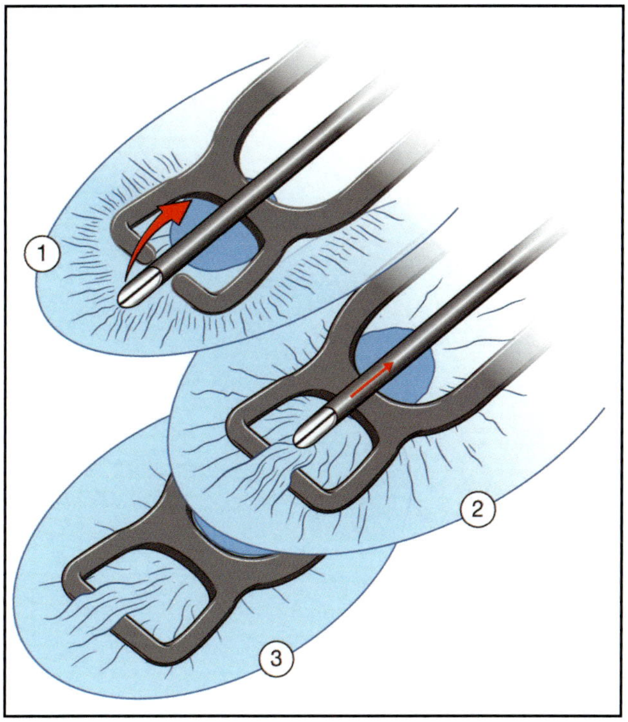

Two-handed microinstrument-assisted Artisan enclavation. Left: A microtyer holds IOL optic in place while an iris forceps grabs peripheral iris tissue. The motion is explained in the diagram (right). (1) Grab a substantial portion of iris tissue in the area of planned enclavation of the nasal haptic. (2) Pull the iris tissue gently toward the pupil and toward the corneal apex, passing iris fibers between IOL claws and using the iris micrograspers to gently splay open the claw. (3) Iris should remain entrapped between claws. Position and pupil size can later be adjusted. Note that the IOL barely moves. Only the iris forceps hand is moving.

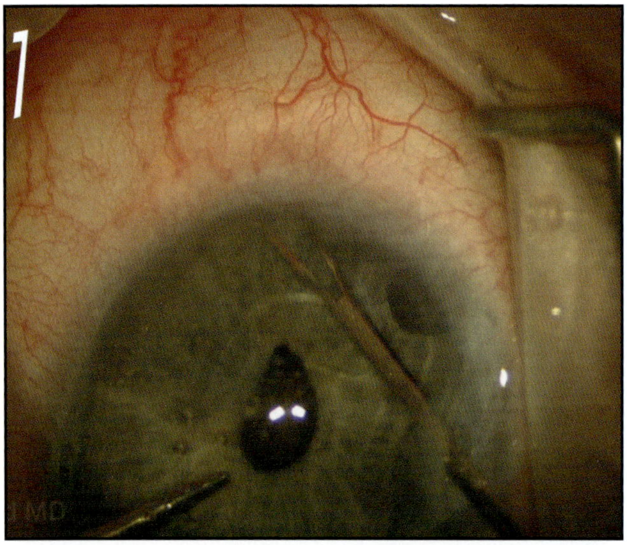

Enclavation of distal haptic (7, 8) and proximal haptics (9). Notice hand position of tyer does not change, stays low, and shaft is parallel to iris plane; this reduces IOL movement and tilt. Distal enclavation can be done through side port with a low pencil grip. For proximal enclavation, we use the main incision, using an elevated overhand grip to allow for a more vertical instrument shaft orientation.

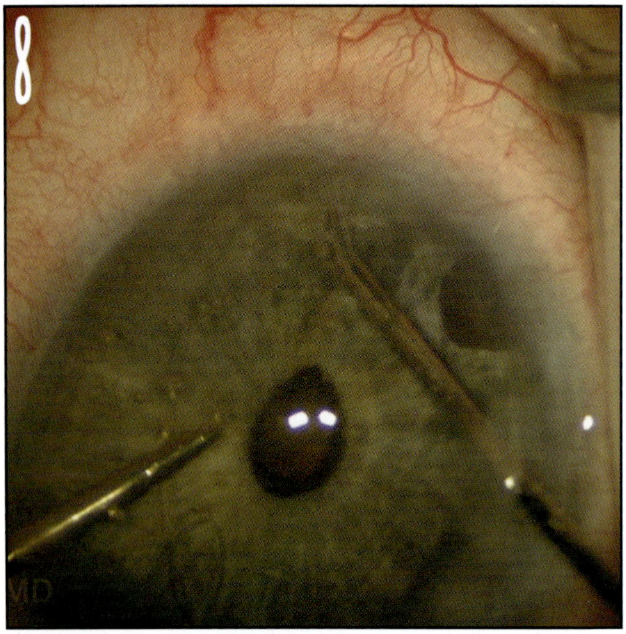

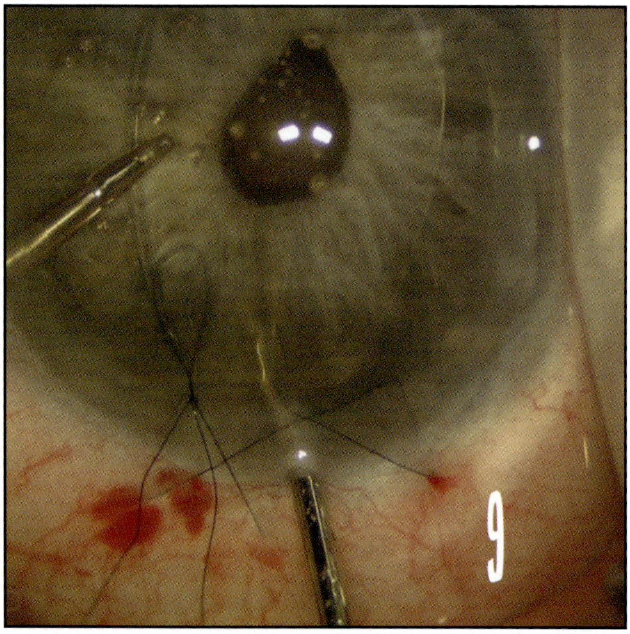

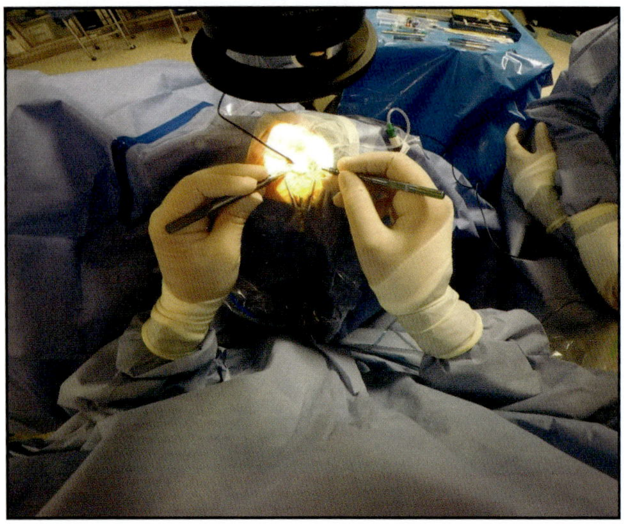

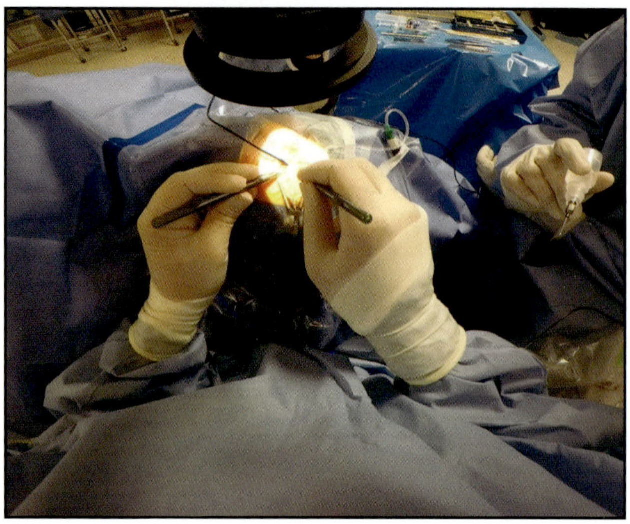

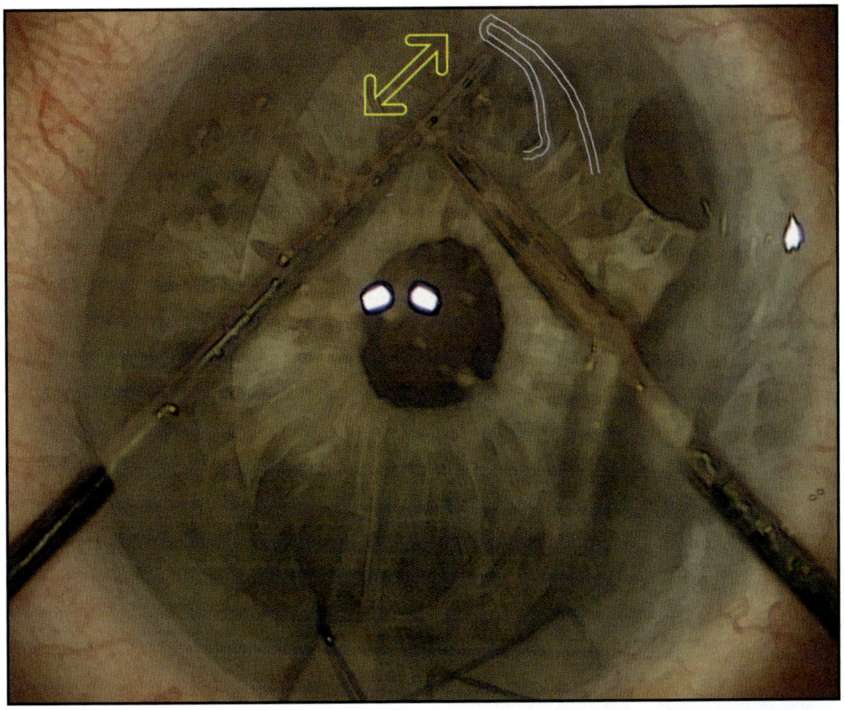

The final position of the IOL can be adjusted by grasping more central iris tissue with microforceps and pushing on the central side or pulling on the peripheral side of the nasal haptic as needed. The IOL has been outlined for identification. The yellow arrows indicate direction of movement of the Sinskey hook.

It is not uncommon for the pupil to be ovalized after successful haptic enclavation. To correct this, the pupil margin can be pulled toward the center of the pupil with an iris forceps, while using countertraction on the IOL optic edge or the central edge of the nasal haptic with a Sinskey hook. Arrows indicates direction of movement of instruments.

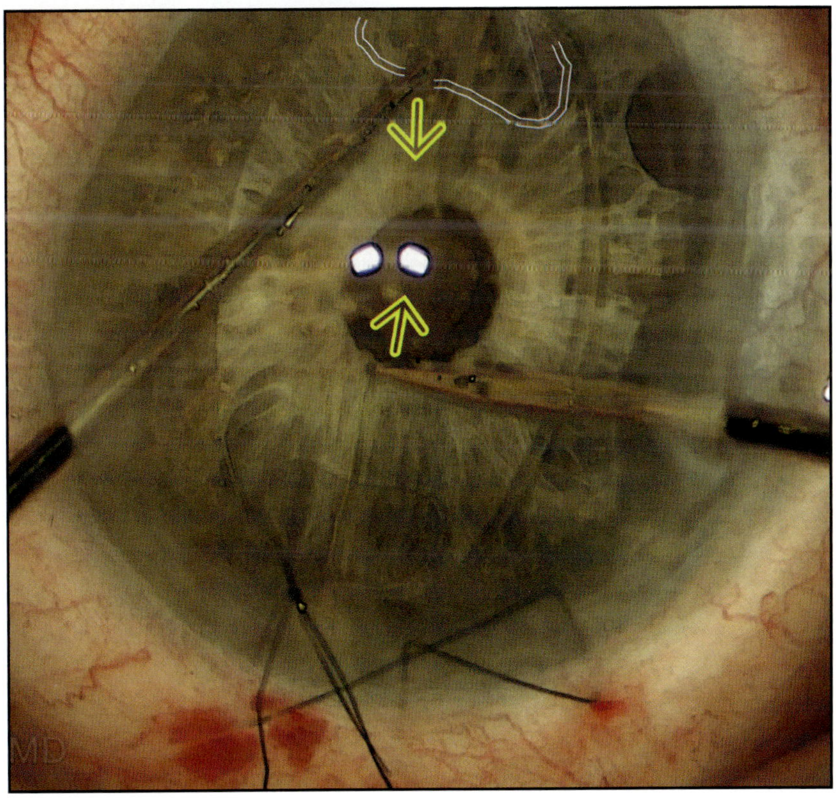

A patent iridectomy is necessary to prevent pupil block. If there is none already present, a vitrector can be used to create one. Use the lowest possible cut rate (1 cut per minute) with moderate vacuum. Engage peripheral iris and achieve occlusion while allowing vacuum to build (on foot position 2). Engage foot position 3 to initiate a single cut, then ensure that the cut piece of iris has been evacuated. Limited vitrectomy at higher cut rate may be necessary to prevent vitreous block. Another option is to use micrograspers and microscissors.

We prefer manual OVD aspiration in order to prevent anterior chamber shallowing and vitreous prolapse. This can be achieved by injecting small volumes of balanced salt solution and aspirating with a Rycroft cannula (Beaver-Visitec) on a 3-mL syringe. Exhaustive removal may risk vitreous presentation, so a slight amount of retained OVD is tolerated. Postoperative intraocular pressure spikes can be managed with topical or oral medications, and are typically short lived. The suture is tied and the knot buried with a 2-handed push-pull technique, where one hand pushes one strand and the other one pulls.

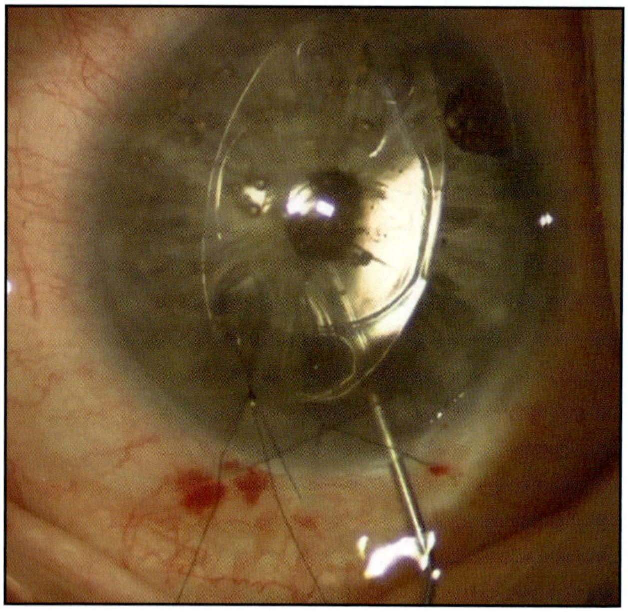

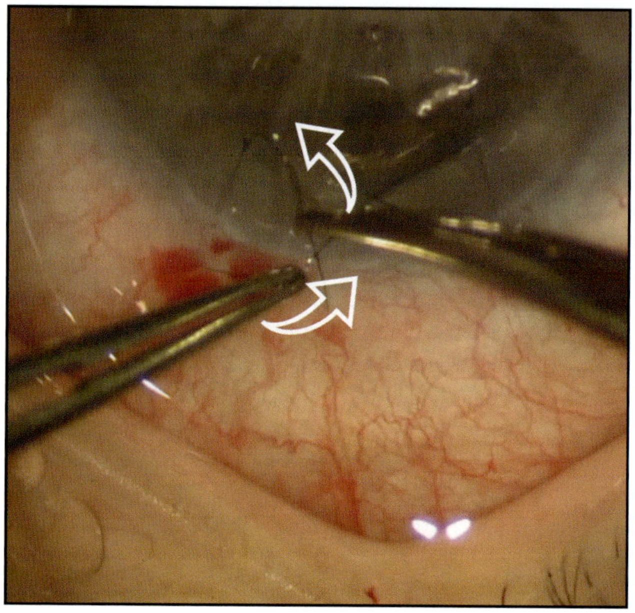

CHAPTER 19

HOW TO SUTURE AN INTRAOCULAR LENS TO IRIS

INTRODUCTION

Suture iris fixation is a good option for patients without capsular support, especially with poor endothelial cell function. Scleral suture fixation requires scleral passes and conjunctival incisions, whereas iris fixation does not. Intraocular lenses (IOLs) sutured to sulcus should be targeted for in-the-bag placement. It is not the procedure of choice in young patients or those with long life expectancy as sutures can break over time. Small pupil diameters are ideal; otherwise, a pupilloplasty may be performed to reduce the pupil size, or a lens glide should be used to support the IOL while it is sutured to iris.

KEY POINTS

- The IOL must be folded in half such that the haptics are both on the same side.
- Placing the IOL in a warm balanced salt solution (BSS) bath can facilitate folding—cold IOL material makes folding difficult, as it is stiff. Stiff material requires more force that risks the IOL slipping out of the forceps.
- Para placement should be 1 clock hour away from where iris will be engaged oriented tangentially. If this is placed too far away from the planned point of entry of the needle into the iris, the initial pass can be difficult.
- Perform a thorough vitrectomy.
- Sweep Miochol (acetylcholine) by brushing over the iris with minimal injection of the medication. This prevents burping viscoelastic and places the medication on the surface of the iris, where it helps constrict the pupil.
- Do not lock the sutures until the IOL has been positioned behind the pupil so that pupil centration can be achieved. Avoid overly tightening the first throw; this will incarcerate iris.
- Avoid suturing too close to the pupil margin as it can limit dilation.
- To prevent sun-setting of the IOL, suturing the haptics at 12 and 6 o'clock is preferred.

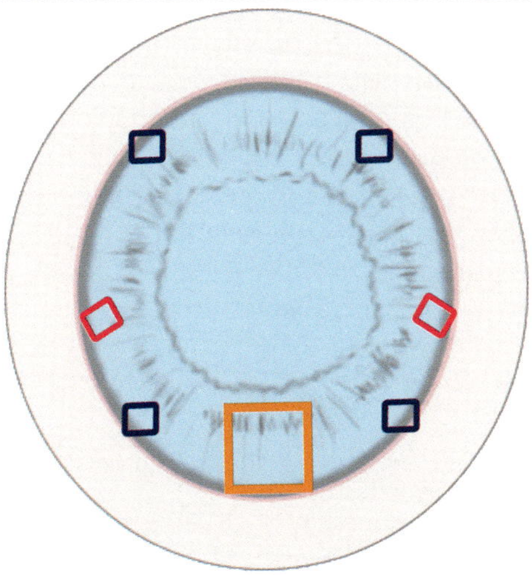

- Knife and fork
- Paracentesis incisions for iris suture passes

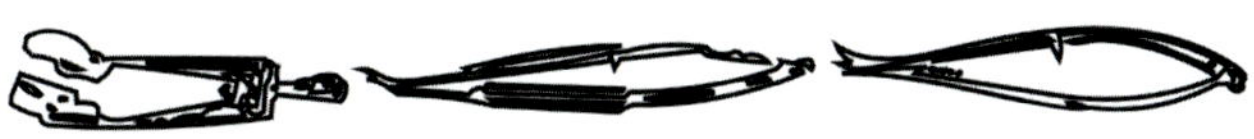

- Microsurgical Technology, Inc microforceps
- Angled Kuglen hook
- Angled Sinskey hook
- 9-0 Prolene (Ethicon, Inc) on a CIF-4 or PC-7 needle, cut single-armed
- Microsurgical Technology, Inc microscissors
- 27-g cannula for docking (the viscoelastic cannula works well for this)
- IOL-folding forceps, such as the Steinert folding forceps
- Buratto IOL grasping forceps (ASICO)
- Miochol

Ahmed IK, Campos-Möller X, Shah M, Sheybani A. *Illustrated Advanced Anterior Segment Surgery: A Step-by-Step Guide for Challenging Cases* (pp 127-139).

SECTION 1: SECONDARY IOL IMPLANTATION WITH IRIS SUTURING

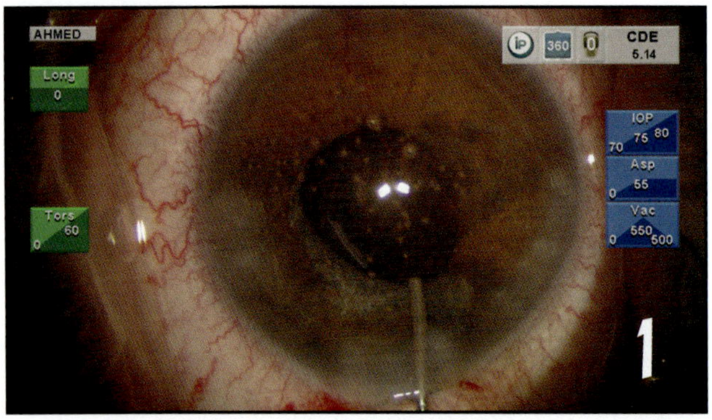

If the pupil is greater than 5 to 6 mm, Miochol should be injected into the anterior chamber prior to viscoelastic placement to constrict the pupil. If viscoelastic is already present, brushing Miochol with a blunt cannula over the iris can also constrict the pupil, as injection of the medication will not work.

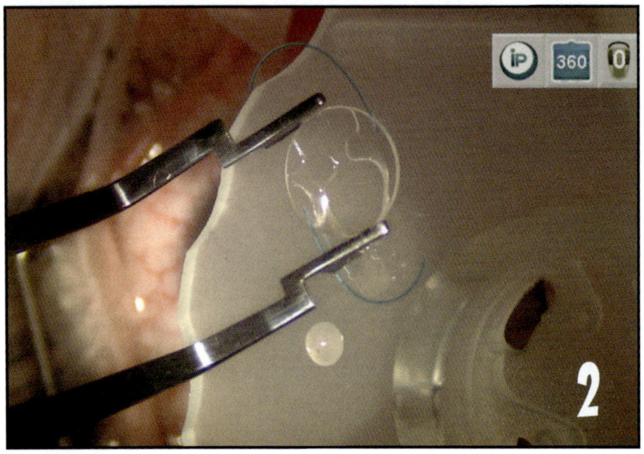

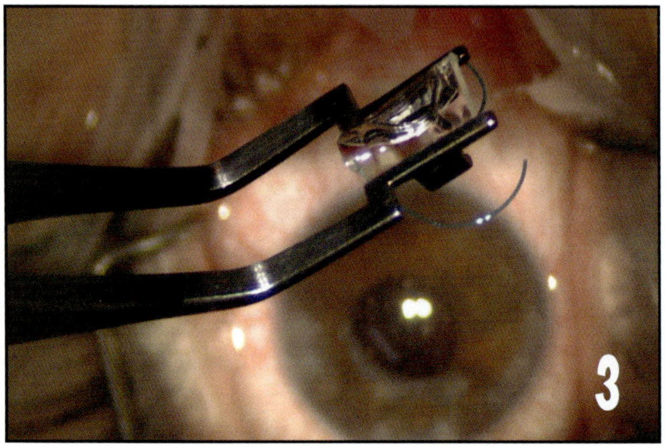

- The IOL is placed in a warm BSS bath for several seconds.
- The IOL is then grasped by the folding forceps, with each haptic near against the forceps footplate.
- The IOL is folded along an axis that bisects the 2 haptics so that one haptic folds onto the other. The optic is now folded in half in the forceps, and the haptics are crossing each other, forming a moustache curled up toward the optic at the tips. With the IOL in proper orientation, the fold occurs with the distal haptic being folded BACK, not forward, against the leading haptic.
- The IOL is then handed off to an IOL forceps so that the leading haptic is ON TOP. Usually, this means that the fold of the optic is to the right and the moustache haptics to the left.

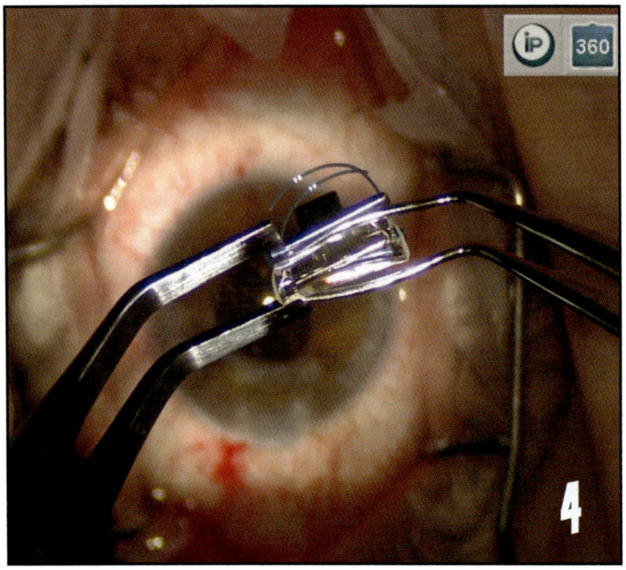

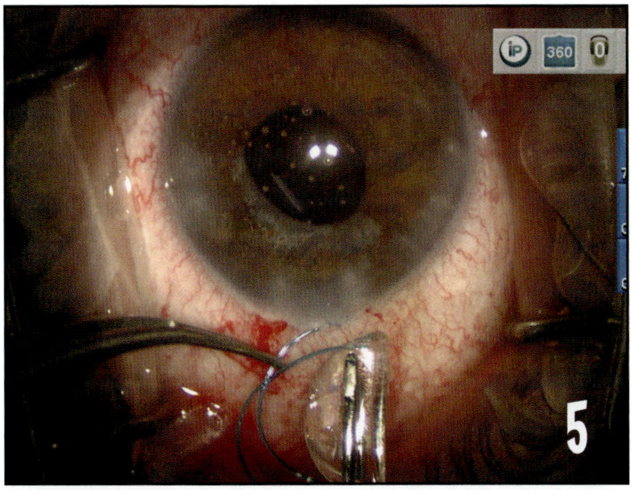

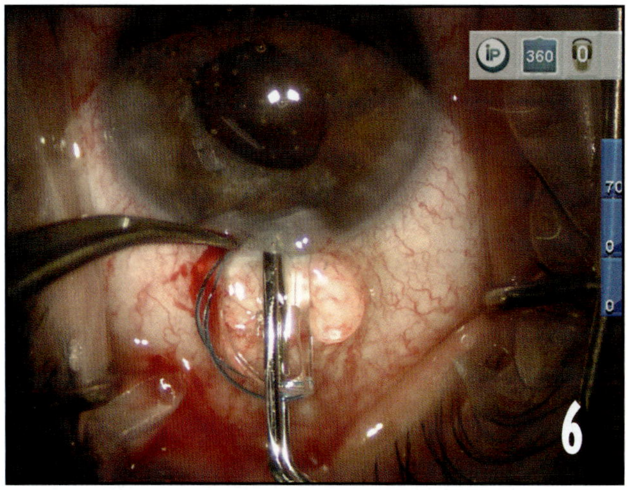

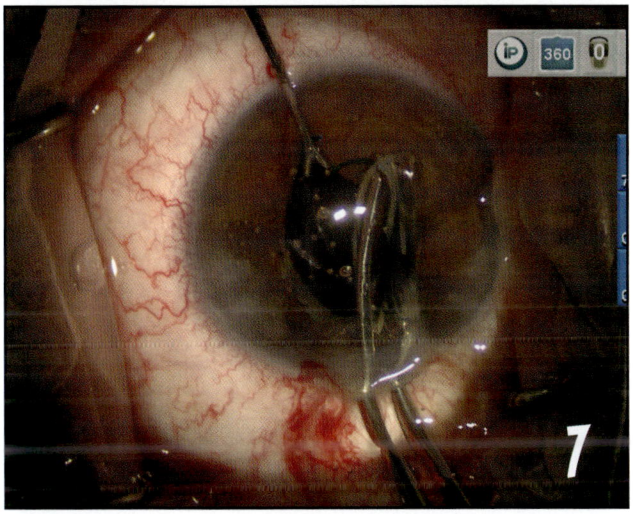

- The IOL is inserted into the eye through the main incision, using tyers to facilitate the insertion of the IOL haptics, which can get stuck at the would. Once in the anterior chamber, the hand is rotated counterclockwise so that the haptics are through the pupil and the optic fold is pointed to the endothelium.
- The forceps are opened slowly, allowing the optic to remain above iris plane while the haptics are below iris in the proper orientation of the IOL.
- Iris suture fixation is performed.

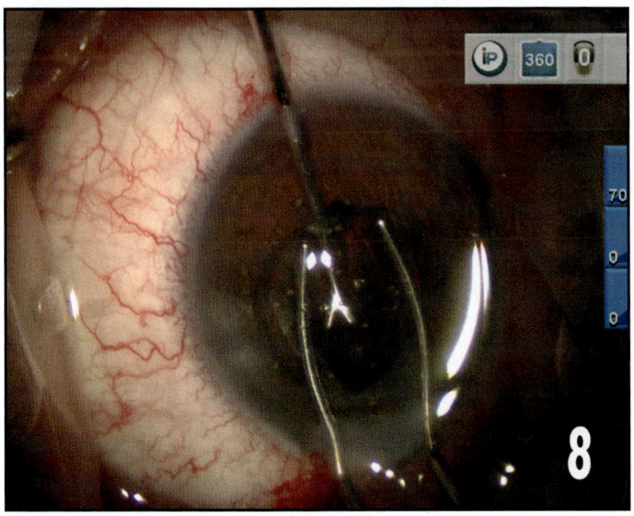

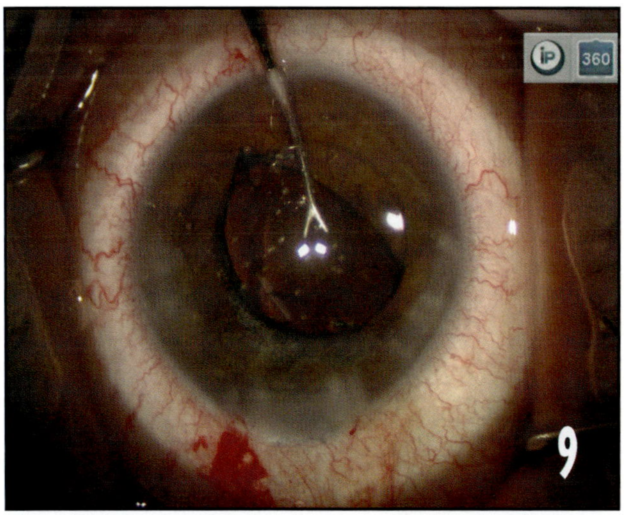

SKIP TO SECTION 3 (STEP 9) FOR SUTURING TECHNIQUE

SECTION 2: IOL REPOSITIONING WITH IRIS SUTURING

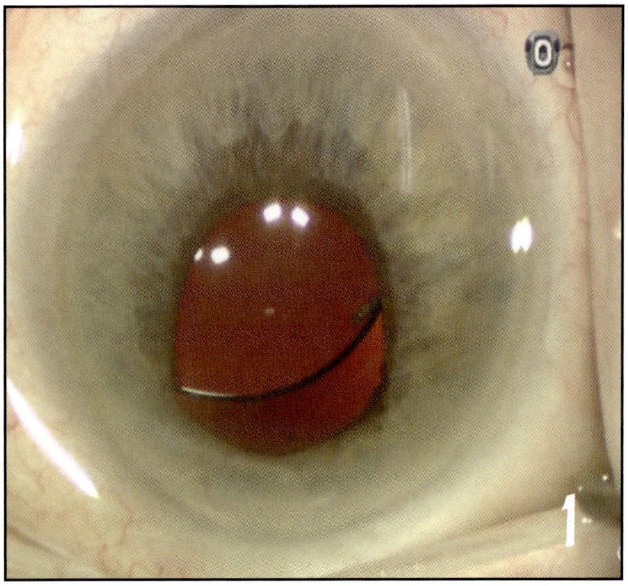

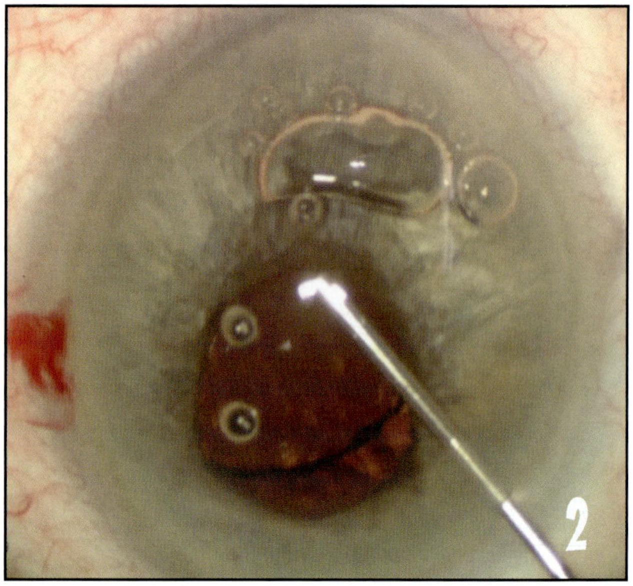

In this case, we will reposition a subluxed 3-piece IOL that was placed in the ciliary sulcus after complicated phacoemulsification (1). Dispersive viscoelastic is used to protect the corneal endothelium and to prevent anterior vitreous prolapse (2). A Kuglen hook can be used to visualize the extent of remaining capsular support and IOL haptic orientation (3). Triamcinolone can be used to stain vitreous. A limited vitrectomy should be performed to ensure that there is not vitreous in the anterior chamber. The pars plana approach has the advantage of drawing vitreous posteriorly, while the anterior chamber approach can be used to clear any remaining vitreous in the anterior chamber (4, 5).

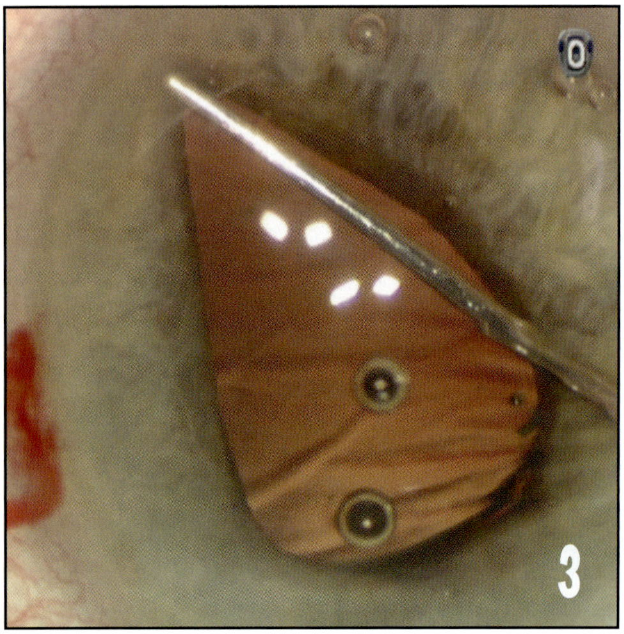

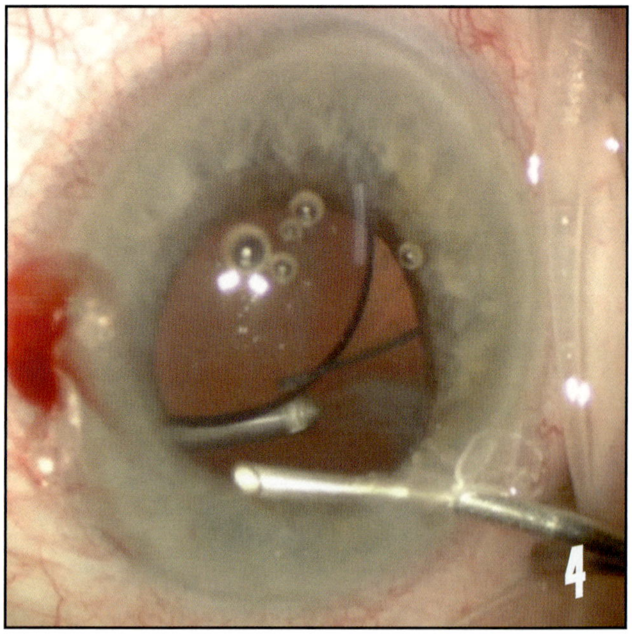

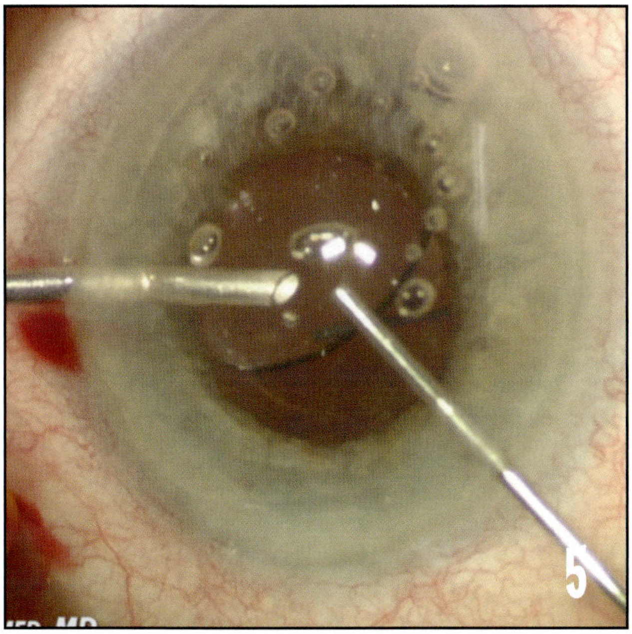

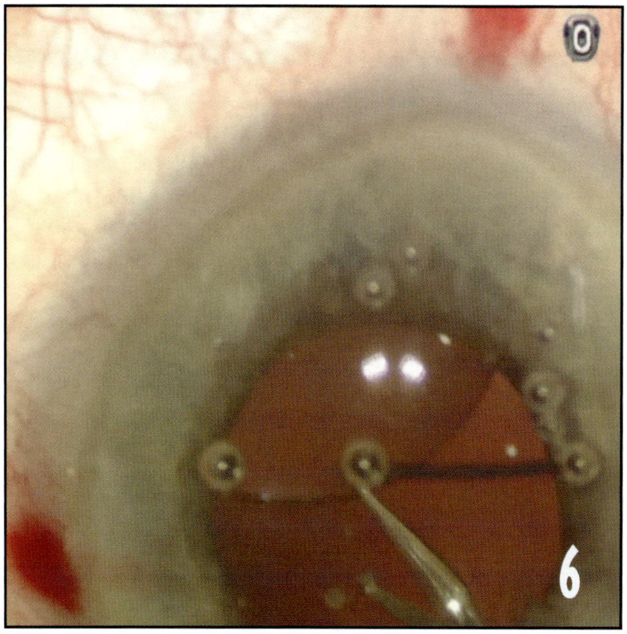

Prevent vitreous prolapse by injecting dispersive ophthalmic viscosurgical device (OVD) prior to coming out with the vitrectomy irrigation cannula (5). The IOL should be captured through the pupil, with haptics posterior to the iris and the optic in the anterior chamber. Use a micrograsper to position the IOL. Alternatively, a Kuglen and Sinskey hook can be used to chopstick the IOL upward (see Chapter 16). Rotating the IOL above iris plane does not work as well since the haptic can follow anteriorly above the iris. The goal is to place the haptic behind the iris and the optic above the iris. Miochol is swept over the iris once the IOL is captured through the pupil.

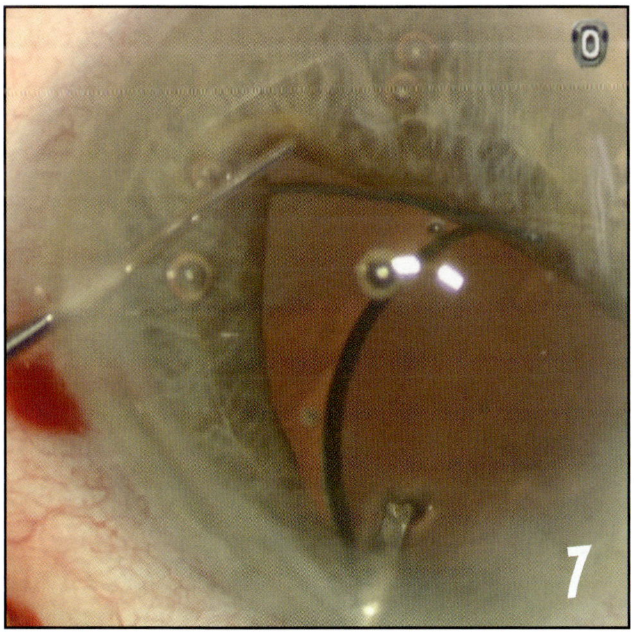

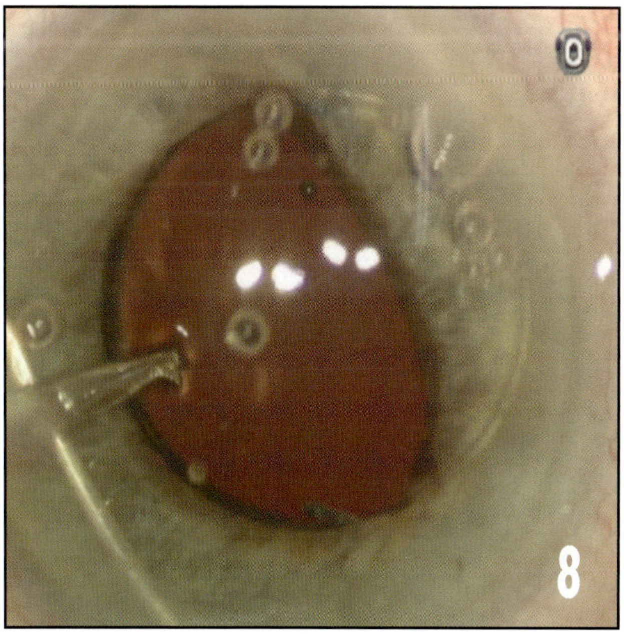

SECTION 3: SUTURING THE IOL TO IRIS

The position of the haptics can be revealed by using a blunt instrument like a Beckert manipulator or an OVD cannula to lift on the IOL optic from behind (9). This will indent the iris (arrow), revealing the haptic position and also facilitating the needle pass. "Wiggle" the needle laterally when entering through the paracentesis to avoid catching corneal stromal fibers. Avoid taking a large bite with the needle to prevent pupil irregularities. The needle pass must go posterior to the IOL haptic and then out the iris again. Lifting of the needle should indent the iris with the haptic. The needle can then be docked into a 27-g cannula for externalization through the opposite paracentesis (10). Docking the needle instead of attempting to pass it directly through the paracentesis prevents catching of stromal fibers at the incision and the accidental creation of another wound.

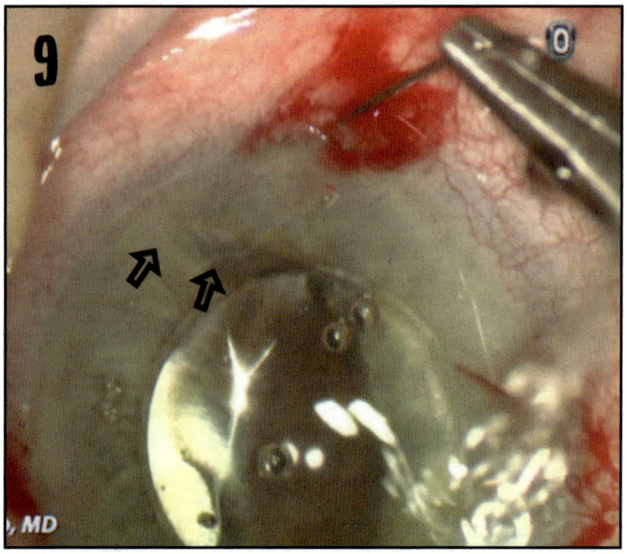

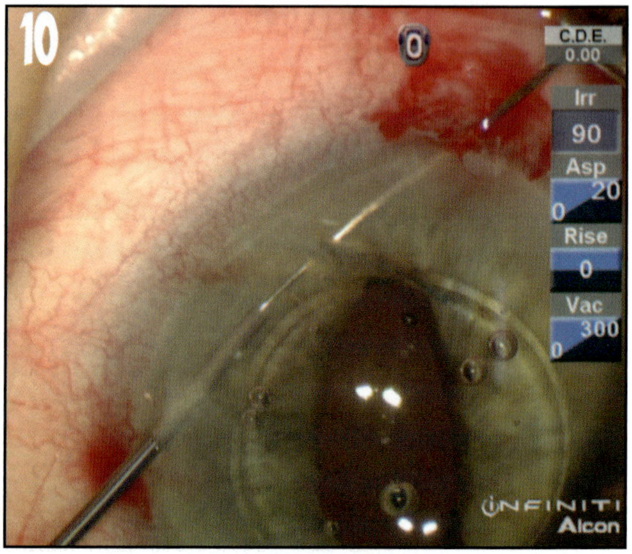

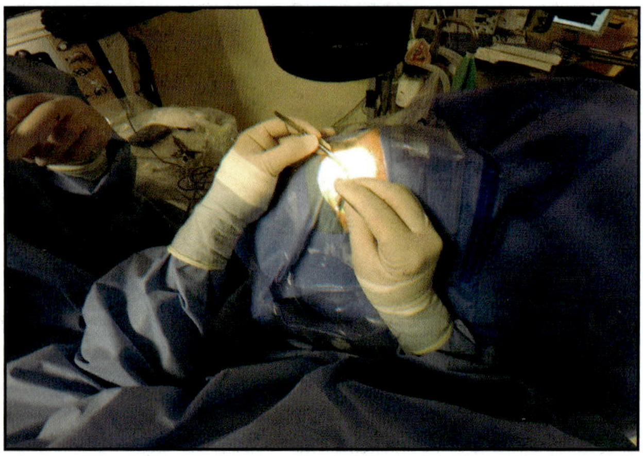

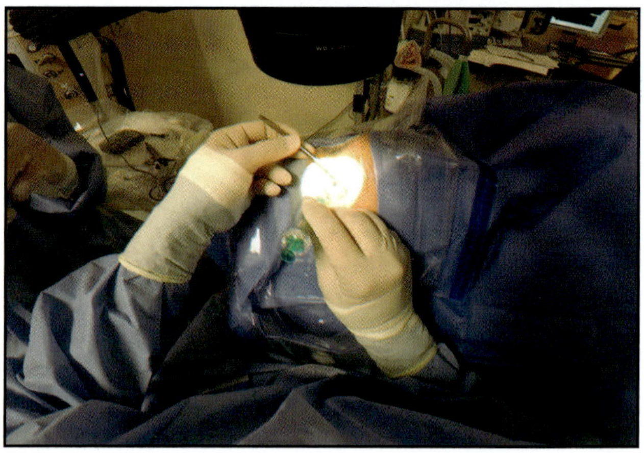

Hand positioning should be such that the needle driver hand remains still during instrument exchange from Beckert spatula to 27-g cannula for docking. Once the OVD cannula is in the eye, a twist of the needle driver wrist will usually suffice to dock the needle.

The suture is cut from the needle and, before tying any knots, a new suture is used to repeat steps 9 to 10 for the second haptic, using the corresponding paracentesis. Image 11 shows an alternative method of revealing the haptic position with a micrograsper. This also helps in obtaining a better final centration of the IOL.

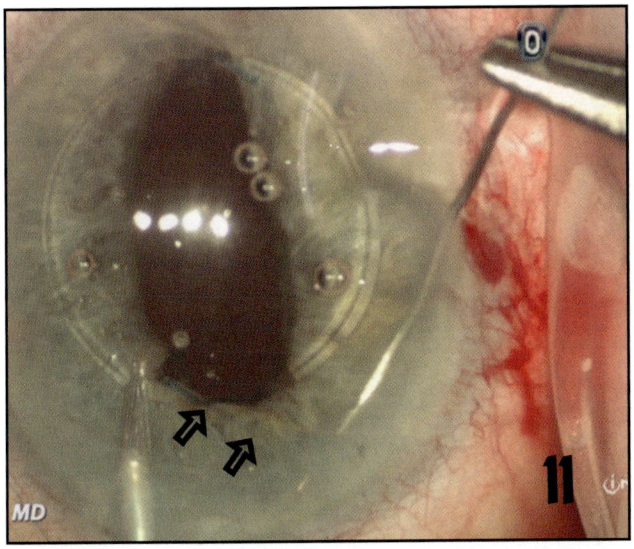

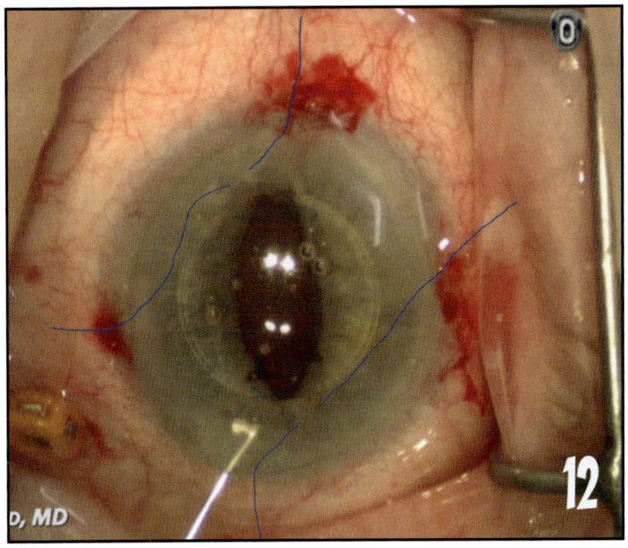

Sutures outlined in blue.

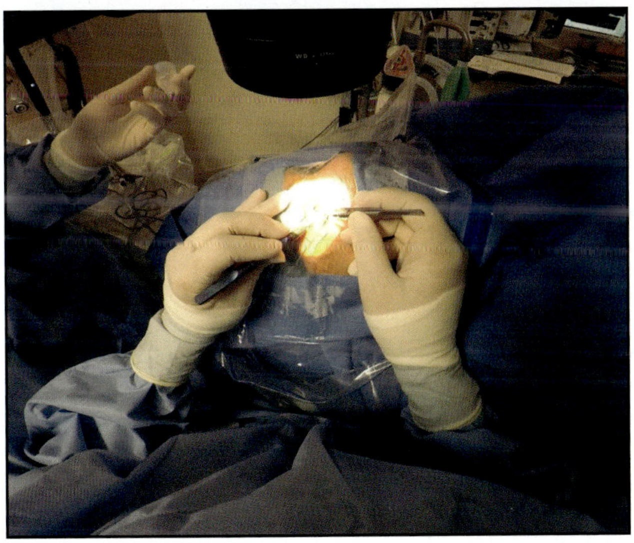

Knot-tying technique of choice can be used to tie a double throw on each haptic, without locking the sutures. This will allow for pupil shape adjustment after the IOL has been placed posterior to the iris. Here, we show a modified Siepser sliding knot for the temporal haptic (inferior in the images) and an intraocular suturing technique for the nasal haptic (superior in the images). See Chapter 26 on iris suturing for detailed explanations of these knots.

SIEPSER SLIDING KNOT

The Siepser sliding knot has the advantage of not requiring intraocular microinstruments like iris forceps or micrograspers. Identification of the 3 proximal strands is the key to a successful knot. This technique is presented in more detail in Chapter 26 on suturing iris defects.

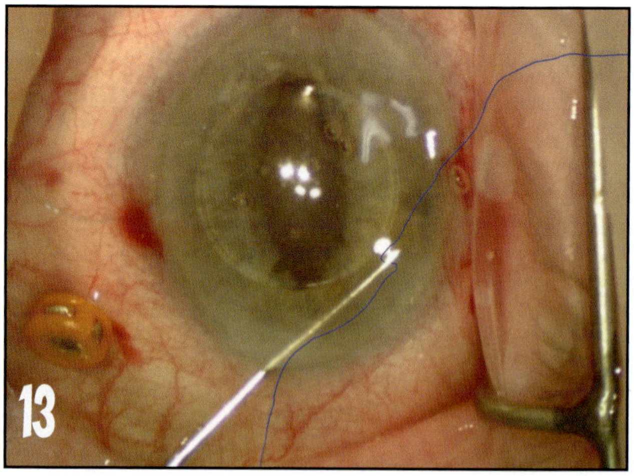

Use a Kuglen hook to bring a loop of the distal suture out through the proximal paracentesis.

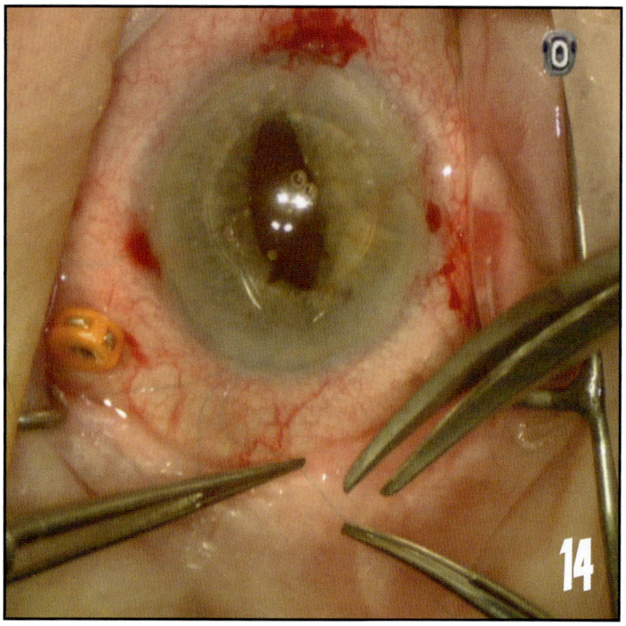

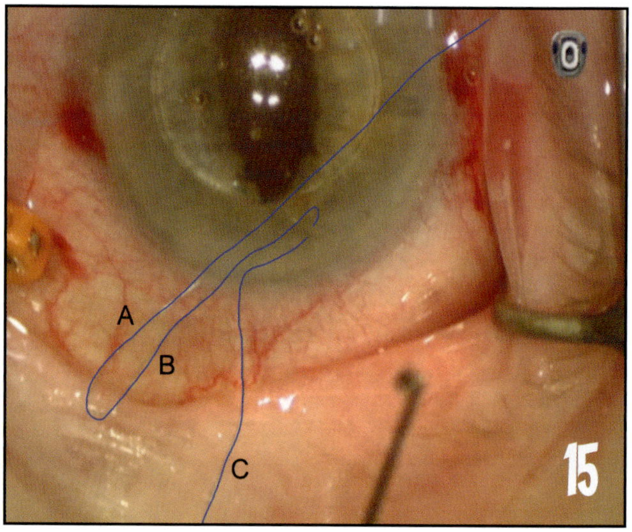

Correct suture configuration: Distal loop (A) goes out through distal paracentesis, and this is the end that will be double-thrown around the tyer. Proximal end (C) will be grabbed after the loops are thrown around the tyer.

Loop end "A" is double-thrown around tyer on right hand (16). Tyer on right hand then grabs proximal end "C" as shown in Image 17. The knot is finalized by pulling on the proximal and distal ends simultaneously to slide the knot into the eye. It is sometimes more comfortable to switch the proximal end to the left hand after the loops have been thrown and the proximal end has been grabbed, but this will depend on IOL orientation and surgeon preference.

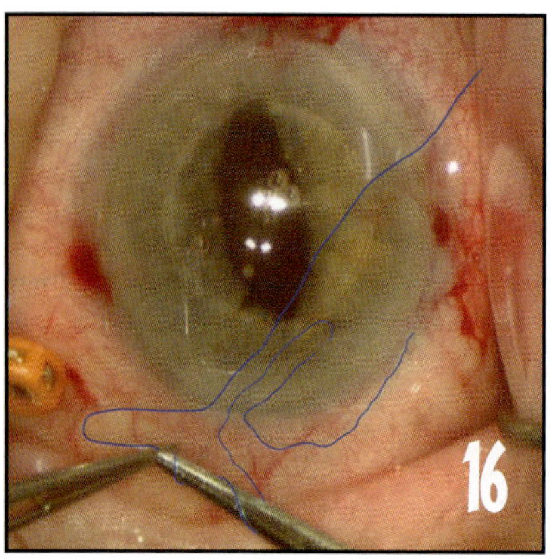

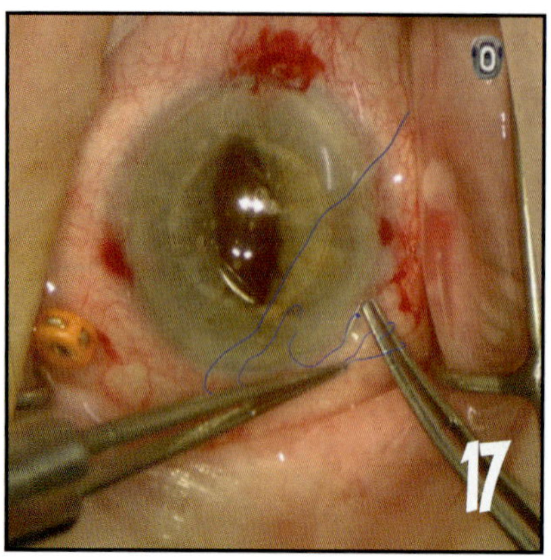

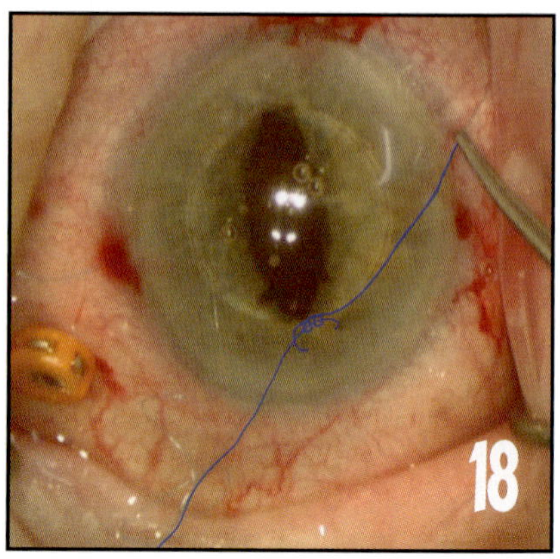

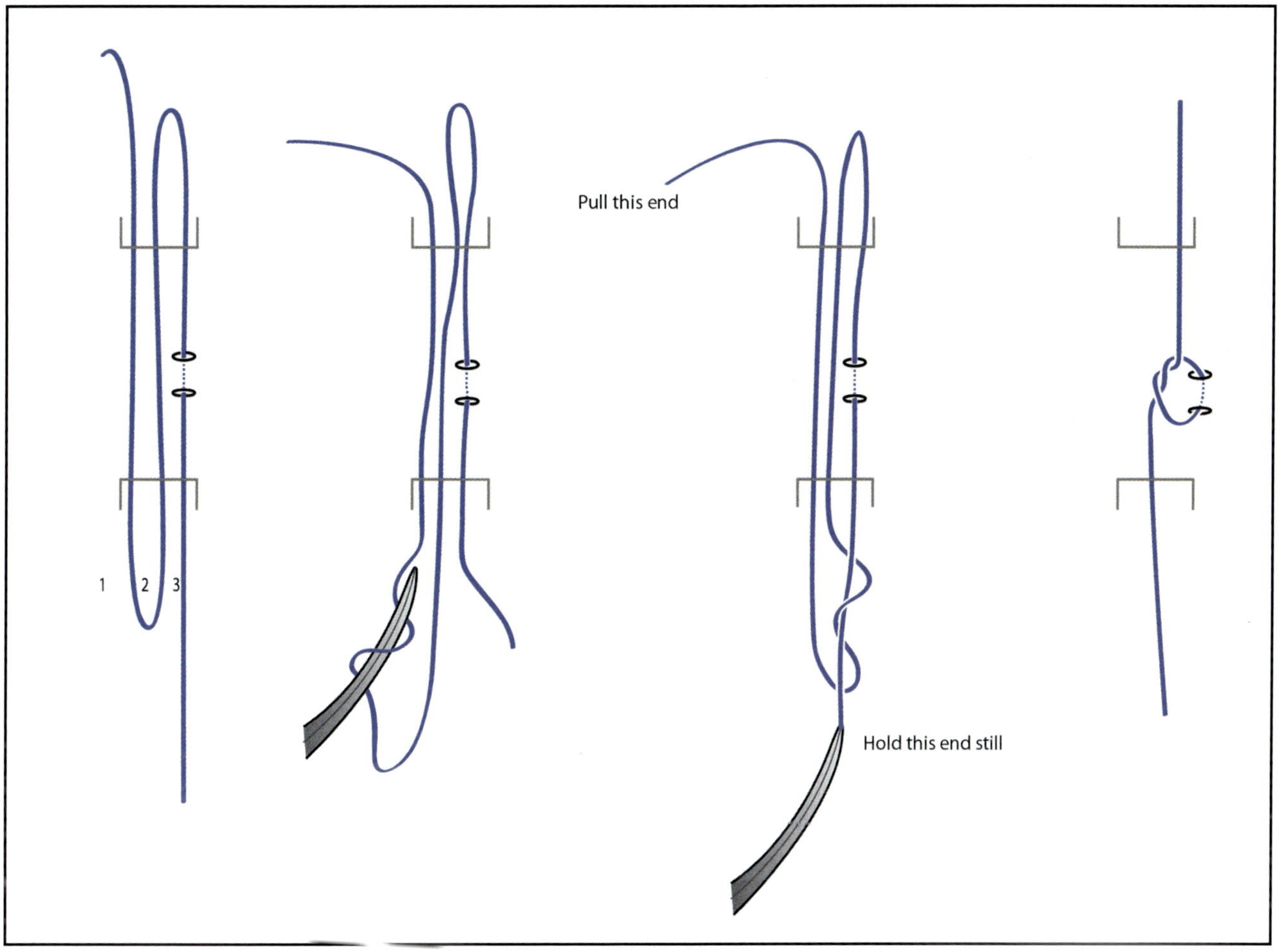
1
2
3
Pull this end
Hold this end still

INTRAOCULAR IRIS SUTURING

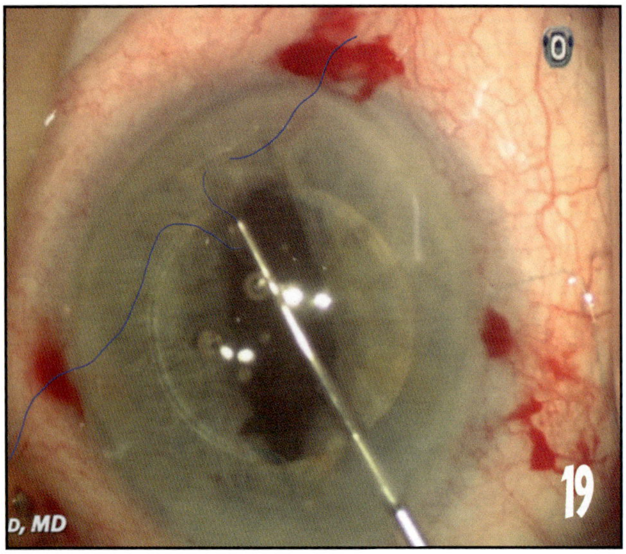

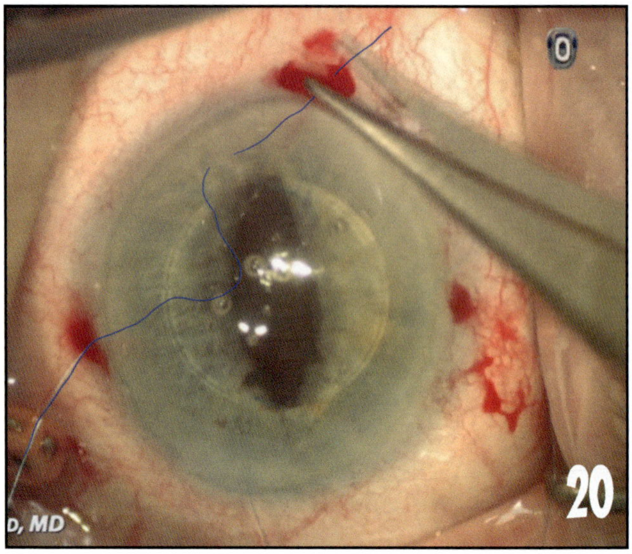

For intraocular suturing, a small loop of the proximal suture is pulled into the anterior chamber with a Kuglen hook (19). The distal end is then cut short (20).

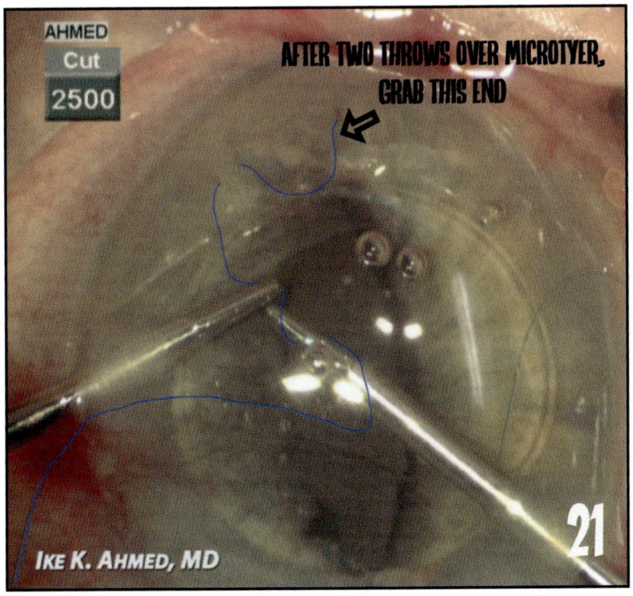

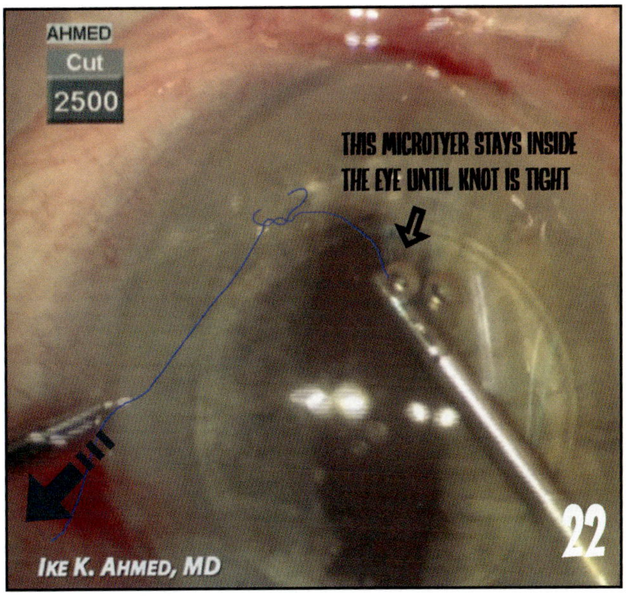

Using microtyers, 2 forward throws of the proximal end are wrapped around the right hand microtyer (21) and the short distal end is then grabbed with this tyer. Tightening the sutures is achieved by pulling the proximal end out of the eye while leaving the microtyer with the distal end inside the anterior chamber. When suturing an IOL to iris, our preference is to tie with a 2-1-1 throw configuration. However, we suggest tying the first double throw first, then pushing the IOL behind the iris, adjusting pupil shape and size and then tying the remaining single throws.

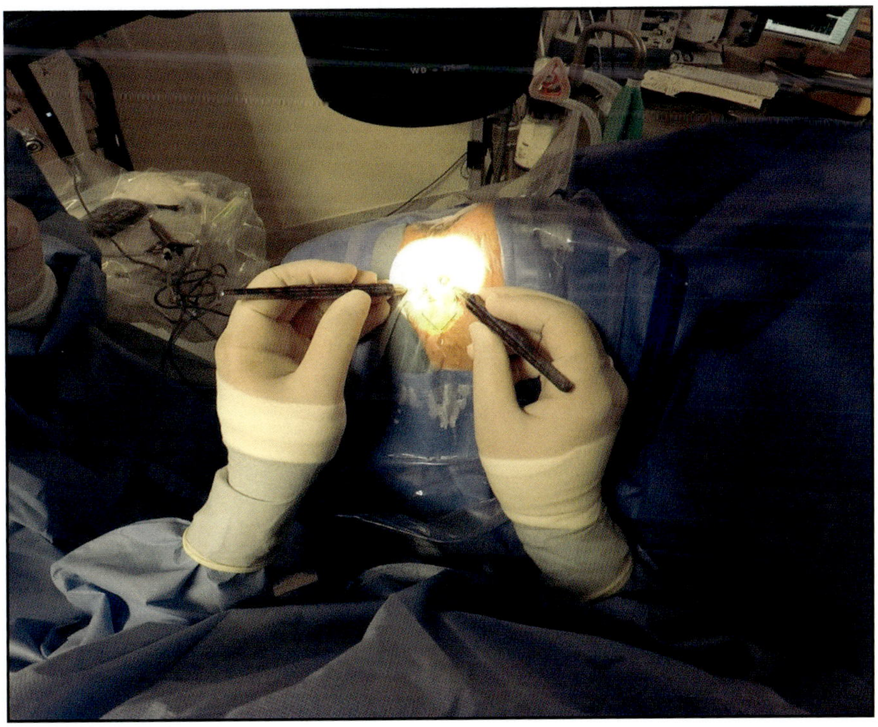

With a blunt instrument, place the optic behind the sulcus with very gentle pressure. A Kuglen can be used to push the iris aside and gently place one side of the IOL behind the pupil at a time.

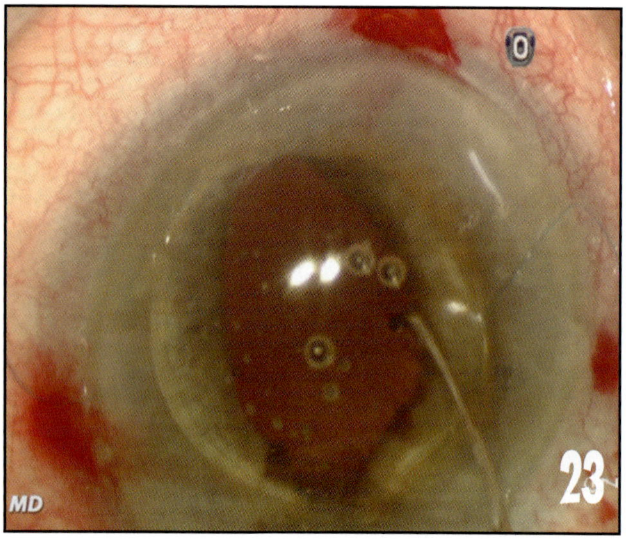

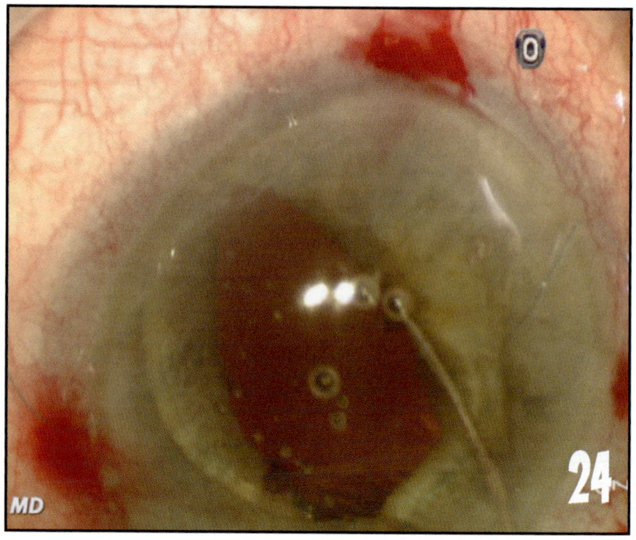

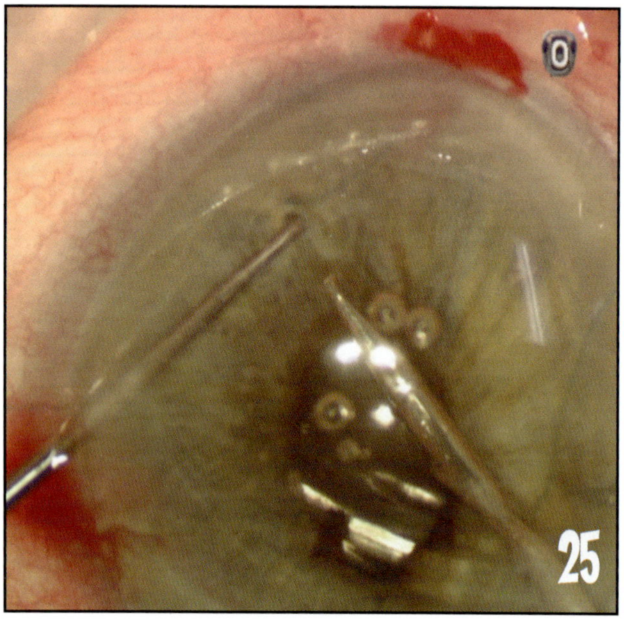

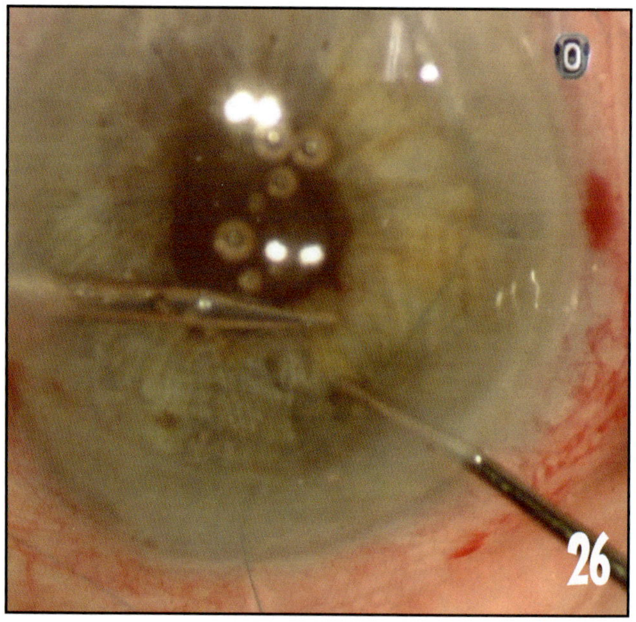

Round out the pupil by drawing iris through the knot, gently pulling centrally with a micrograsper. Sometimes, it will require countertraction against the knot with a Sinskey hook.

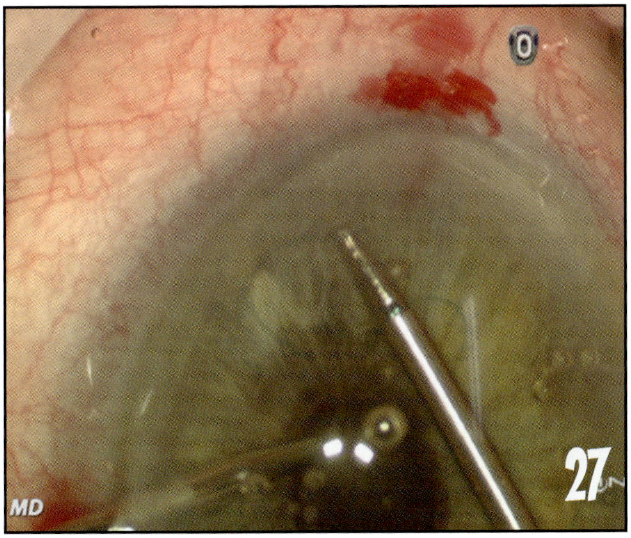

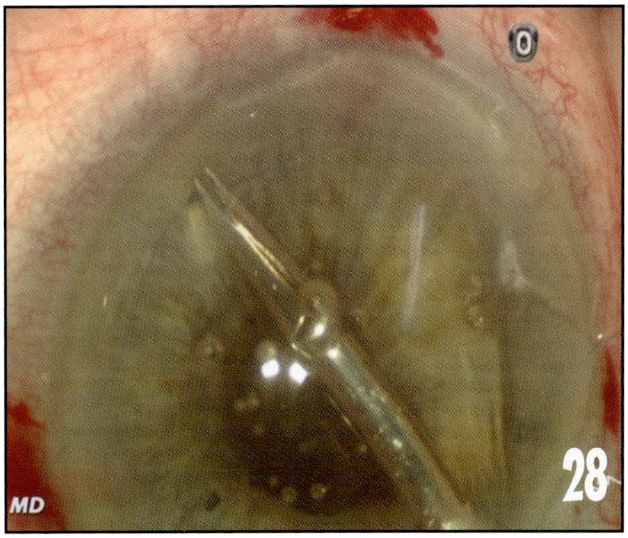

Finish tying the suture (one reverse single throw followed by a forward single throw). Lock the knots and cut them short with microforceps and microscissors once the pupil is round. Evacuate viscoelastic manually with a blunt cannula. Intraocular pressure reduction with medication or Diamox (acetazolamide) for 2 to 3 days may be required.

CHAPTER 20

HOW TO PERFORM INTRASCLERAL HAPTIC FIXATION OF A THREE-PIECE IOL

INTRODUCTION

Described initially by Scharioth and later modified by Agarwal, intrascleral haptic fixation (ISHF) of an intraocular lens (IOL) is also called the *glued-IOL technique*. We prefer the term ISHF because the IOL itself is not glued. Rather, fibrin glue is used to close scleral flaps. This technique can be used to scleral fixate a 3-piece IOL without the need for scleral suture passes. Many techniques have been described, including ones that do not create scleral flaps. We recommend creating scleral flaps to reduce the risk of conjunctival erosion.

KEY POINTS

- Beware of long eyes: The increased width of larger eyes may preclude adequate haptic fixation.
- Inadequate haptic length means that the externalized haptic is not long enough to tuck into a scleral tunnel and may risk future dislocation of the IOL.
- Measure from scleral spur as this is the most consistent landmark. Long eyes have a more posteriorly placed ciliary body, and short eyes have a more anteriorly placed ciliary body. Measuring from the limbus increases the risk of placing the haptics too close to the ciliary body, causing vitreous hemorrhage or tissue chafing.
- Fibrin glue is used for scleral flap closure but does not hold the haptic in place. The intrascleral tunneling of the haptic is what holds the IOL into position. If fibrin glue is unavailable, the scleral flaps can be sutured.

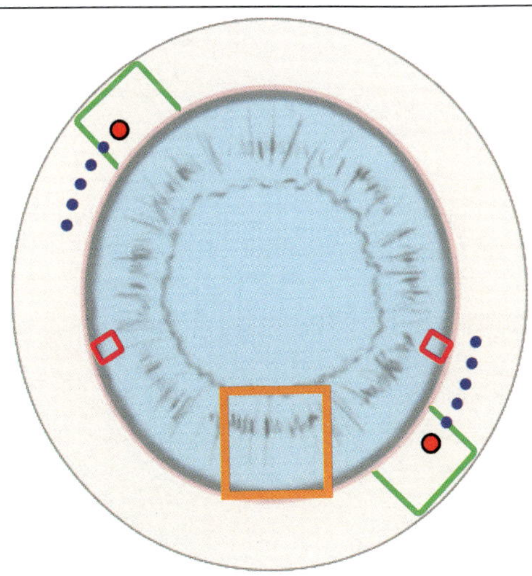

- Knife and fork
- 3.2-mm main
- 23-g sclerotomies
- 30-g scleral tunnels 180 degrees apart beneath L-shaped conjunctival peritomies

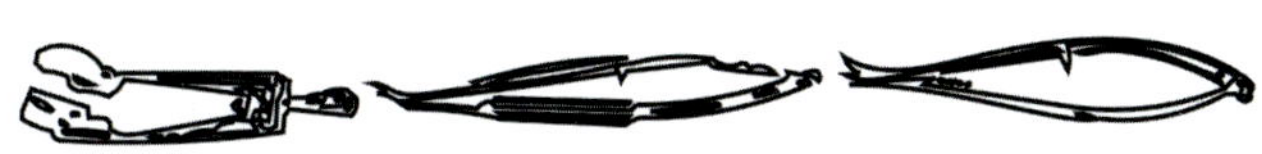

- Two Microsurgical Technology, Inc microtyers
- Anterior chamber maintainer or pars plana infusion
- 30-g needles (2x)
- 23-g trocar (microvitreoretinal [MVR] blade)
- Fibrin glue (TISSEEL, Baxter International Inc)

Ahmed IK, Campos-Möller X, Shah M, Sheybani A. *Illustrated Advanced Anterior Segment Surgery: A Step-by-Step Guide for Challenging Cases* (pp 141-150).

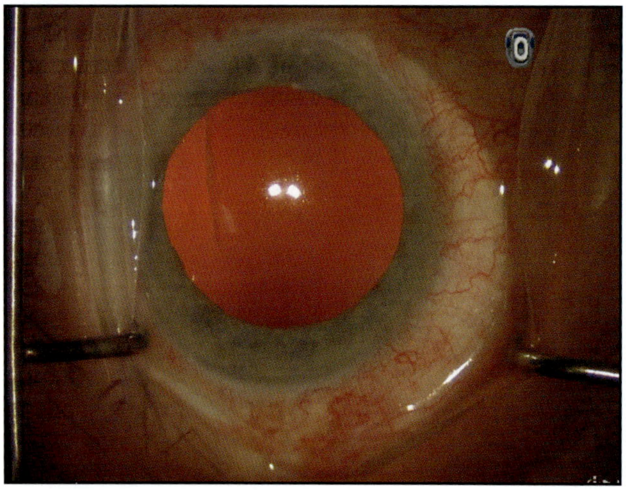

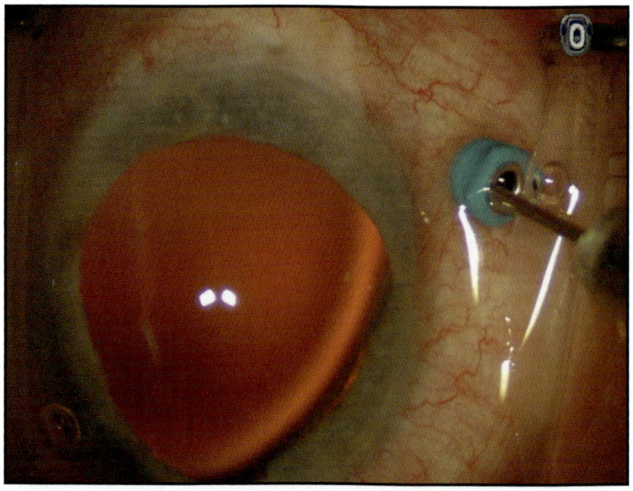

In this case, we are implanting a 3-piece acrylic IOL with ISHF to correct aphakia secondary to trauma. The patient had vitrectomy and lensectomy prior to this surgery. A pars plana infusion port or anterior chamber maintainer is crucial for this technique, and it should be placed before paracentesis incisions are made. L-shaped conjunctival peritomies are made 180 degrees apart from each other. For a right-handed surgeon, aligning the proximal peritomy just to the right of the main temporal clear corneal wound can make the handshake maneuver easier (incision template).

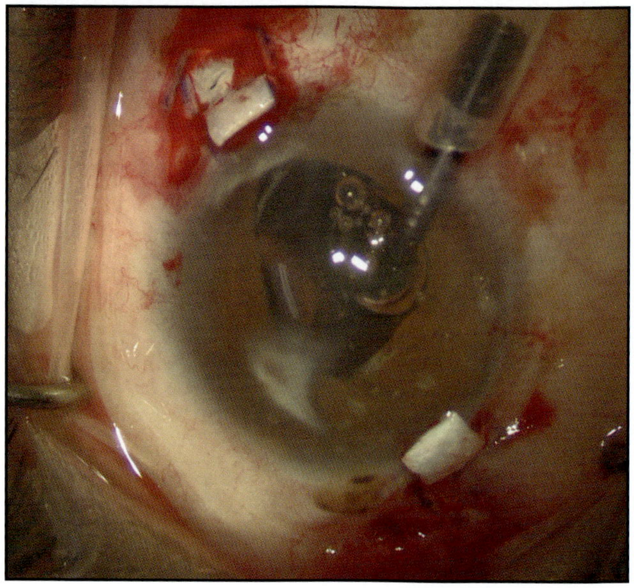

An alternative to the pars plana vitrectomy infusion is an anterior chamber maintainer.

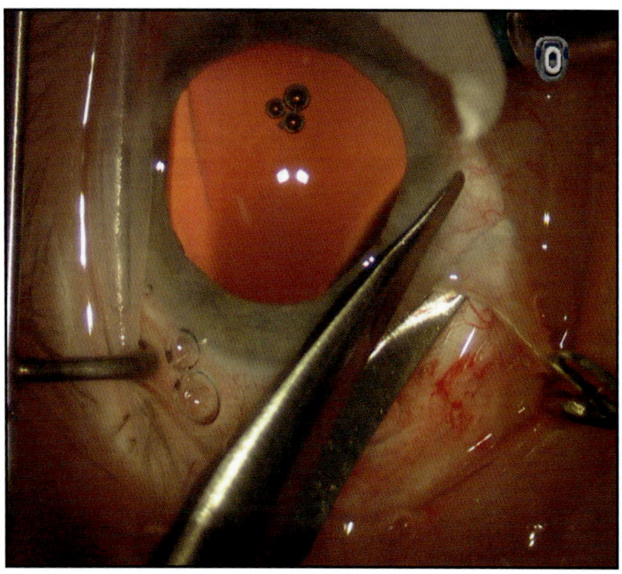

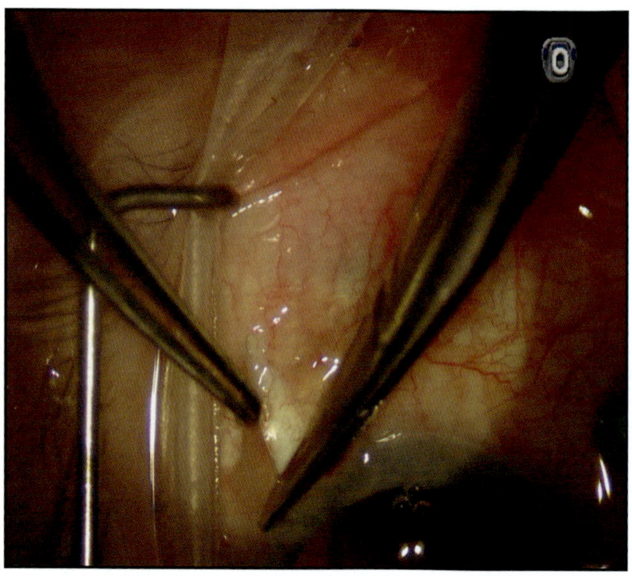

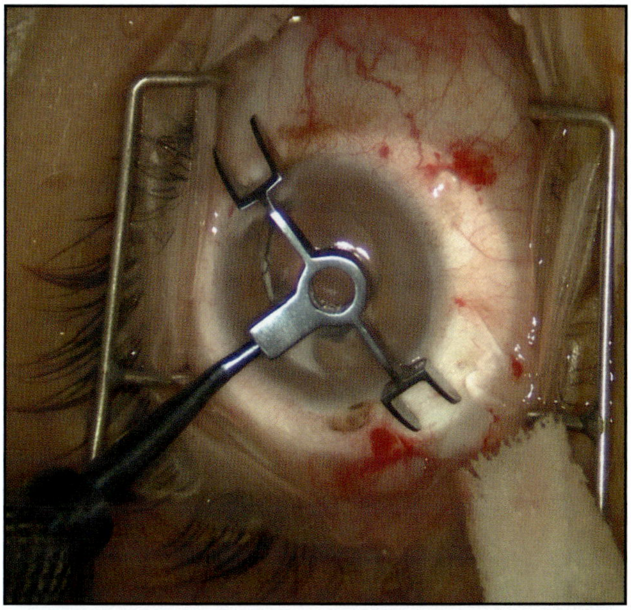

Limbal-based, square scleral flaps measuring approximately 2.5 mm are made 180 degrees apart from each other. They should be about 50% scleral depth. The outline can be traced with a 1-mm blade, and the flap can then be generated with a crescent blade. A specially designed marker can be useful to ensure that the flaps are positioned exactly 180 degrees apart from each other.

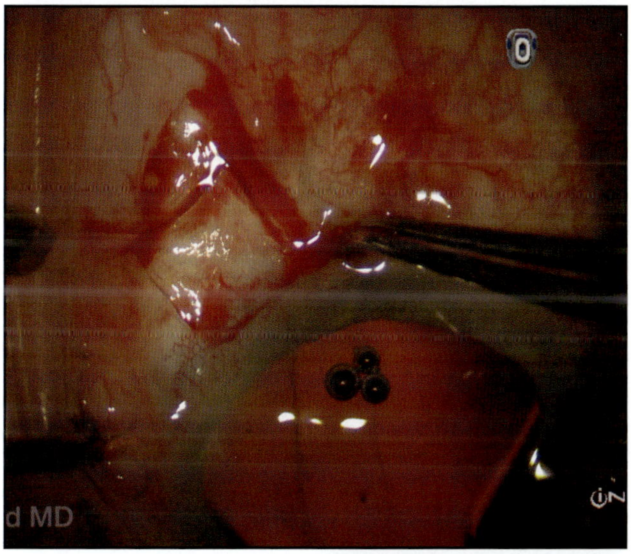

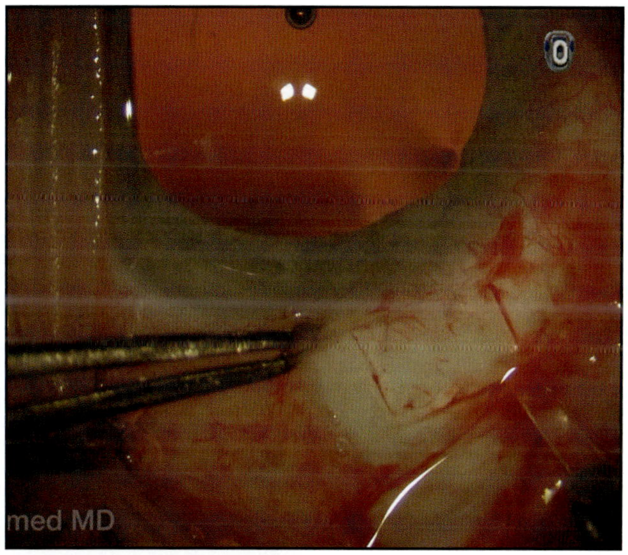

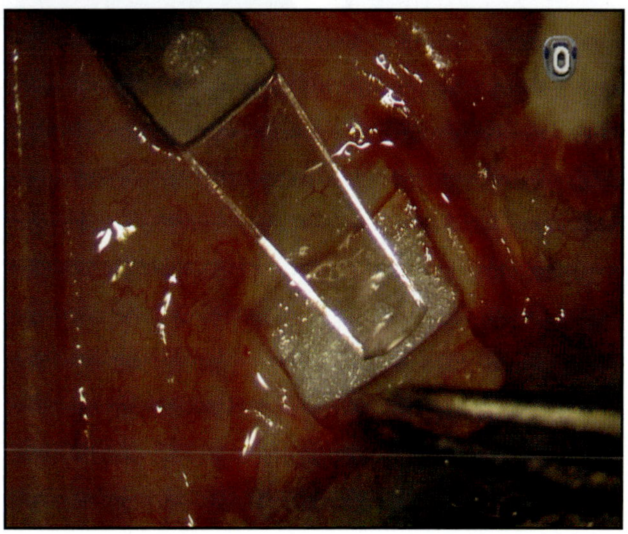

A 20-g MVR blade is used to make sclerotomies for haptic externalization. They are 0.5 to 1 mm posterior to the scleral spur (where the blue limbal fibers meet the white scleral fibers). Instead of incising the sclerotomies at the center of the scleral beds, they should be shifted toward the site of haptic tunnel entry (incision template). This ensures that the externalized haptic travels through a longer scleral tunnel (illustration). A limited anterior vitrectomy should be performed to remove anterior vitreous and reduce risk of vitreous incarceration at the sclerotomies.

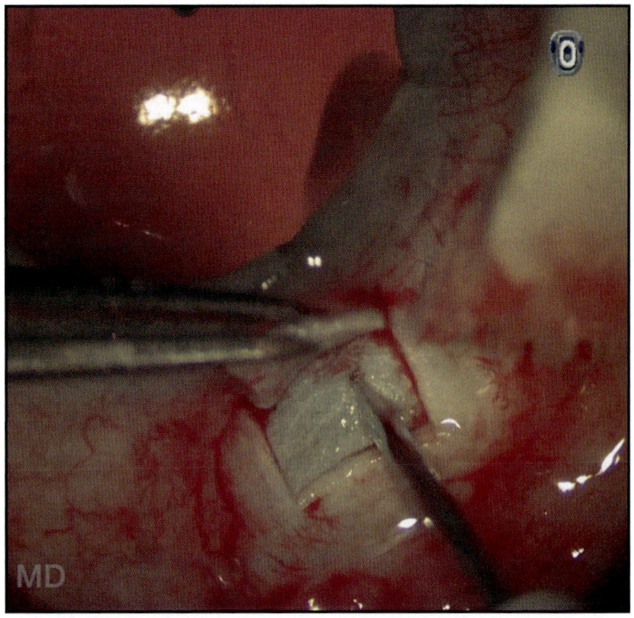

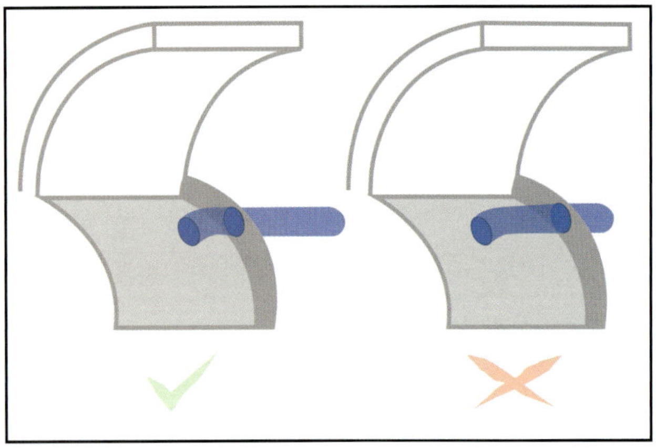

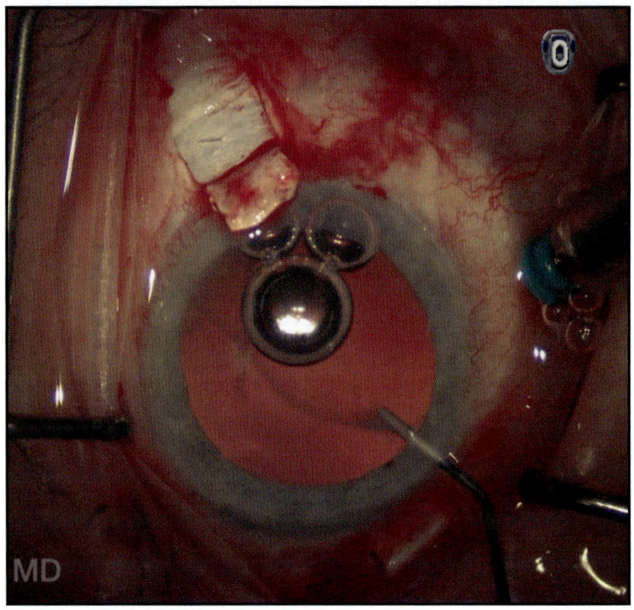

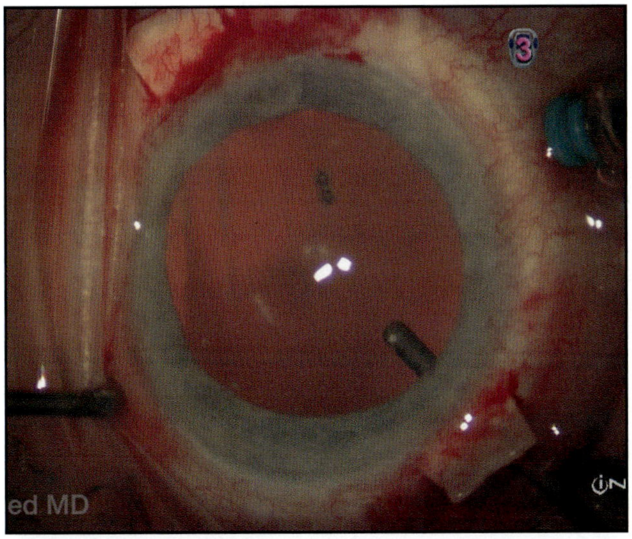

A 26-g hypodermic needle is used to create a tunnel for haptic insertion. This starts at the same distance from the limbus as the sclerotomy and is tunneled parallel to the limbus for approximately 1 mm. This step is repeated for the opposite scleral flap. Using ink to "paint" the needle can mark the trajectory of the tunnel and can facilitate identification later on in the case. A 3.2-mm clear corneal incision is then created to allow for IOL cartridge insertion. Next, a 3-piece IOL is folded into a cartridge.

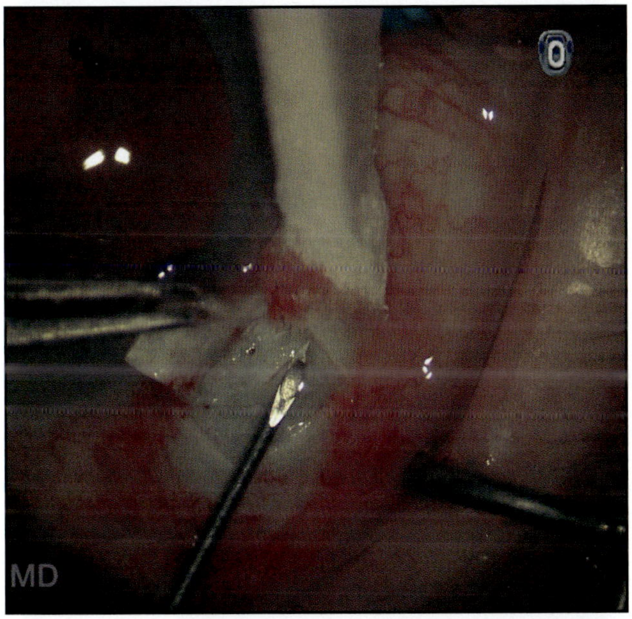

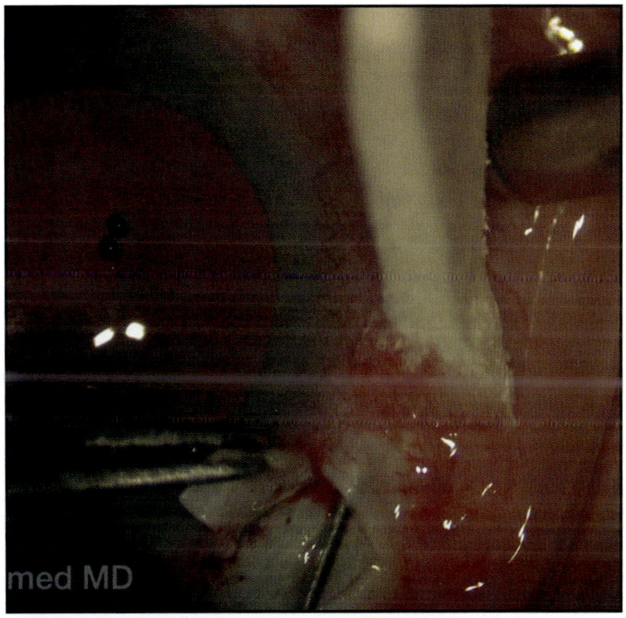

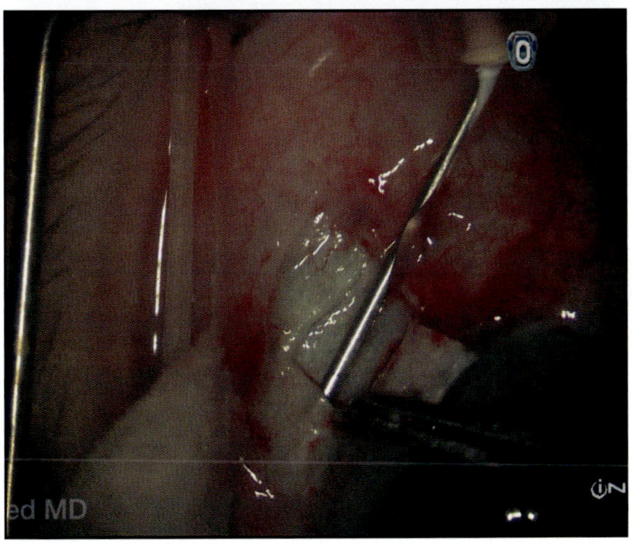

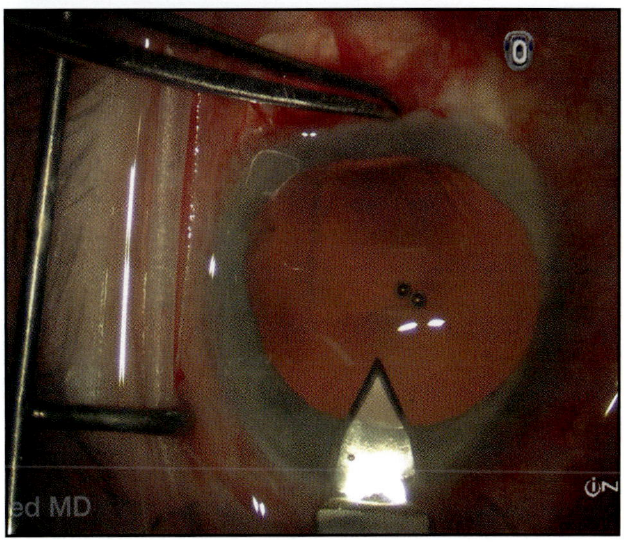

The cartridge is fully inserted in the anterior chamber. The aid of an assistant to turn the screw on the injector is valuable here. The surgeon should maintain control of the injector itself, and be prepared to grasp the leading haptic with a micrograsper in the left hand.

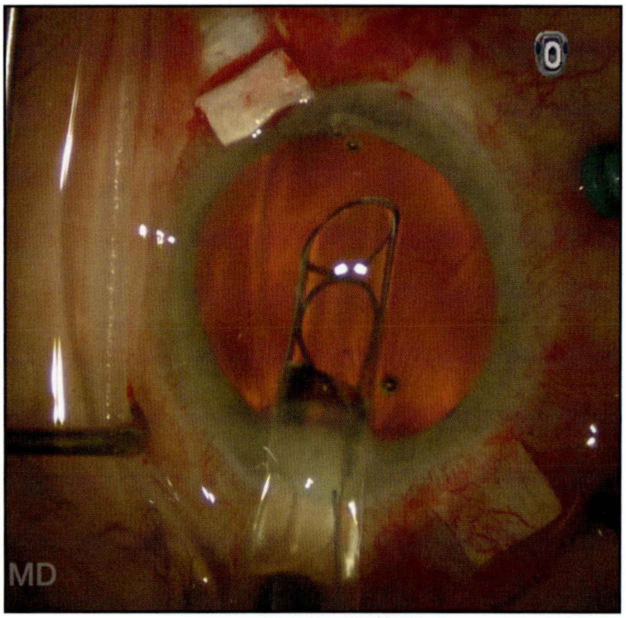

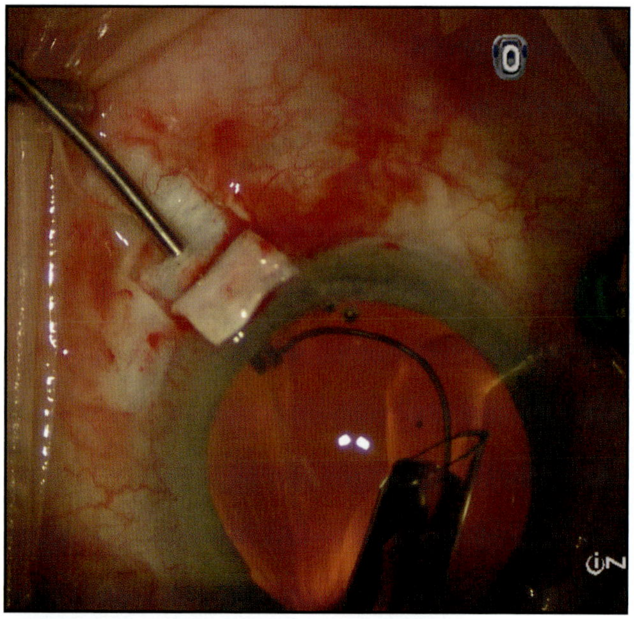

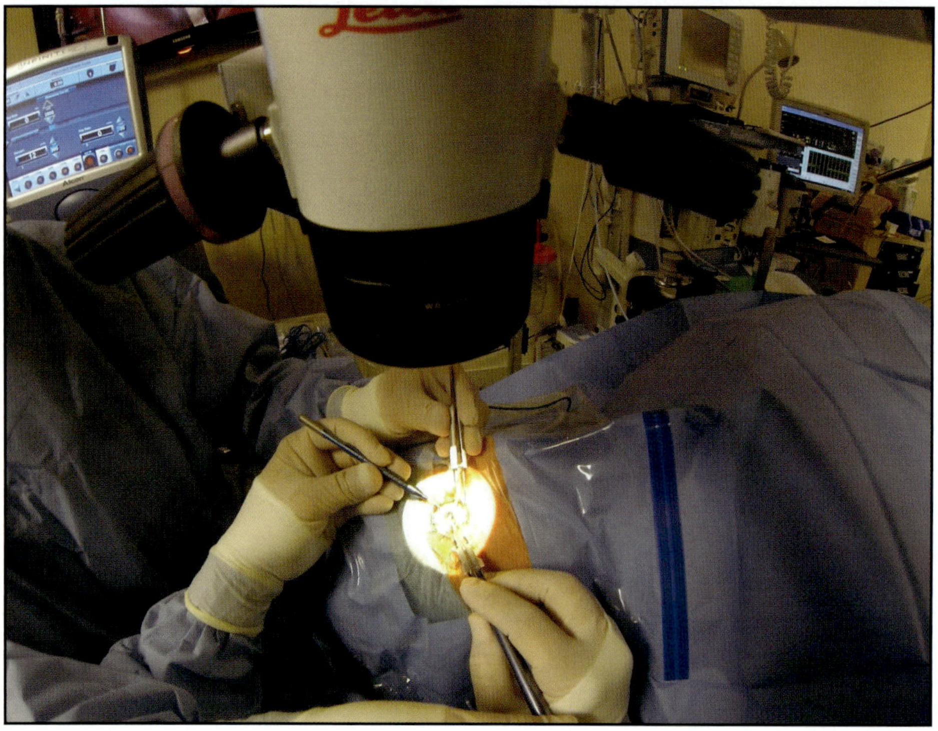

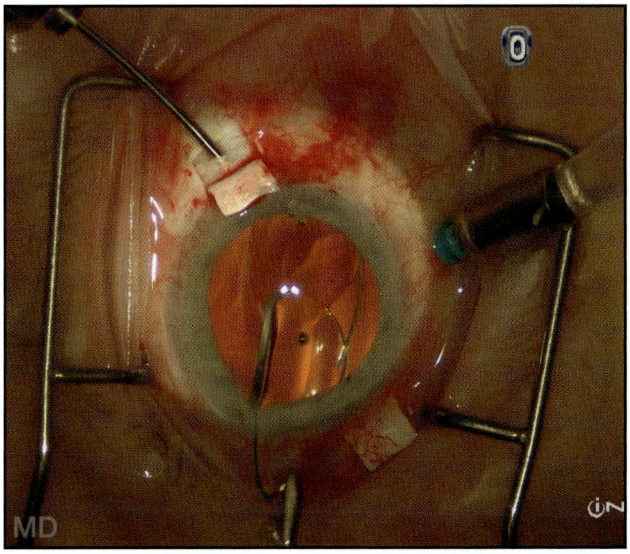

The trailing haptic should remain outside the main incision. Holding it with a tyer will prevent accidentally pulling it into the eye when externalizing the opposite haptic.

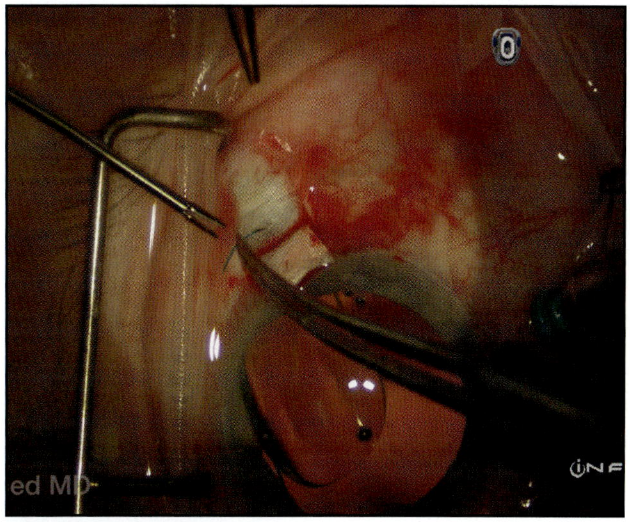

Avoid using microinstruments outside the eye as they are fragile. We suggest switching to a regular tyer to position and hold the haptic outside of the eye.

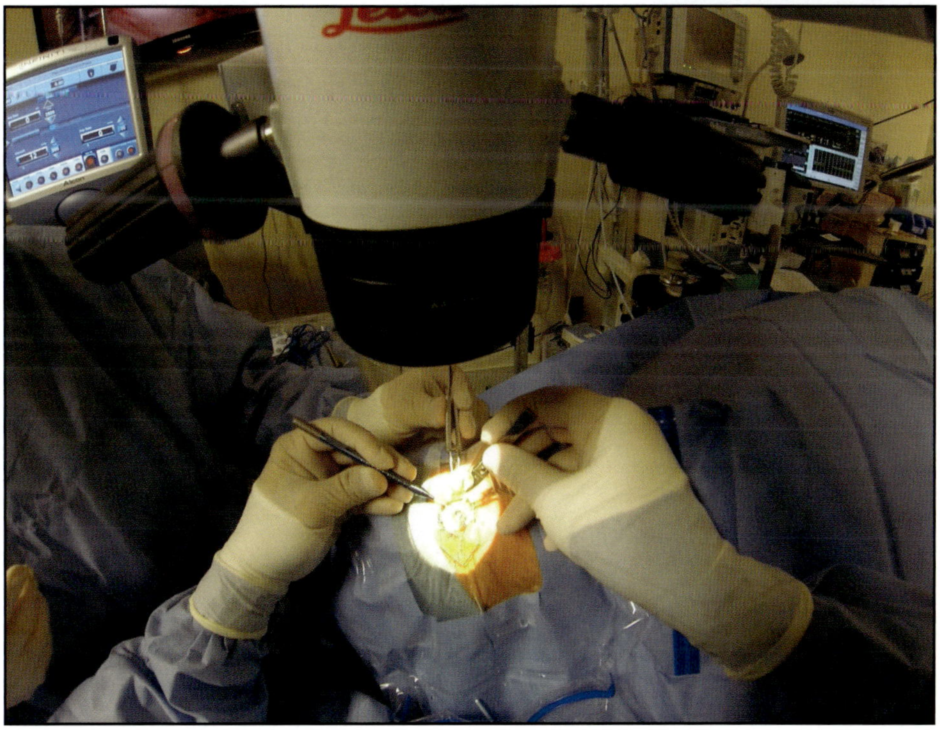

An assistant holds the leading haptic that has been externalized, as the next maneuvers can accidentally draw the haptic back into the eye. If no assistant is available, the sleeve of an iris hook can be used to keep the externalized haptic from retracting back into the eye.

A microtyer is used to insert the trailing haptic into the anterior chamber, grasping in such a way that the distal third remains free. Another microtyer, placed through the sclerotomy, is used to grab the tip of the haptic and externalize it through the proximal sclerotomy.

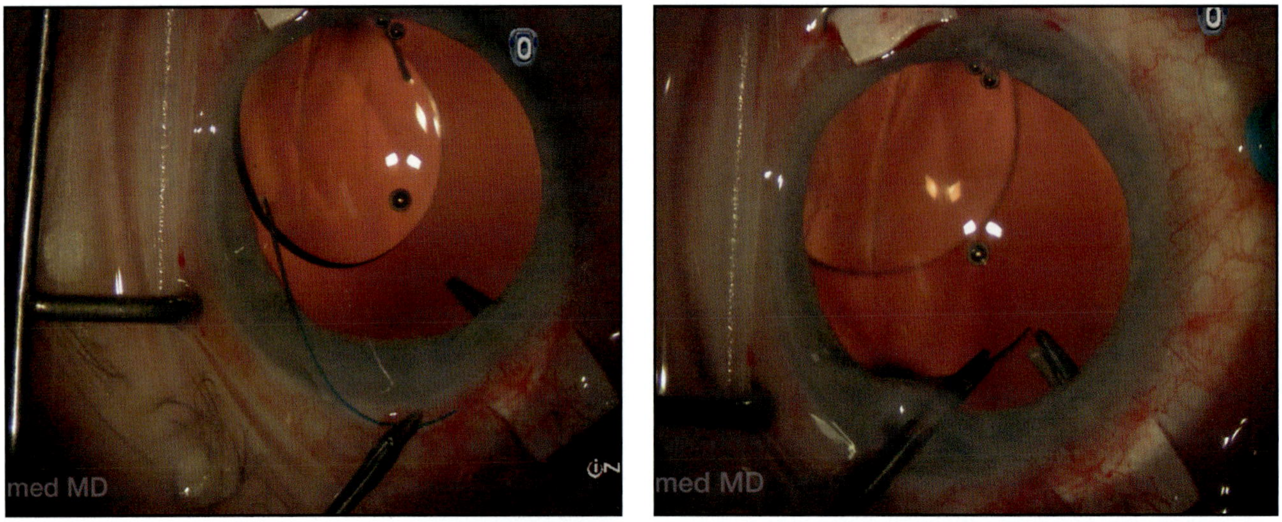

Assistant holding leading (nasal) haptic while the surgeon performs the "handshake" maneuver with the proximal (temporal) haptic.

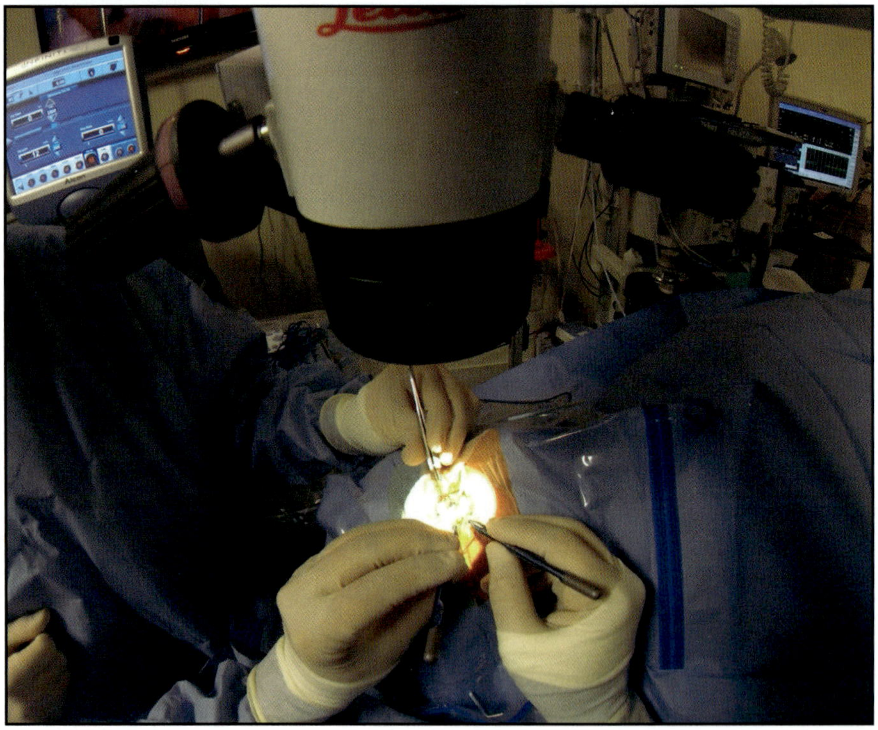

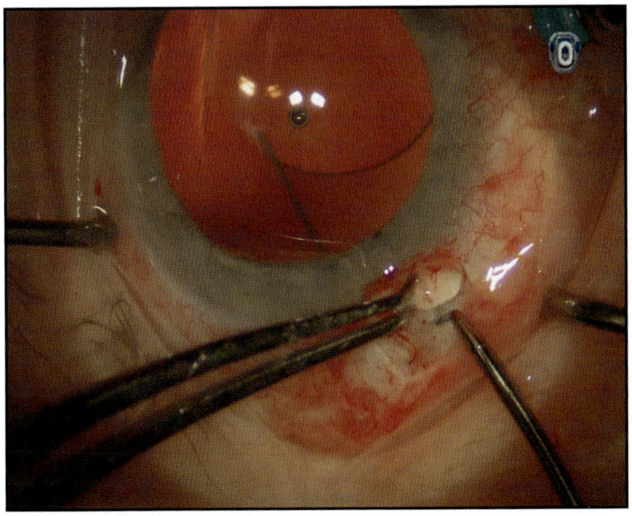

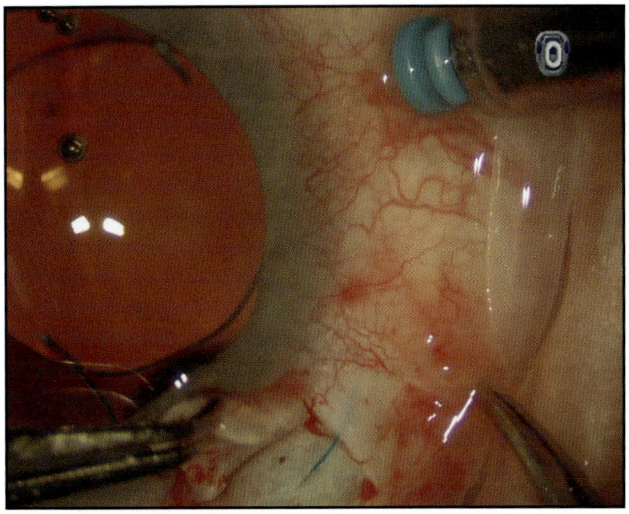

Both haptics are then placed into the pre-tunneled scleral passes made with the 26-g needle. The haptic positioning into the tunnel is adjusted at both ends in order to center the IOL. Suturing of the main wound is advisable to prevent anterior chamber shallowing and vitreous prolapse. The scleral flaps are then placed back and can be sealed down with fibrin glue, and the conjunctiva is sutured or glued closed.

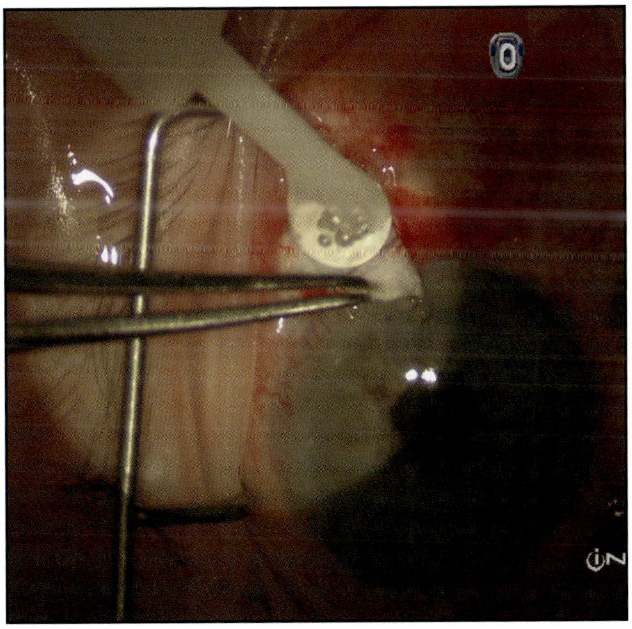

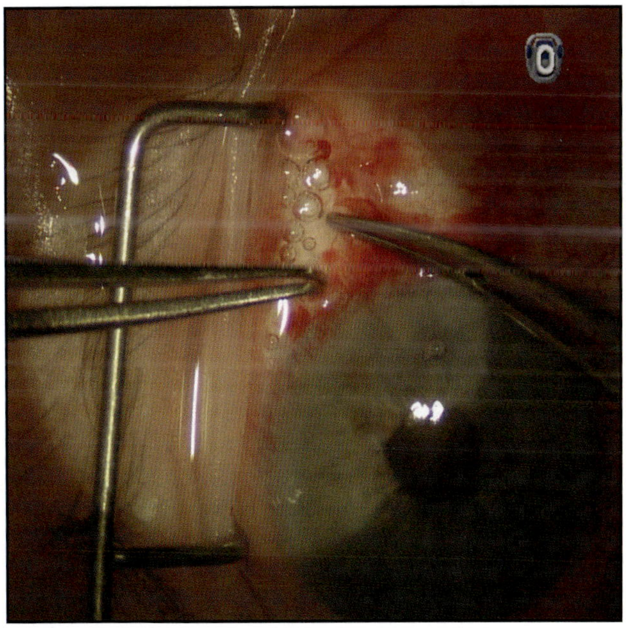

Our fibrin glue of choice comes as 2 separate reagents that mix into the common cannula. The area must be thoroughly dried prior to application. Only a small amount of glue is needed. Slow injection will result in a slightly thicker mixture, which is preferable as it is less likely to flow to other parts of the ocular surface. Place the scleral flap directly on top of the glue and hold in place for 5 to 10 seconds. Follow prepackaged instructions as sealing times can differ. Do not pull on excess glue; instead, cut this using Westcott scissors (Acme United Corp).

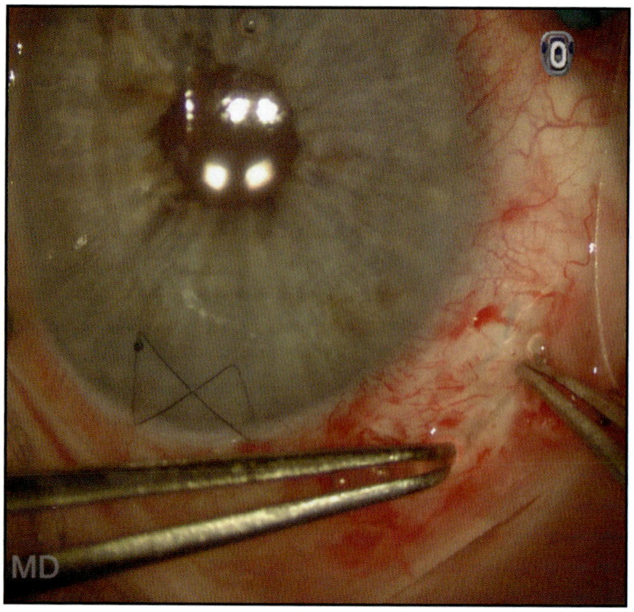

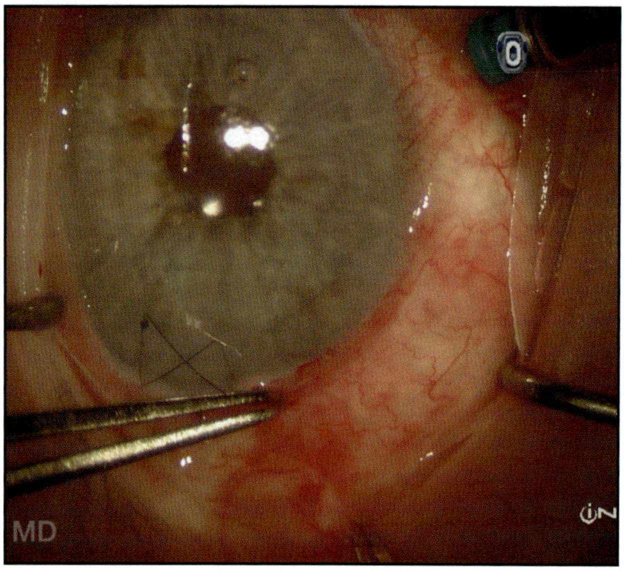

CHAPTER 21

HOW TO FIXATE AN IOL TO SCLERA WITH THE YAMANE DOUBLE-NEEDLE FLANGED HAPTIC TECHNIQUE

INTRODUCTION

The Yamane technique is a modification of the intrascleral haptic fixation technique described in Chapter 20. It allows for stable scleral fixation without the need to dissect conjunctiva or create scleral flaps.

KEY POINTS

- Corneal incision configuration should be optimized to allow for easy access to the leading and trailing haptics.
- Marks for sclerotomies must be 180 degrees apart to minimize IOL tilt.
- Consider the use of an anterior chamber maintainer or posterior infusion.
- As with any scleral fixation technique, ensure that needle entries into the sclera are perpendicular to the scleral surface to avoid inadvertent contact with the ciliary body or posterior iris. In this technique, this can be achieved by lifting the heel of the bent needle.
- While any 3-piece IOL will work, certain haptic materials like polyvinylidene fluoride seem to be more resilient to the manipulation required in this technique.

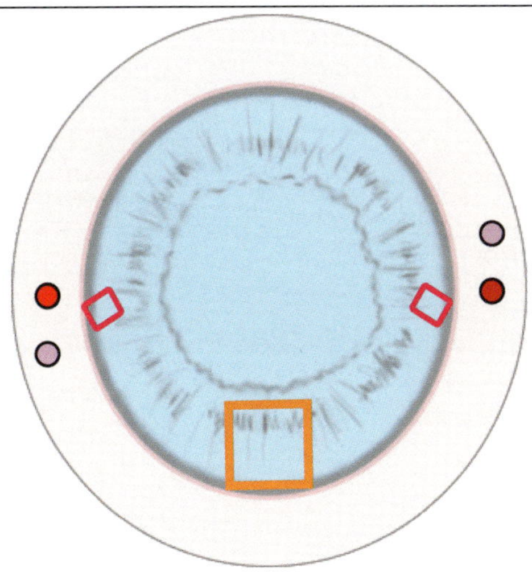

- Main incision (2.75 to 3.2 mm)
- Knife and fork paracentesis
- Tunneled transconjunctival sclerotomies

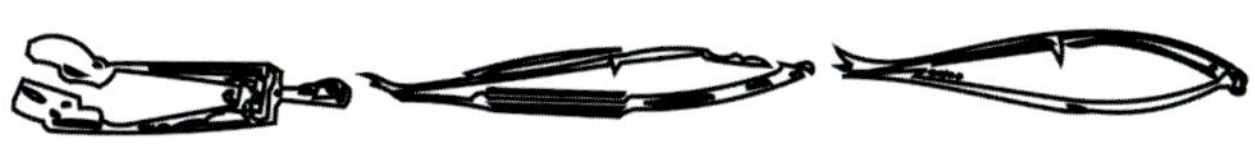

- Microforceps or microtyers
- Two 27-g or thin-walled 30-g hypodermic needles
- Low-temp, handheld cautery

Ahmed IK, Campos-Möller X, Shah M, Sheybani A. *Illustrated Advanced Anterior Segment Surgery: A Step-by-Step Guide for Challenging Cases* (pp 151-162).

Preliminary steps (not shown in images):

- Ensure thorough anterior vitrectomy has been performed to avoid inadvertent traction on the vitreous base.
- Consider placement of anterior or posterior infusion.
- Create 2 paracentesis incisions and a slightly large main clear corneal incision for IOL implantation. Ensure that the main incision is adequately sized to allow for in-the-eye controlled delivery of the IOL.

- Mark the conjunctiva 2 mm posterior to the limbus at 6 and 12 o'clock. If there is an adequate view of the scleral spur without creating a peritomy, use this landmark and mark 1 mm posterior to the spur.
- On the surgeon's left side, create another mark 2 mm temporal to the previously placed mark. On the surgeon's right side, create a mark 2 mm nasal to the previously placed mark. These second marks correspond to the conjunctival entry site and will help guide the creation of the intrascleral tunnels. Adequate length and symmetry of these tunnels ensures IOL centration and reduces tilt.

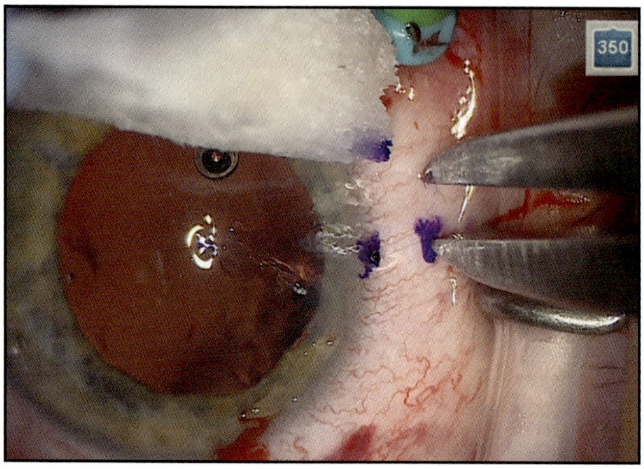

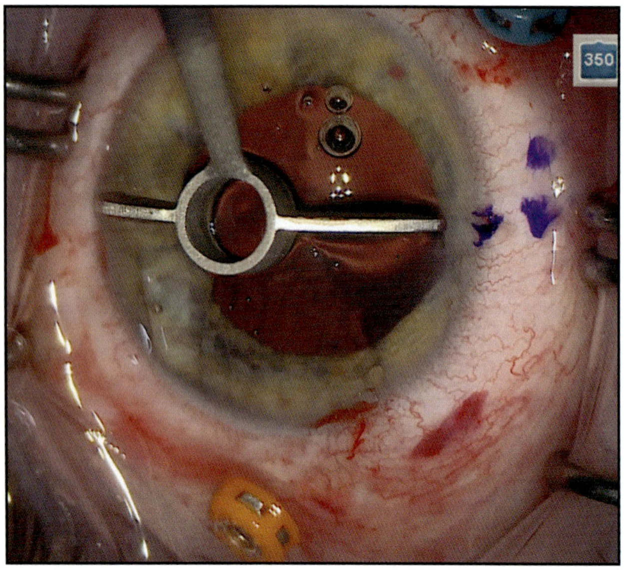

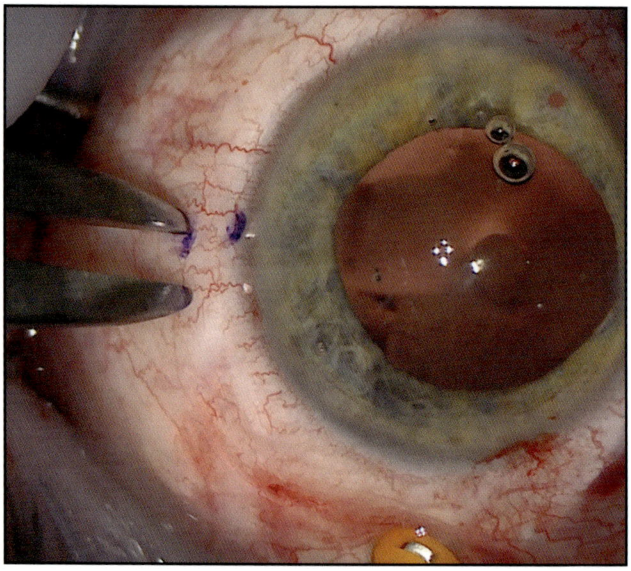

A toric IOL marker can be used to ensure marks are placed 180 degrees apart.

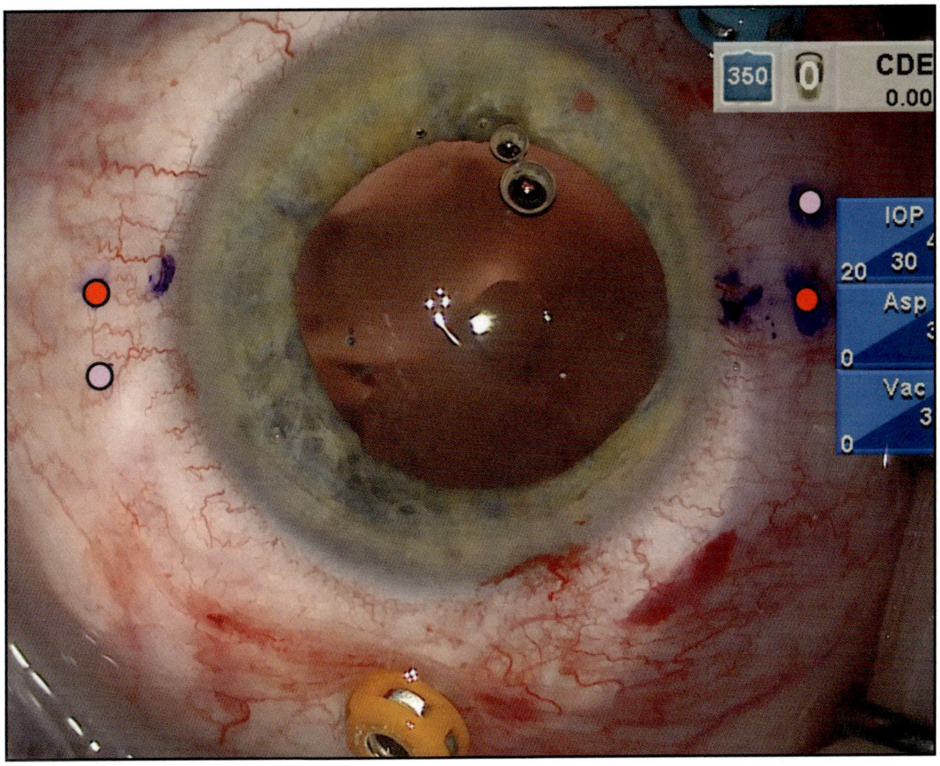

Schematic view of the conjunctival needle entry (pink) and sclerotomy needle entry (red) markings.

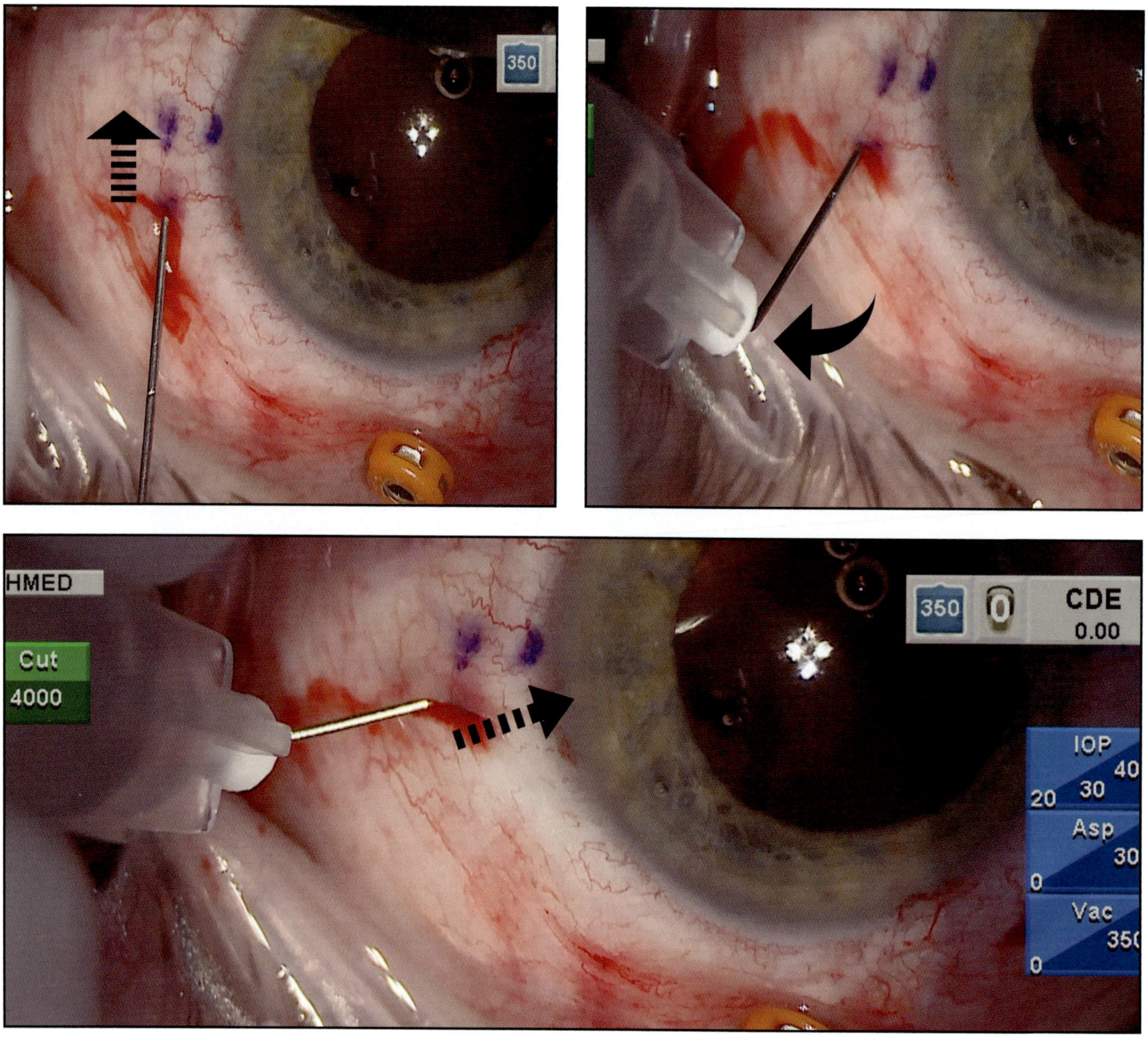

- Using one of the hypodermic needles affixed to a 3-cc, balanced salt solution–filled syringe, create a scleral tunnel by entering the needle through conjunctiva at the mark closest to the surgeon, on the surgeon's left (at the conjunctival entry mark). Advance the needle through sclera for 2 mm until the tip of the needle is at the level of the sclerotomy mark (the one furthest away from the surgeon).
- Once the 2-mm intrascleral tunnel has been created, lift the heel of the bent needle to facilitate a perpendicular entry through sclera into the posterior chamber. Advance the needle until it is visible through the pupil and bring the needle parallel to the iris plane. The syringe can then be gently laid down over the patient's eye and drape, taking care that the needle is not engaging any intraocular structures. The same steps will be repeated for the second needle, 180 degrees apart from the initial sclerotomy.

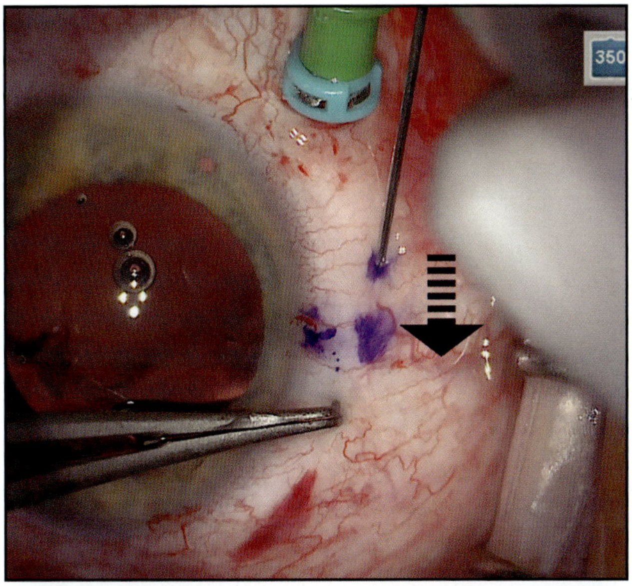

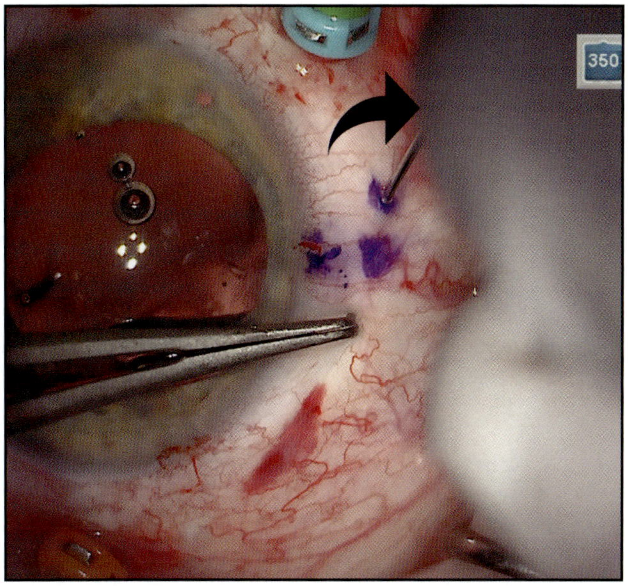

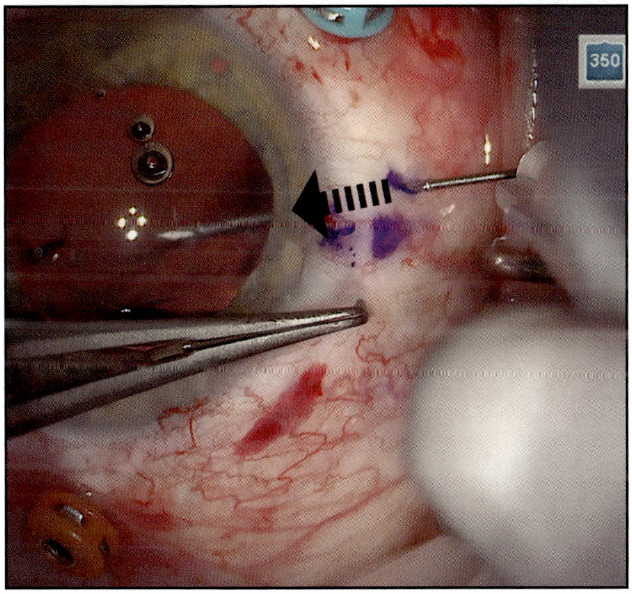

- The Key Point regarding the second needle pass is to create a scleral tunnel by advancing the needle in the opposite direction to the first needle's tunnel (see dotted arrows).
- This will ensure that both haptics will exit at the sclerotomies, which are 180 degrees apart from each other, but the tunnels that will lodge the haptics will be facing away from each other. The needle is advanced until the tip is at the sclerotomy mark (red dot on incisions template) and then the heel of the needle is lifted to enter perpendicular to sclera, aiming toward the posterior pole (in the direction of the optic nerve).

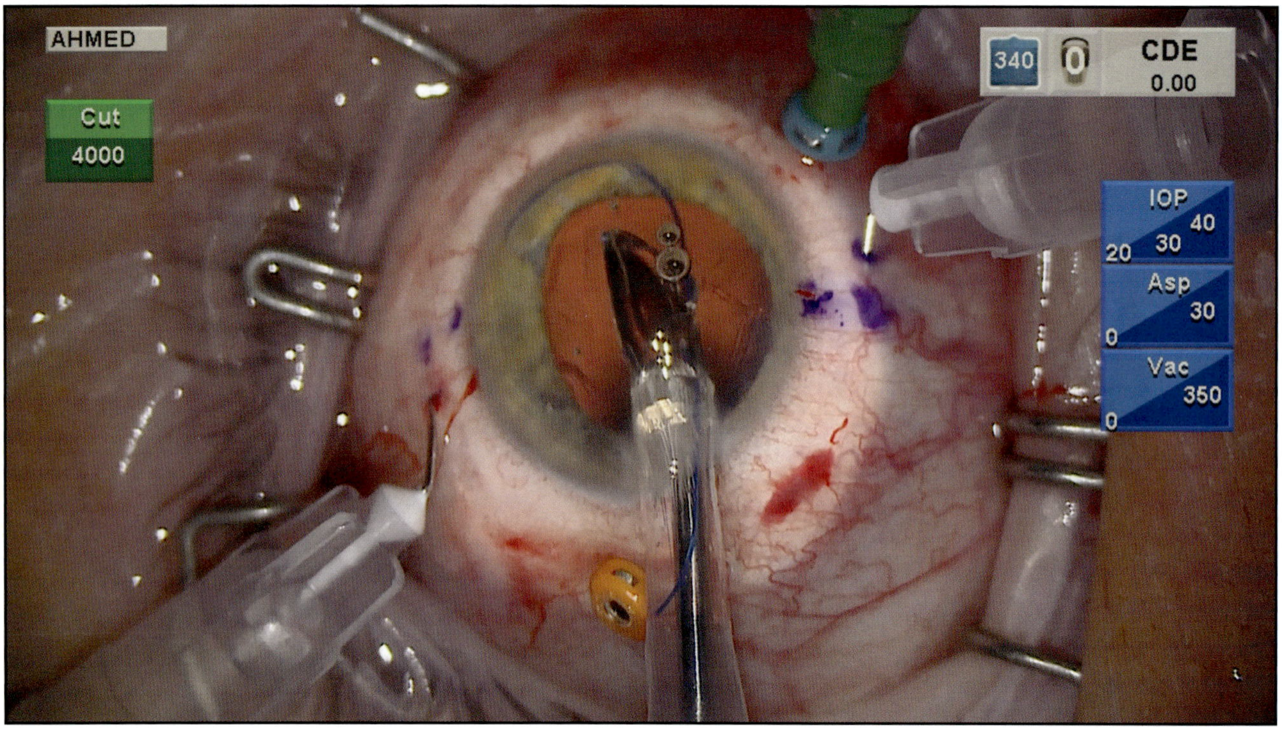

- Notice the placement of syringes over the surgical field, in a configuration where the needles are aiming posteriorly and in opposite directions. With both needles now in place, the IOL can be inserted into the anterior chamber. Place the leading haptic over the iris, allowing the trailing haptic to remain outside the eye through the main incision.

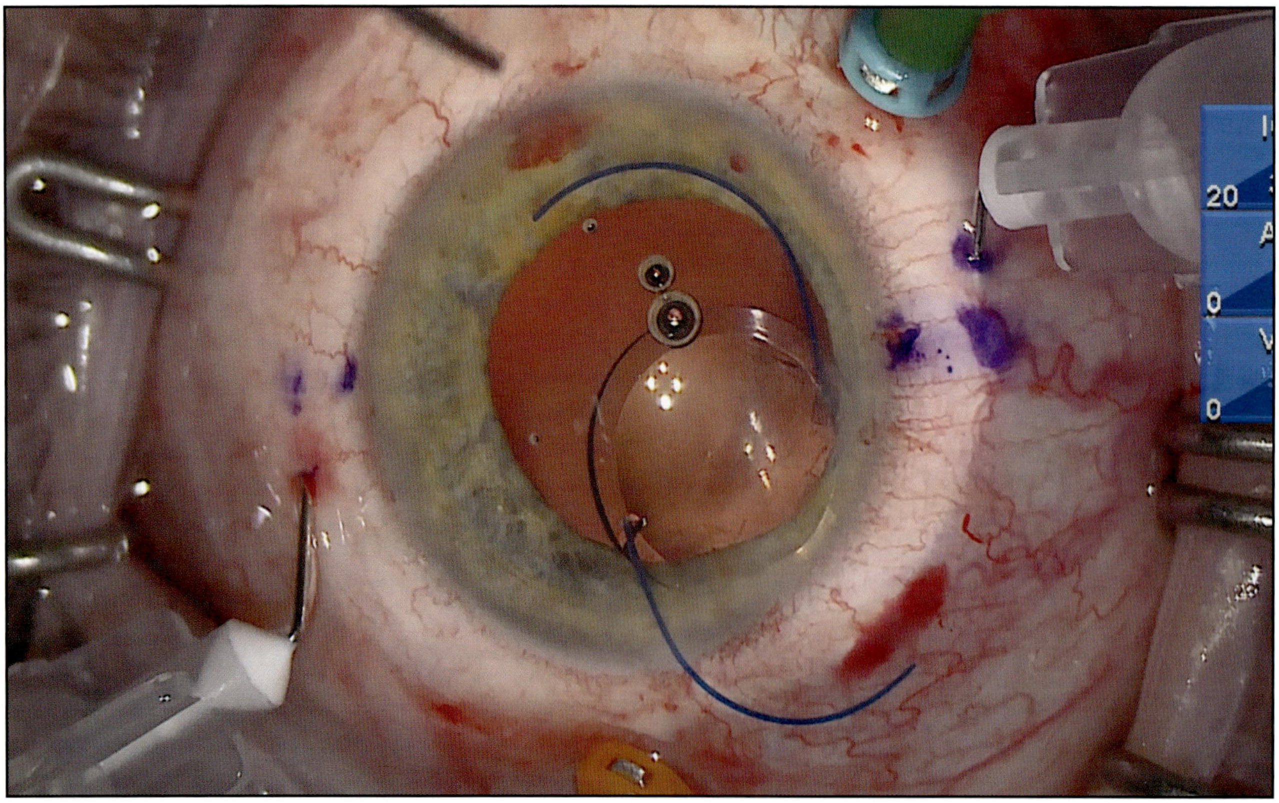

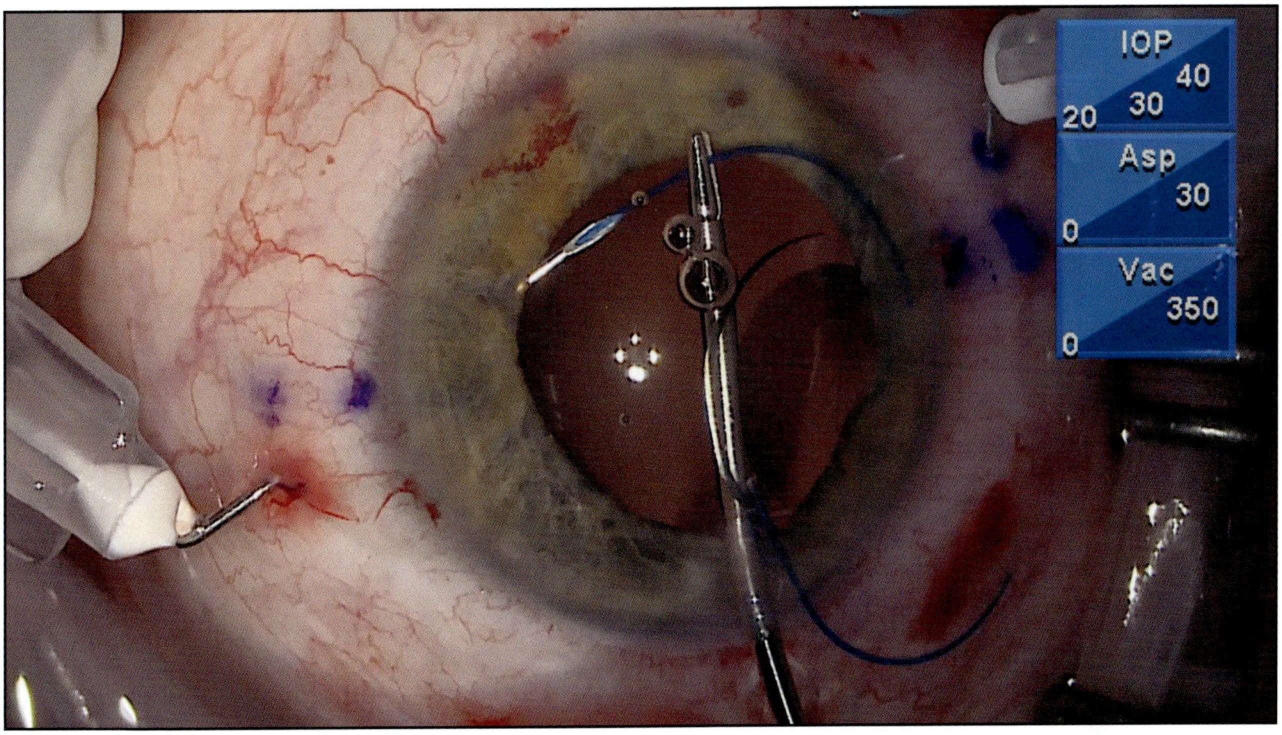

- Use microforceps to grasp the leading haptic and dock it into the lumen of the hypodermic needle on the left. The curve of the haptic will keep the IOL stable and prevent the IOL from dropping.
- Once adequately docked, the syringe can be handed to an assistant, or simply remove the syringe from the hypodermic needle and allow the needle to rest on the ocular surface.

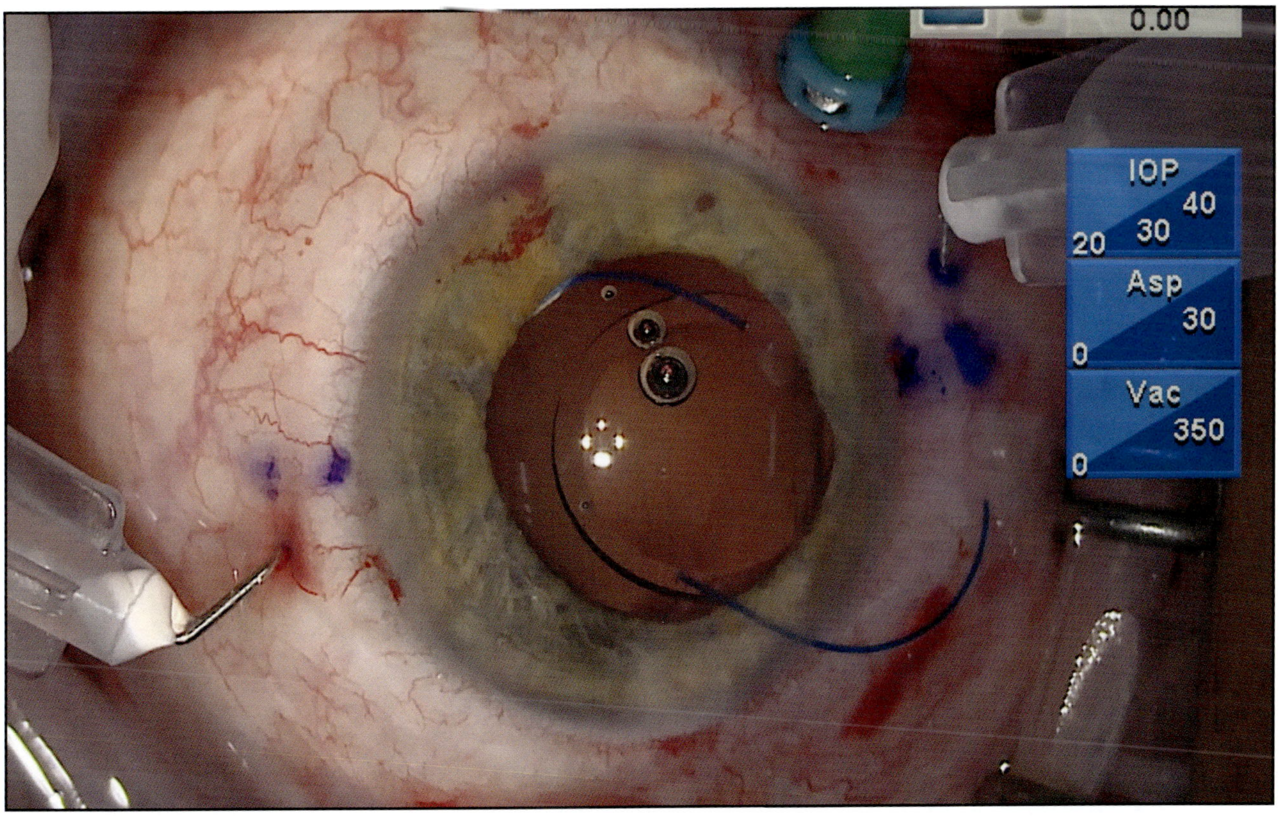

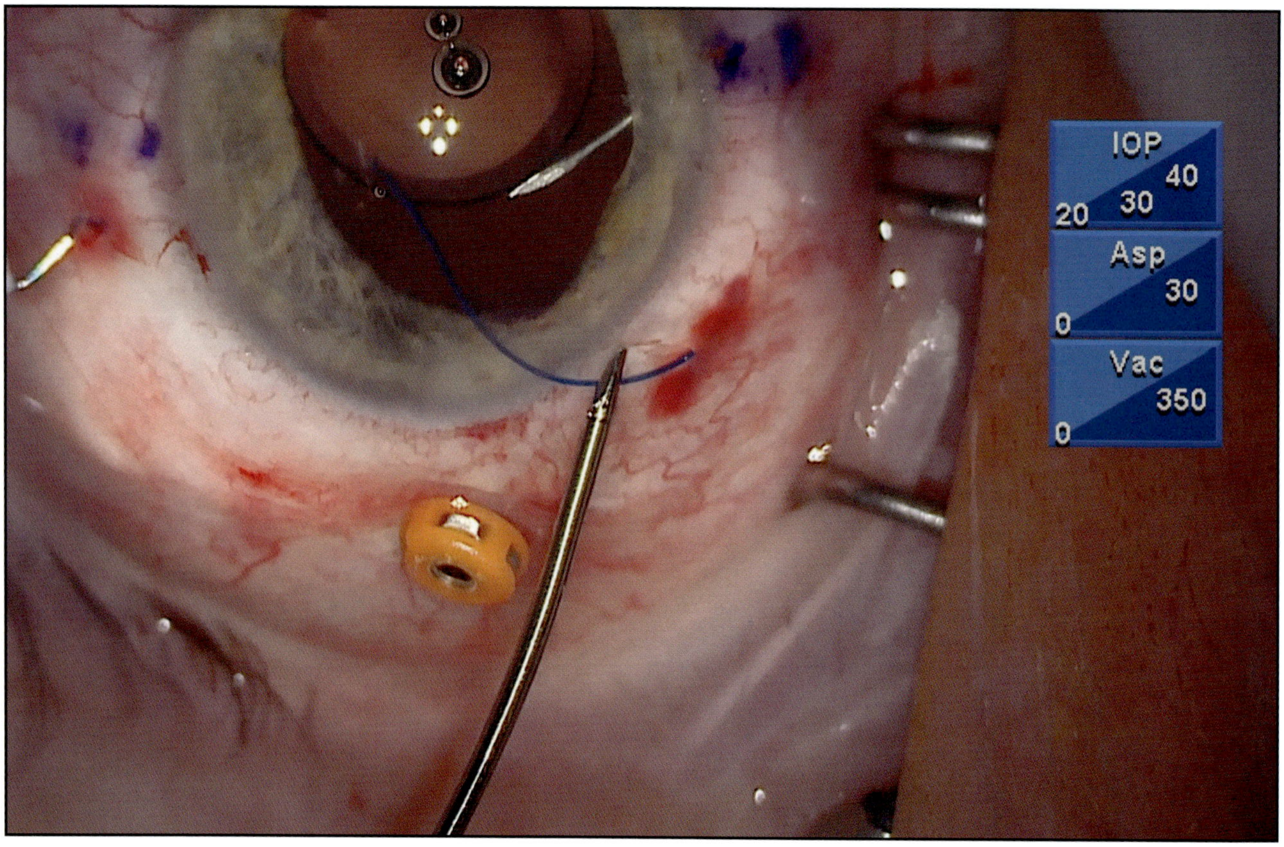

- Docking the trailing haptic can be slightly more challenging. Grasping the haptic outside the eye and utilizing the main incision is an option, as is working slightly more posteriorly. Pay attention to the position of the IOL optic during this maneuver to avoid damaging iris or retina while manipulating the haptic into the needle.

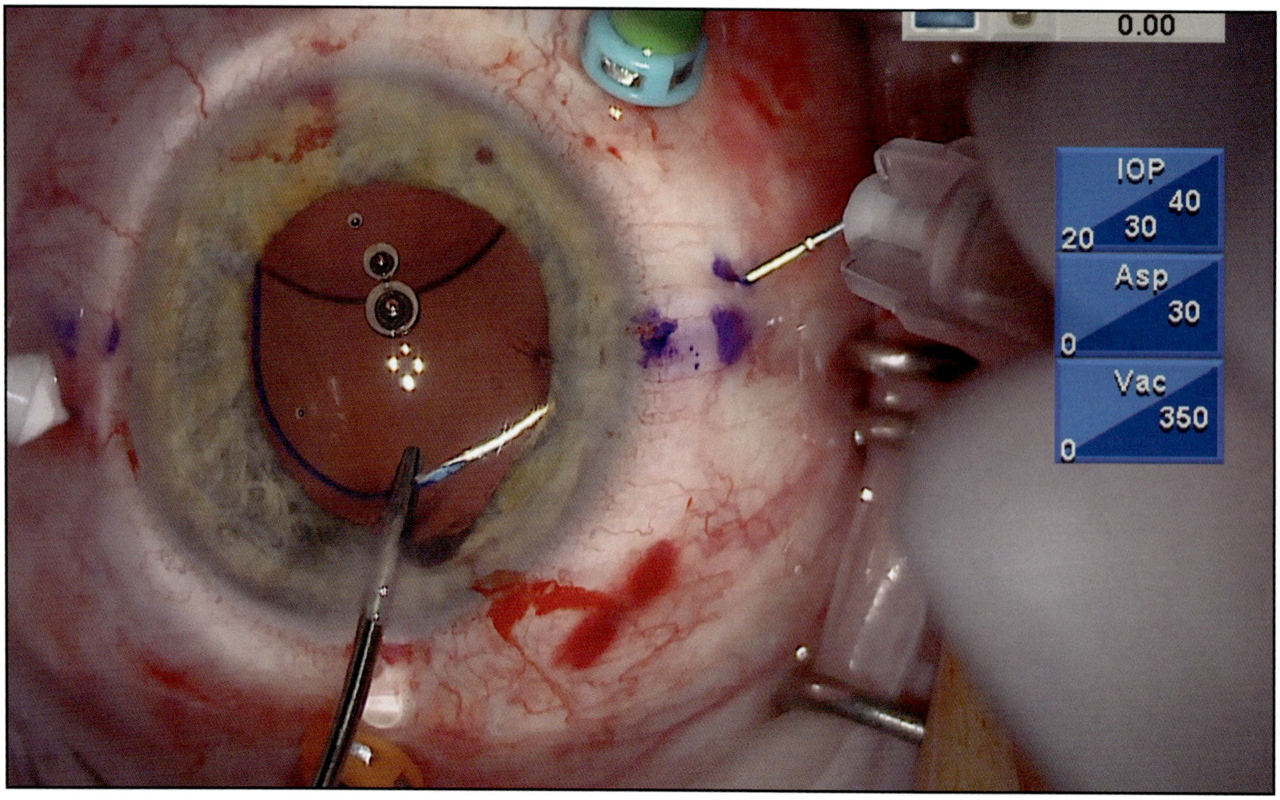

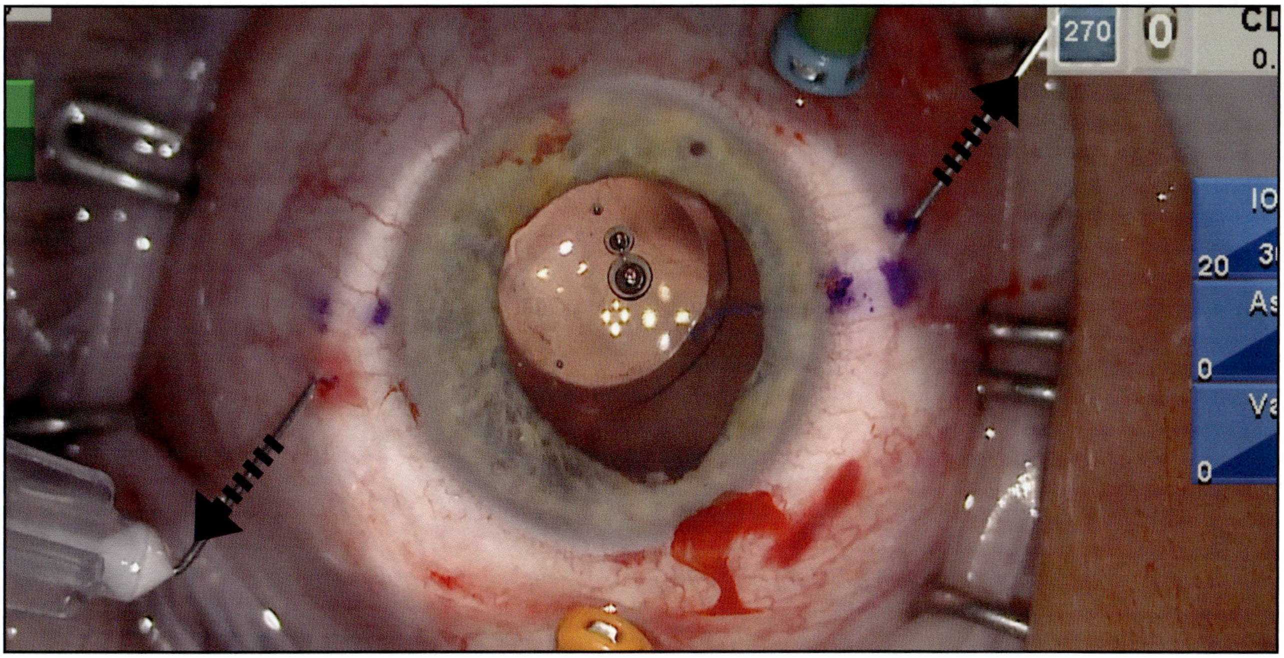

- Once both haptics are adequately docked, the surgeon should grasp the first hypodermic needle again and simultaneously remove both needles from the sclera in a coordinated and simultaneous fashion. The direction of travel should be along the previously fashioned intrascleral tunnels. If performed correctly, the ends of the haptics should now rest on the conjunctival surface.

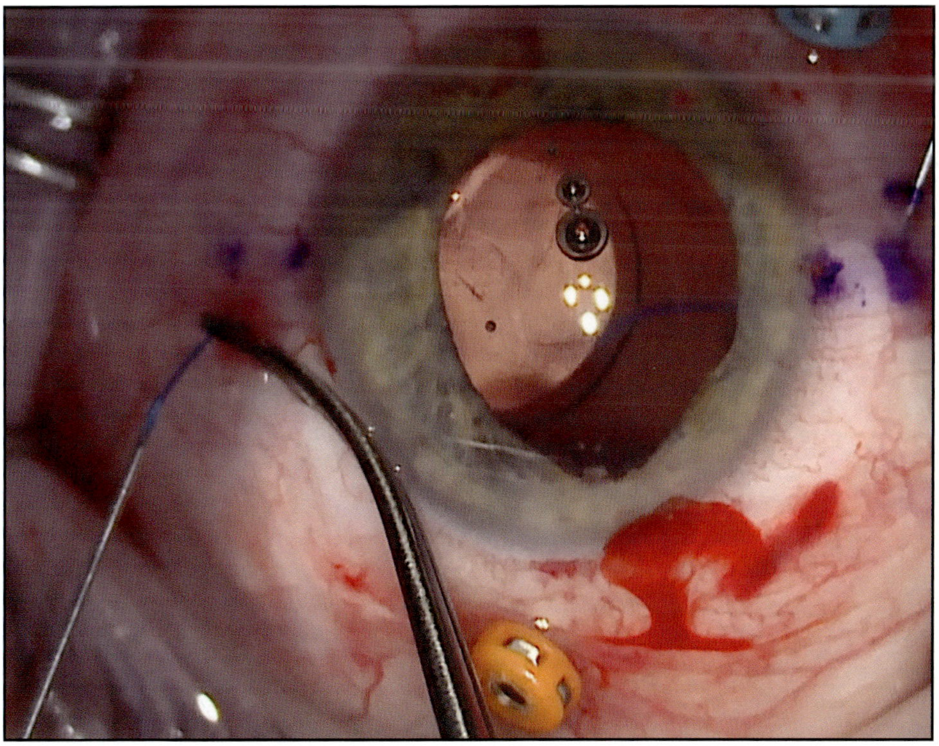

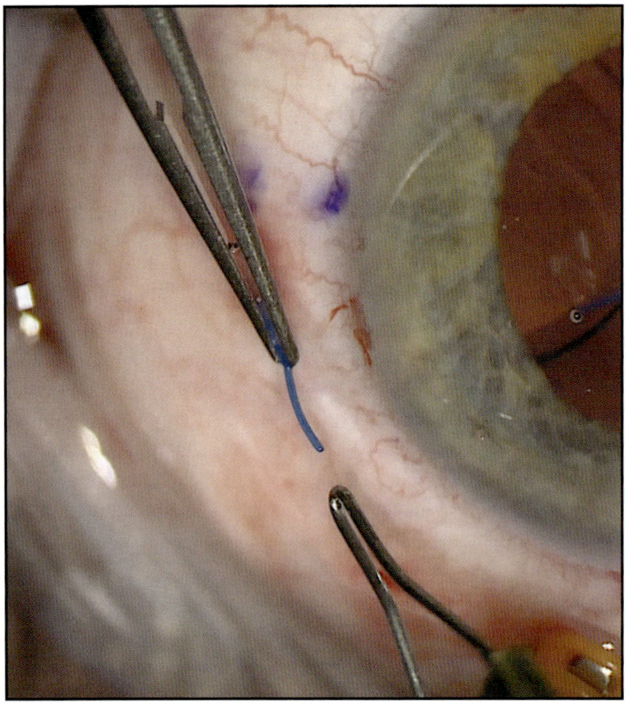

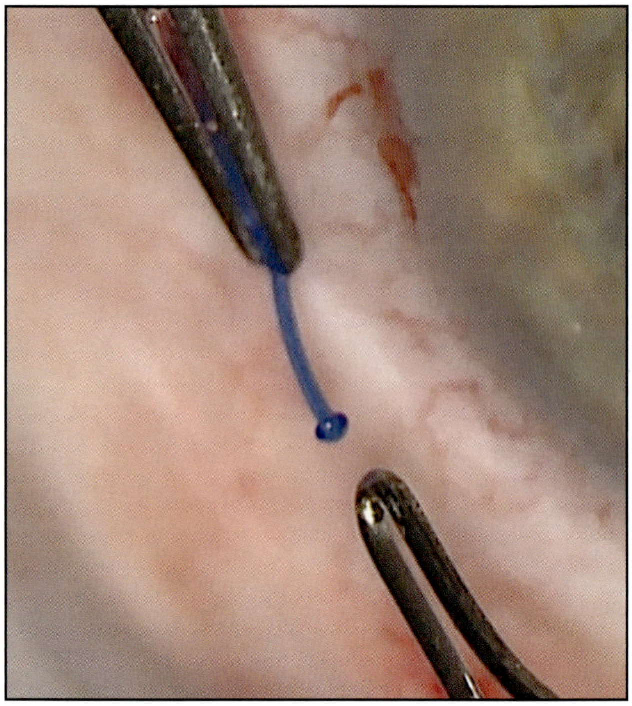

- One haptic at a time, grasp the haptic with tying forceps and use the handheld cautery to heat the tip of the haptic, without touching it. The heat diffusion will creating a mushroom-shaped flange. Be careful not to excessively pull the first haptic until both haptics are flanged.

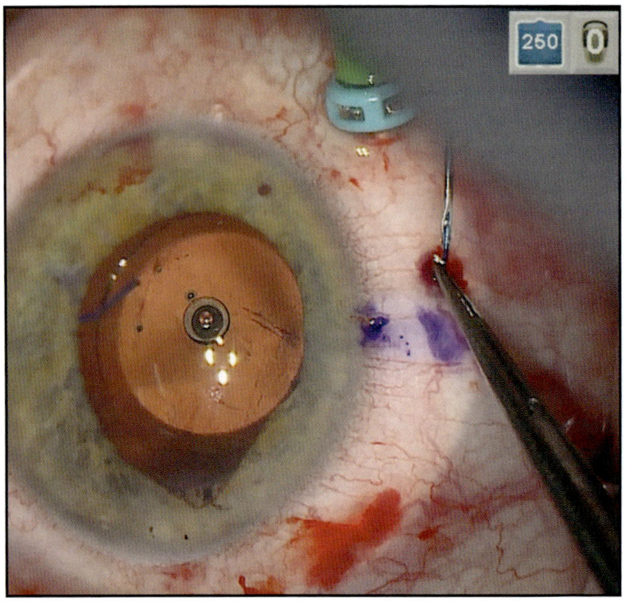

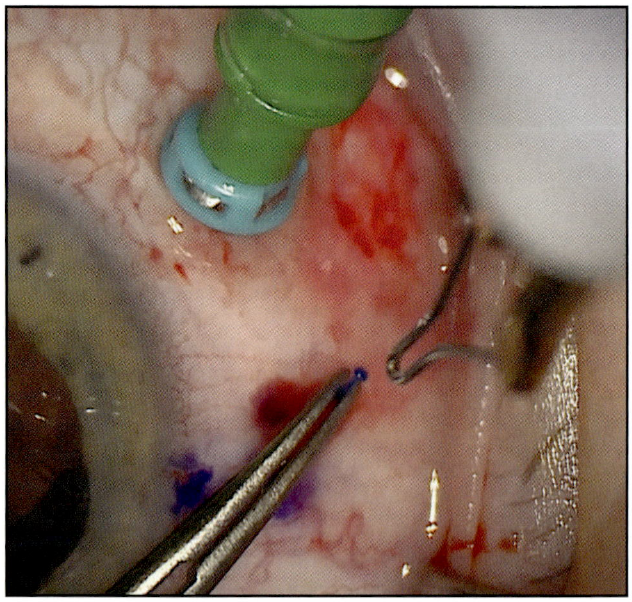

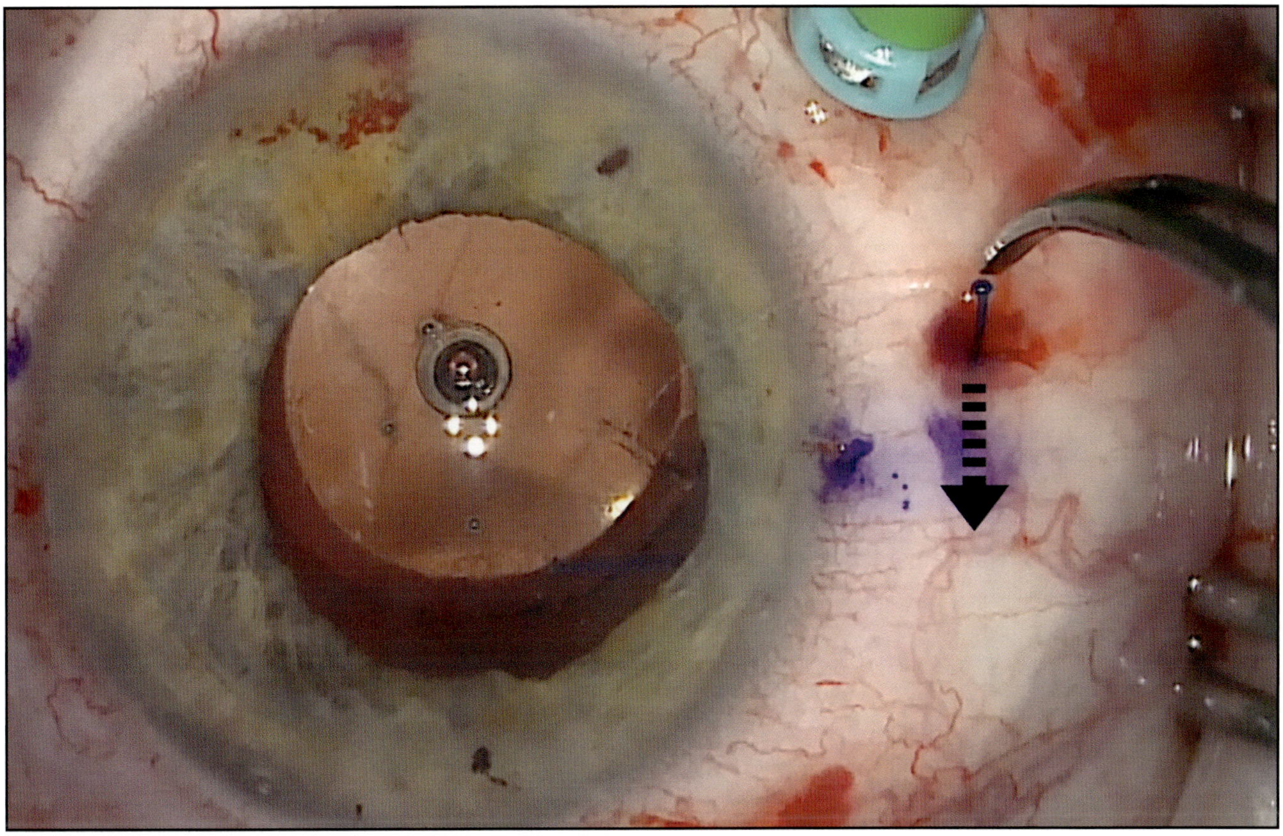

- Once the haptics are flanged, use tying forceps to push the haptic ends through the conjunctival opening and into the scleral tracks. The flanges will prevent the haptic from being pushed all the way through sclera, thus achieving scleral fixation. Ensure that the flanged ends of the haptic are advanced to be deep to the scleral surface to avoid ocular surface irritation or late-term exposure.

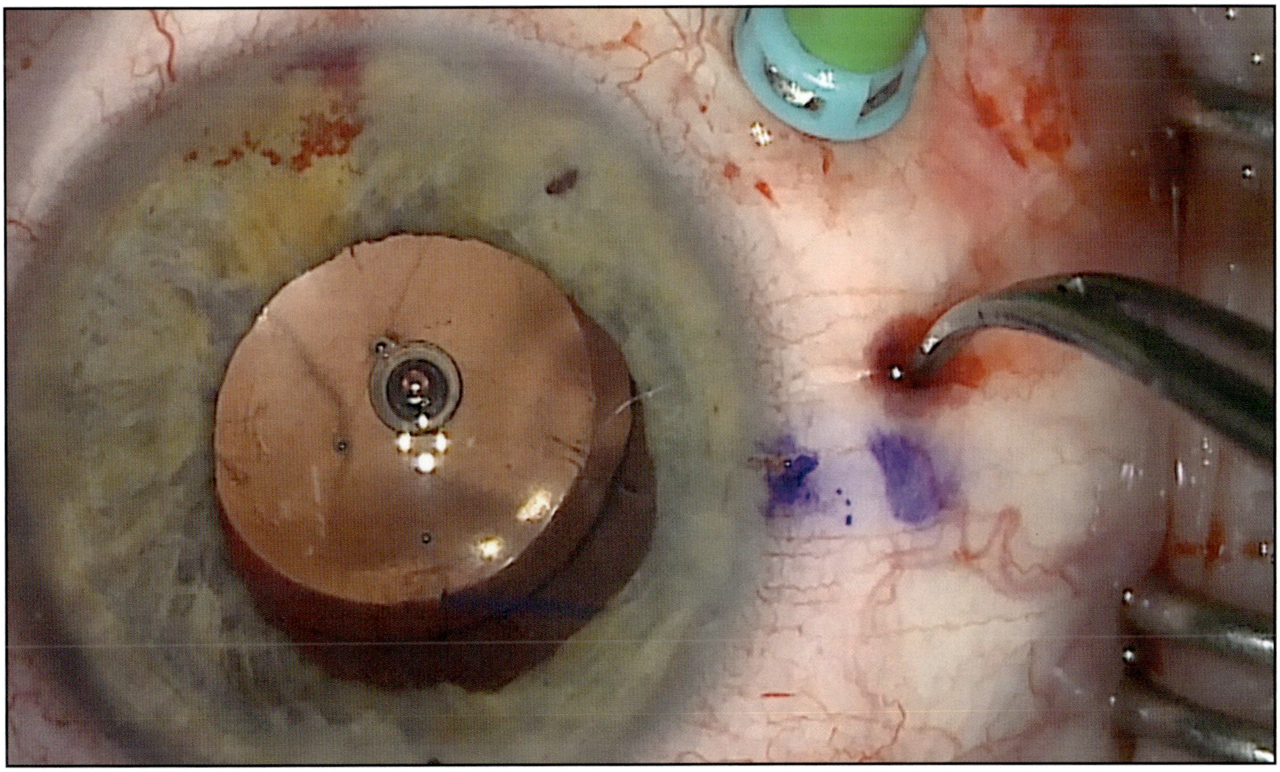

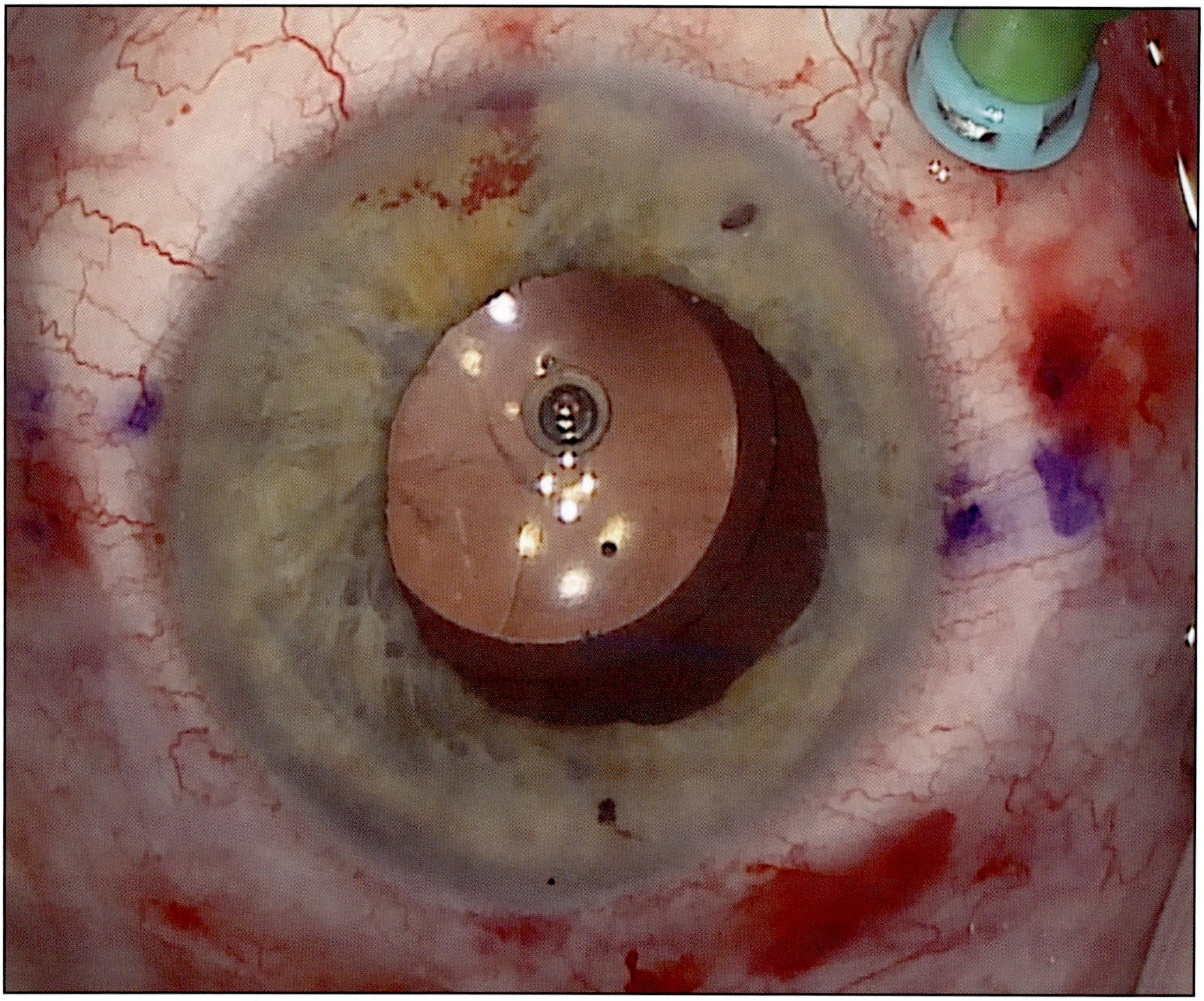

- Ensure the IOL is centered and planar—if it is decentered, there may be an asymmetrical tunnel length or haptic length. Consider slightly shortening a haptic or recreating a more optimal scleral tunnel if needed.

CHAPTER 22

HOW TO SUTURE AN INTRAOCULAR LENS TO SCLERA

INTRODUCTION

When there is no capsule or adequate iris support for intraocular lens (IOL) placement or suturing, scleral fixation is required. This can be done with or without sutures. See Chapter 26 for sutureless fixation. In this chapter, we discuss scleral sutured IOL fixation, in particular using the Morcher 67G prosthesis.

KEY POINTS

- Perform as much work as possible using small incisions.
- Do not irrigate with an anterior chamber maintainer until it is time to place the IOL into the eye. Use viscoelastics to keep the anterior chamber formed to minimize endothelial trauma from moving fluid.
- Measure from scleral spur to minimize the risk of ciliary body chafing due to improperly placed suture passes that can be too anterior when measuring from the limbus.

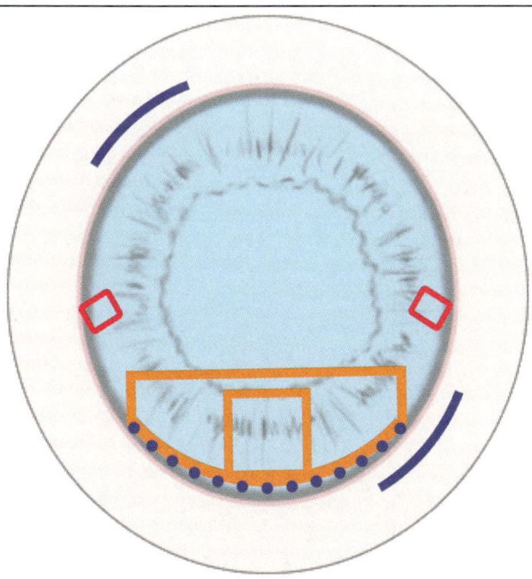

- Anterior chamber maintainer away from main incision or pars plana infusion
- Main incision initially 3 mm enlarged as needed to accommodate the IOL (in some cases, over 7 mm)

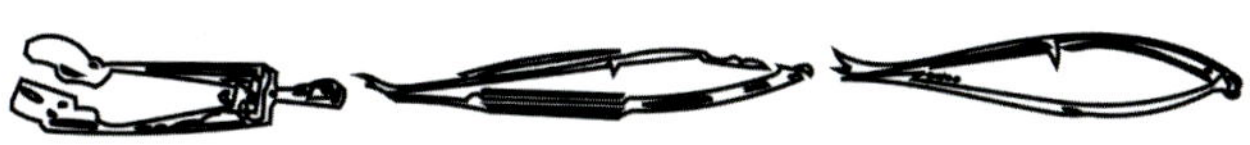

- Microsurgical Technology, Inc microforceps
- Gore-Tex 7-0 suture on CV-8 needle left double-armed
- 0.5-inch, 25-g hypodermic needle for docking the Gore-Tex suture
- If using 9-0 or 10-0 Prolene (Ethicon, Inc) instead, use a 27-g hypodermic needle to dock

Ahmed IK, Campos-Möller X, Shah M, Sheybani A. *Illustrated Advanced Anterior Segment Surgery: A Step-by-Step Guide for Challenging Cases* (pp 163-171).

- An anterior chamber maintainer or a pars plana infusion trocar is placed prior to creating the main wound. At this stage, keep the irrigation off.
- Two conjunctival peritomies are performed 180 degrees apart at the same clock hour as the planned haptic orientation.
- A 2.5-mm, partial-thickness scratch incision is made radial to the limbus. Start this 1 mm back from the scleral spur (where the blue meets the white on the sclera). The incision is 10% to 20% thickness.

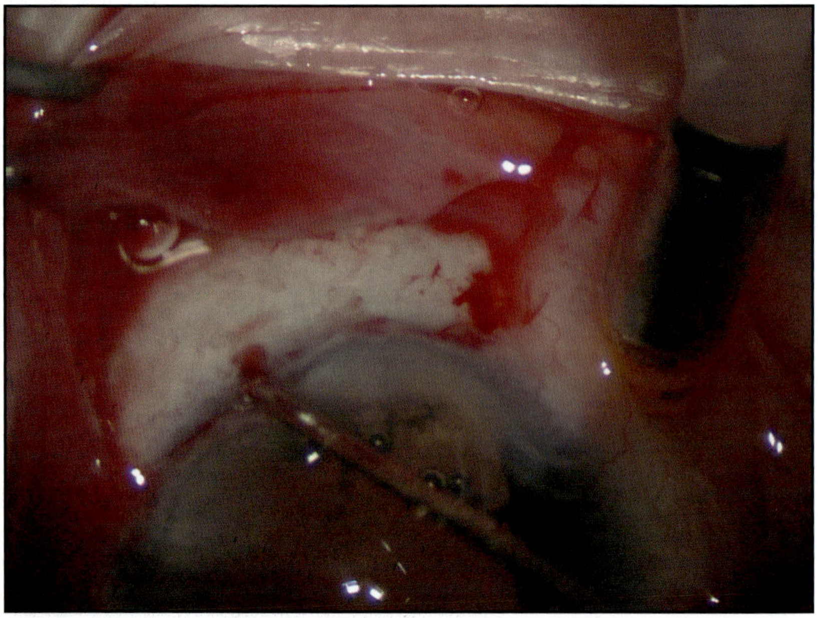

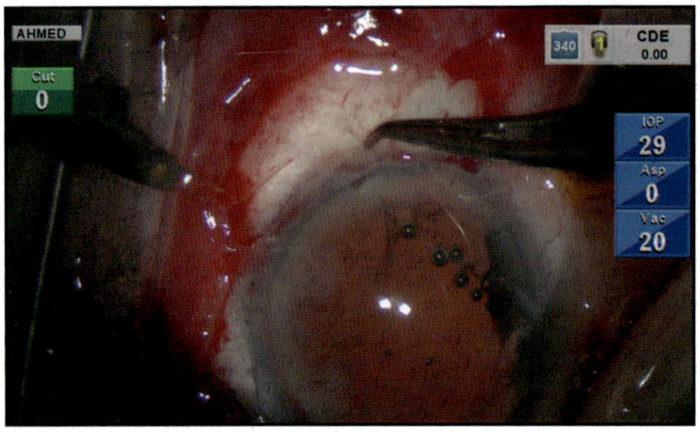

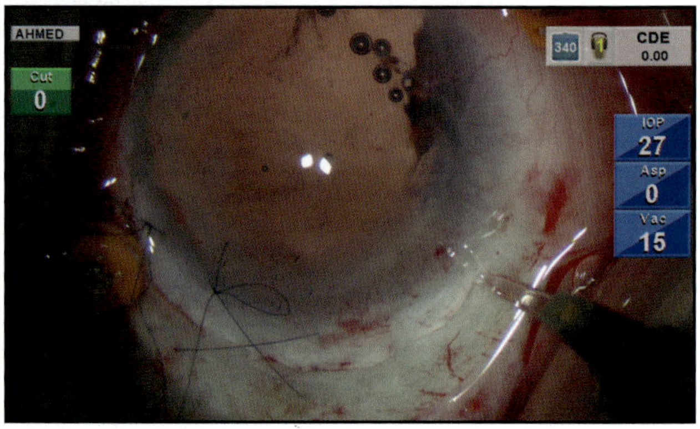

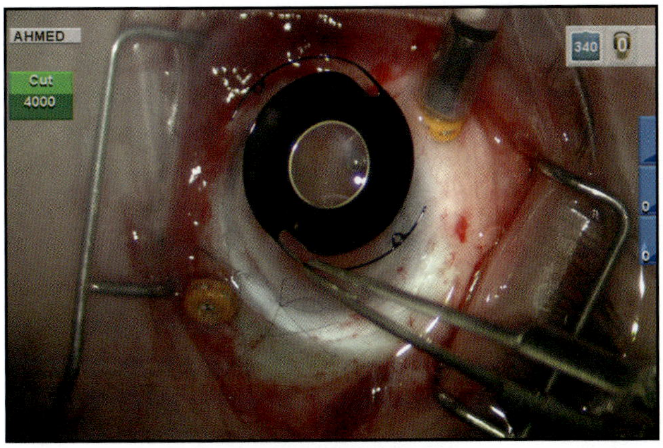

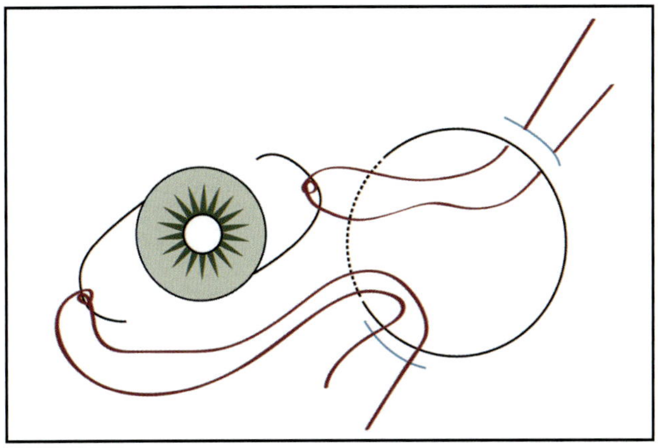

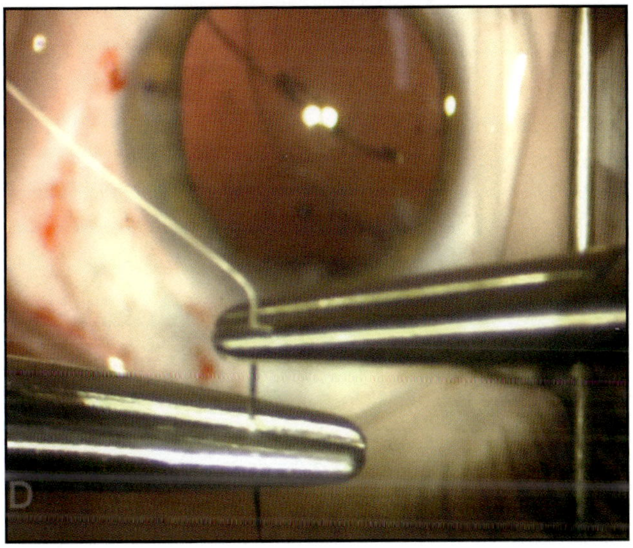

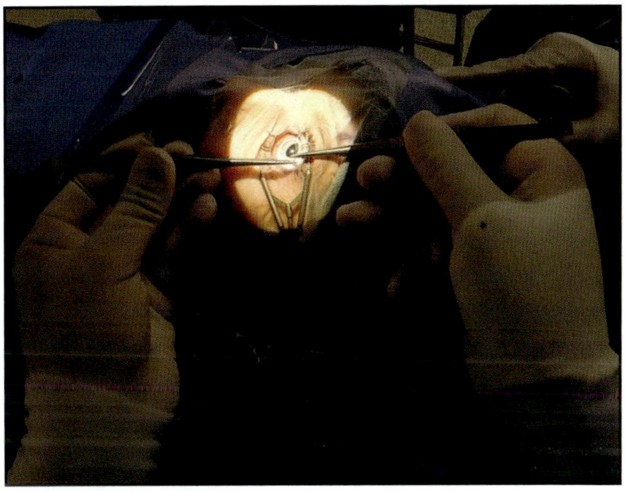

The curved Gore-Tex needle is straightened by 2 heavy needle drivers.

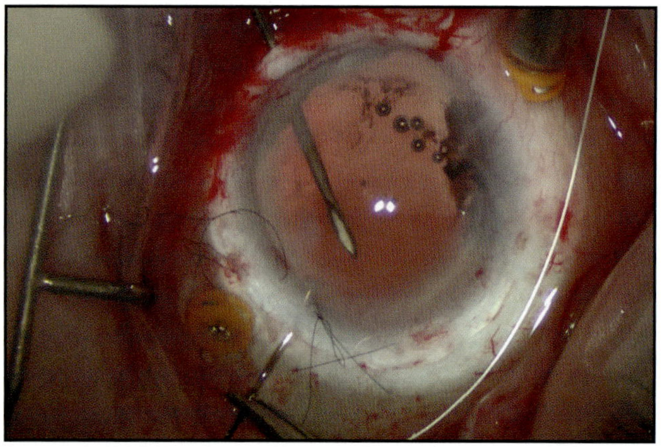

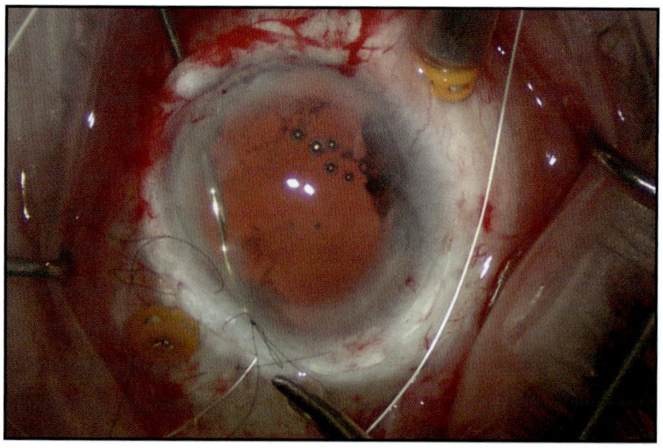

- A 25-g docking needle is inserted through one end of the scleral scratch incision.
- One end of a double-armed Gore-Tex needle is drawn through the main incision and docked into the 25-g needle and withdrawn out of the eye.

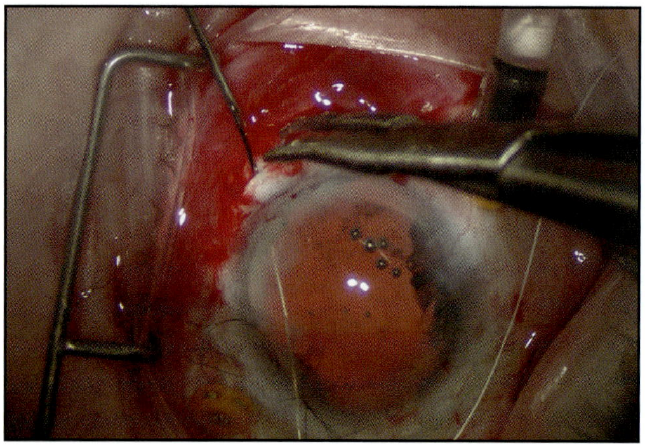

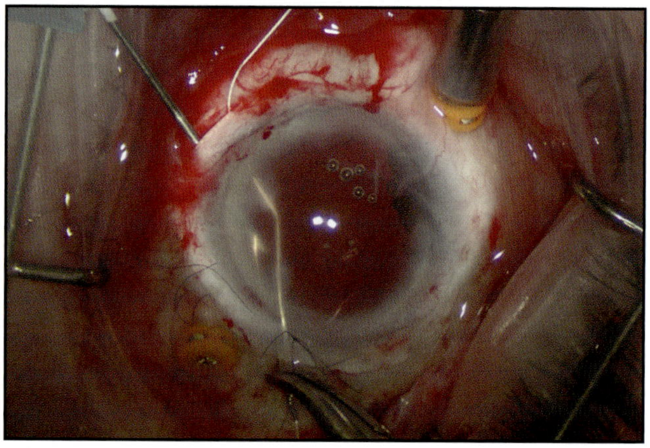

- The second end of the suture is passed through the eyelet of the scleral IOL.
- The second pass of the 25-g needle is made at the other end of the scratch incision.
- The second arm of the suture is then docked to this needle and withdrawn out of the eye in a similar fashion. Avoid rotation of the suture.

- A new Gore-Tex suture is threaded through the remaining eyelet of the IOL.
- Care must be taken to avoid entangling of the 2 sutures at this point.
- The 25-g needle and docking steps are repeated 180 degrees apart for the opposite haptic.

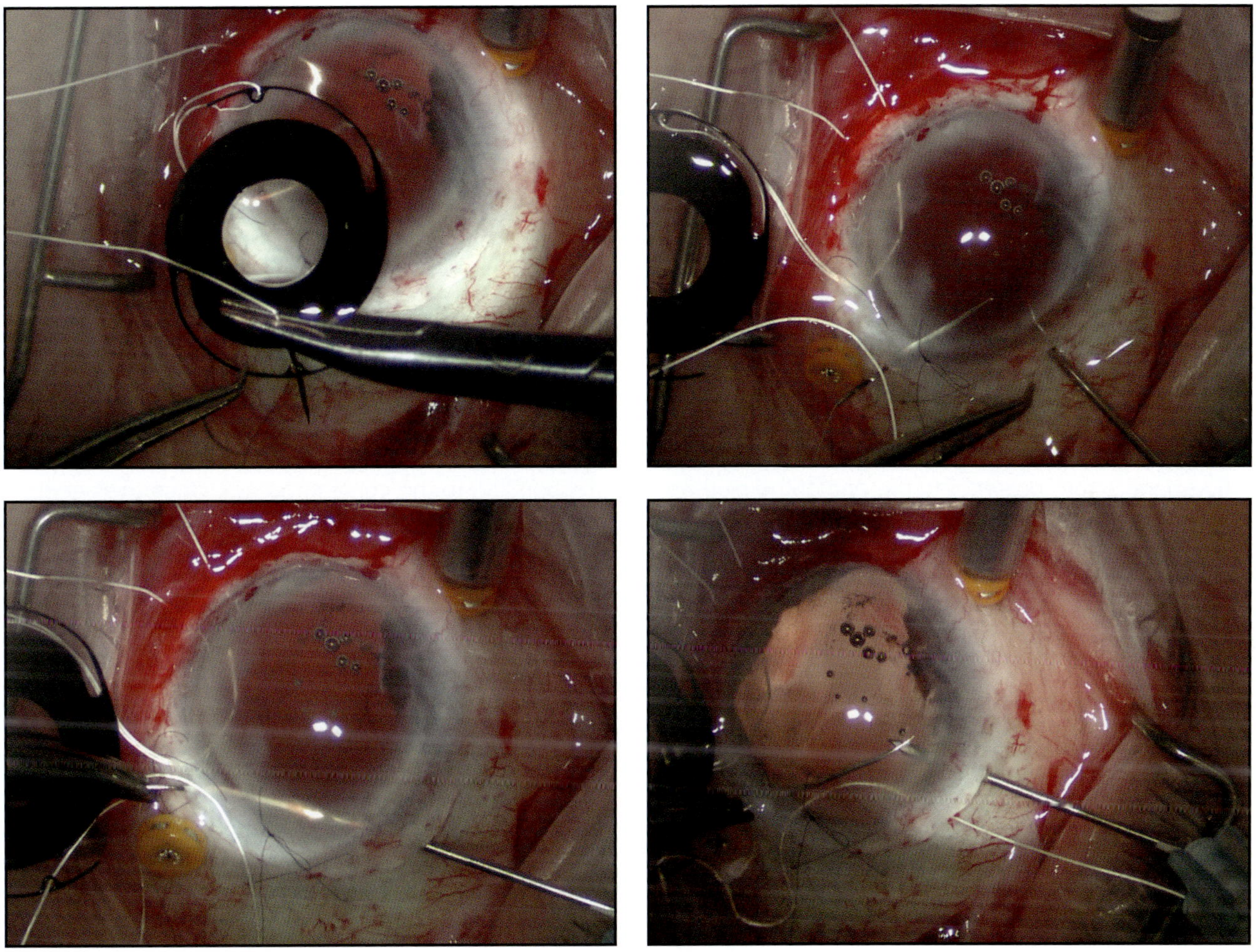

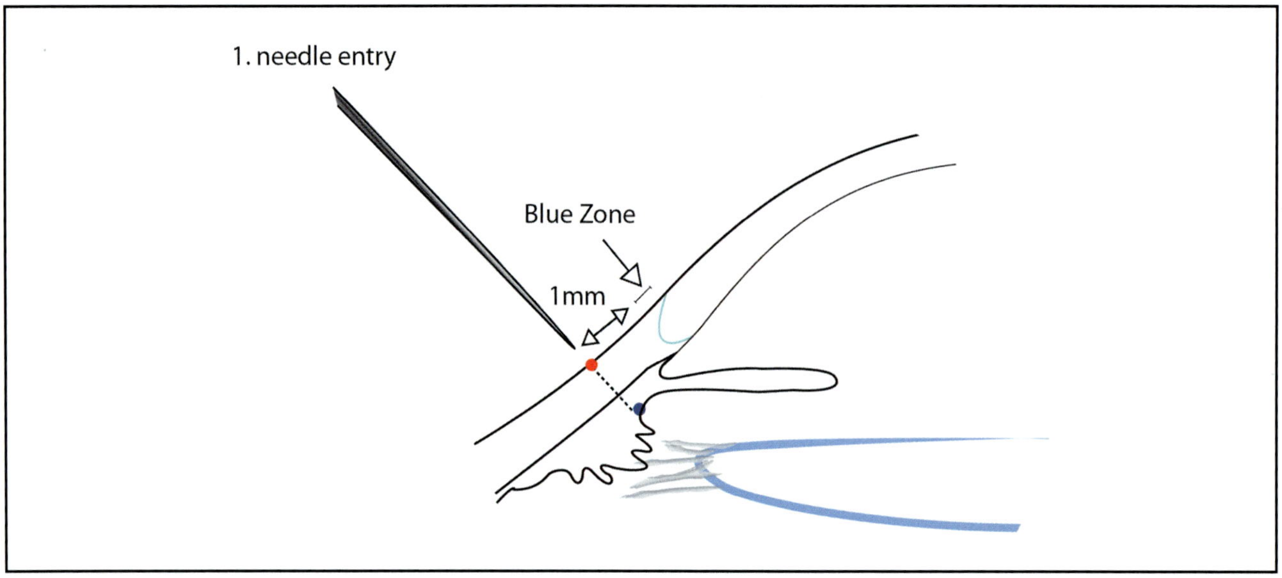

Diagram of needle entry and angle change for sulcus fixation. Needle entry should be done perpendicular to the sclera, 1 mm posterior to the end of the blue zone (corresponding to the corneal wedge). Once the needle has advanced into the scleral thickness, a 45-degree angle change should be carried out in order to enter the ciliary sulcus parallel to the iris plane (dotted arrow).

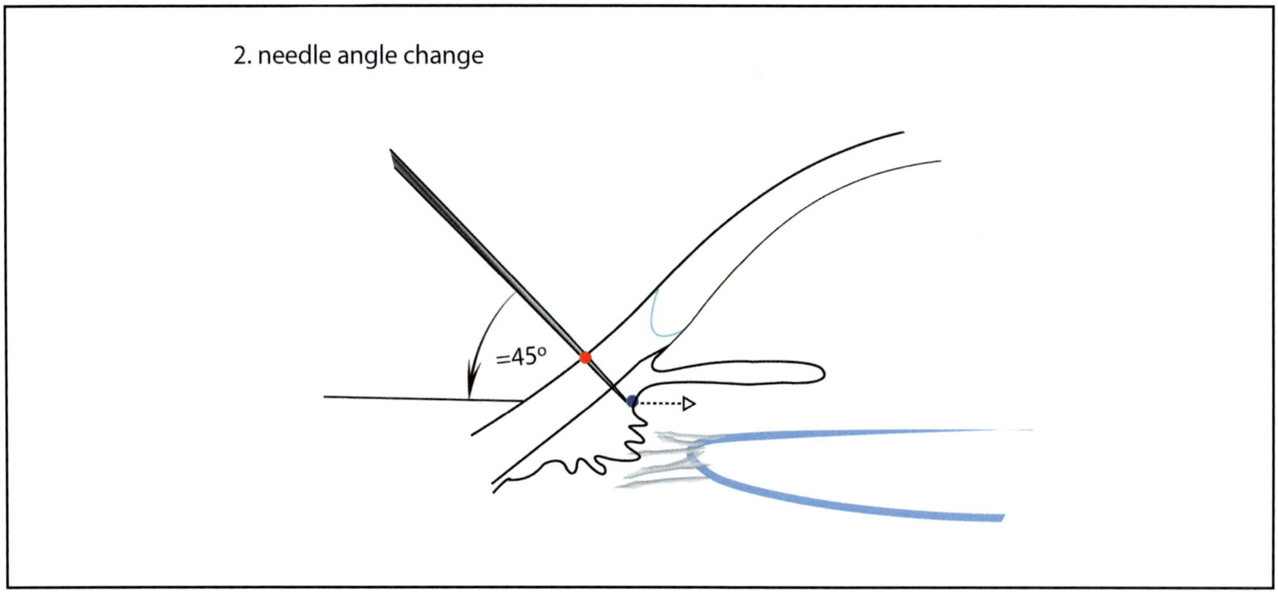

- If the wound was not previously created, it should be enlarged to fit the IOL; in this case, using a Morcher 67G, the wound was enlarged to 6 to 7 mm.
- The anterior chamber maintainer is turned on as the IOL is slid into the eye using a nontoothed forceps (tying forceps) while pulling both ends of the Gore-Tex suture looped through the leading eyelet. Do not leave slack in the system.

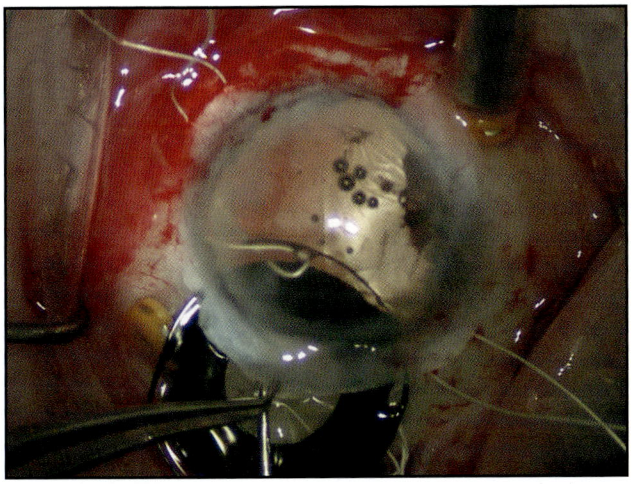

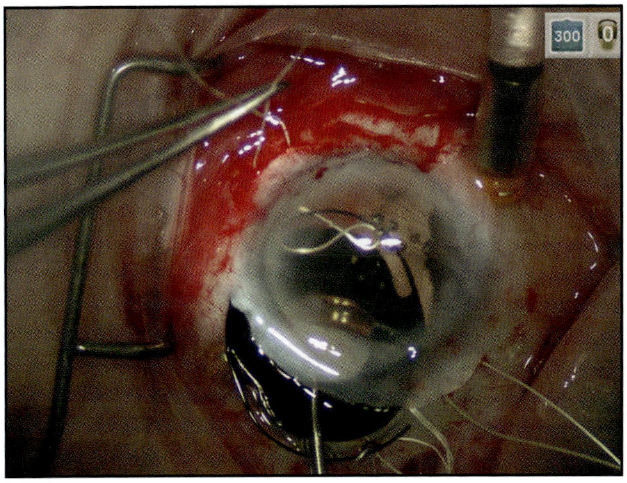

- Ensure the IOL is completely in the eye before pulling both suture ends of the trailing eyelet in order to position the IOL in the sulcus space.

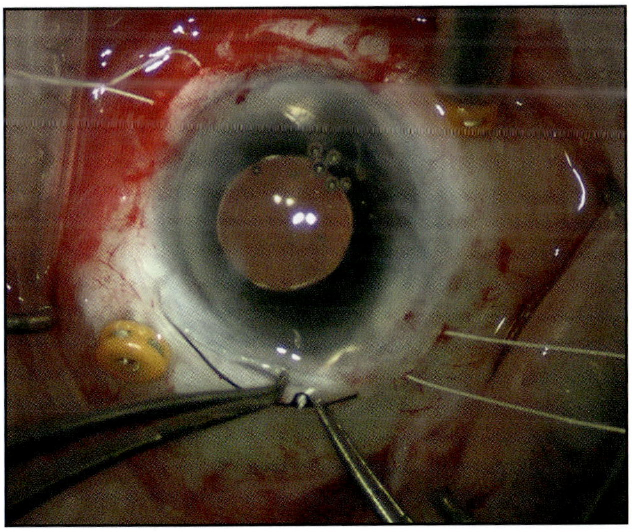

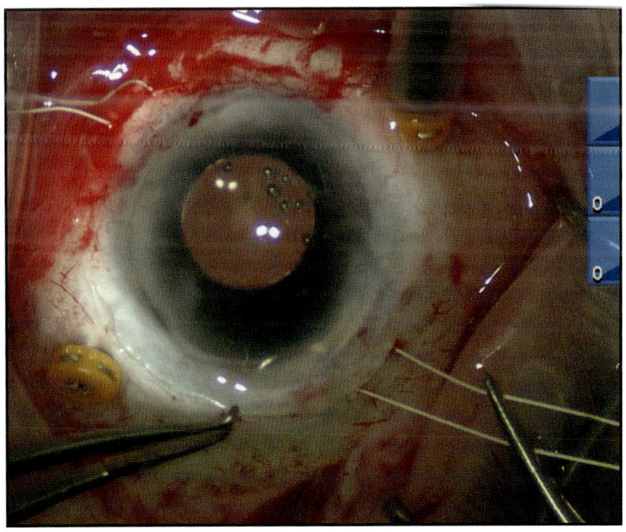

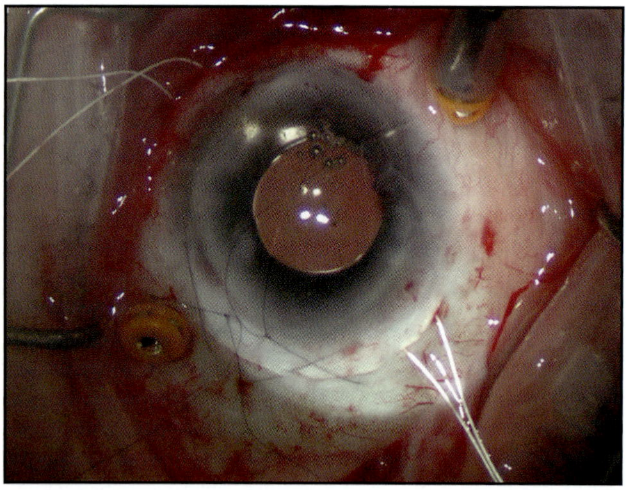

Close the large incision, then shut off the anterior chamber maintainer and use cohesive viscoelastic to maintain chamber.

Close the external sutures using a slip knot (see p 76 for slip knot diagram). In this case, do not overtighten, but loose placement can lead to IOL tilt. Overtightening can potentially cheese-wire the suture through the sclera over time.

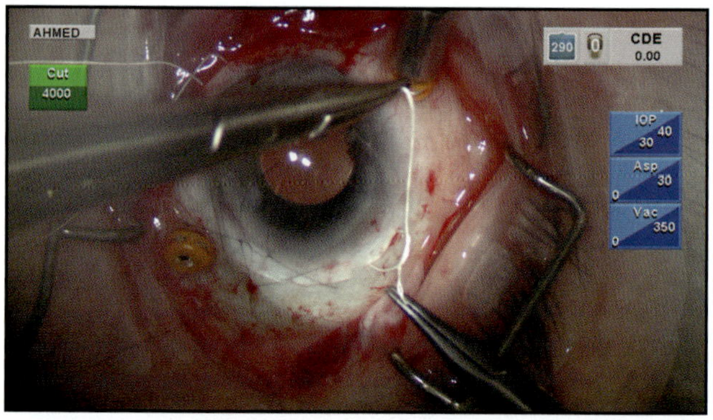

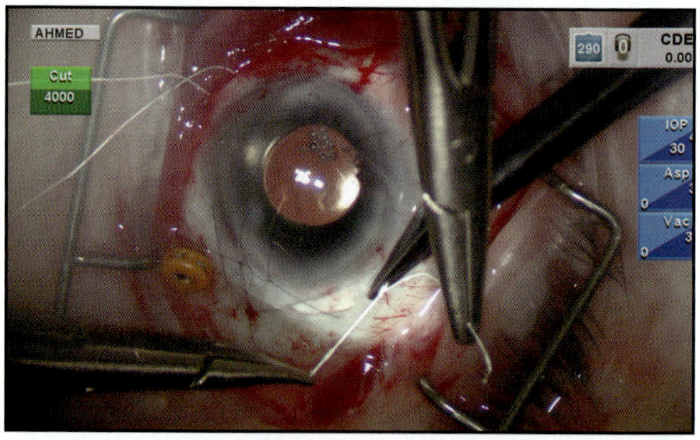

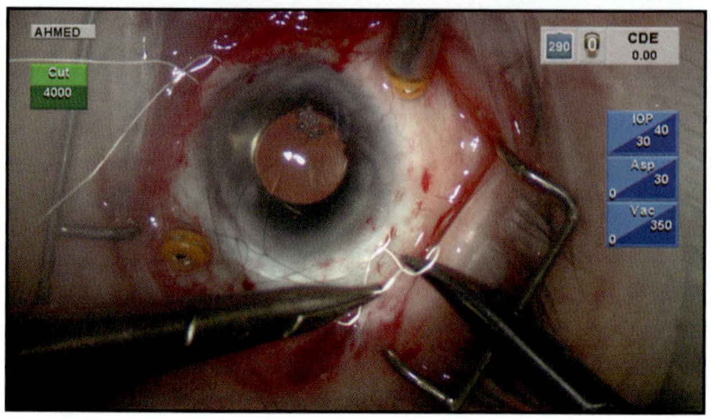

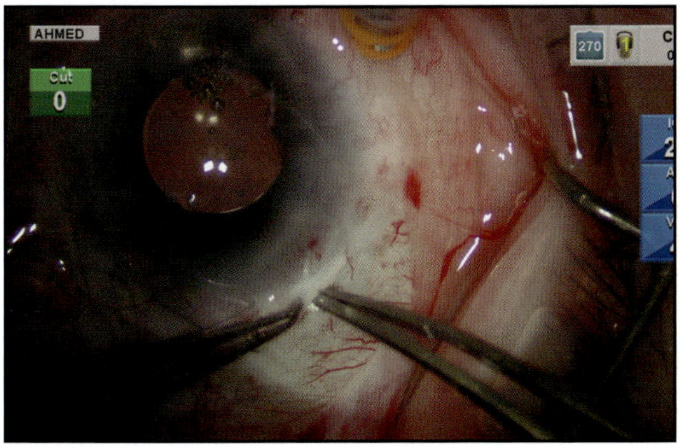

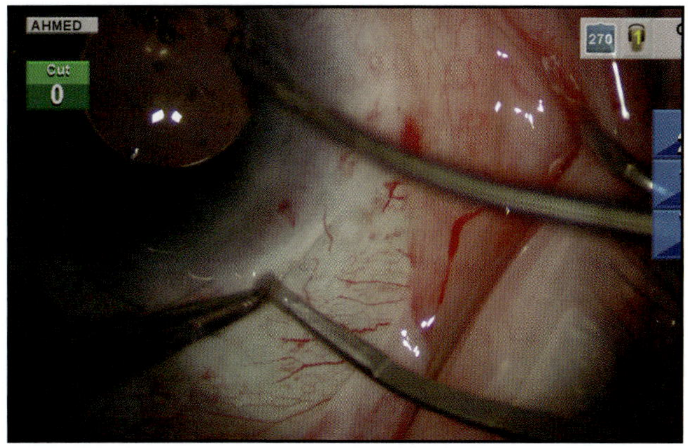

- Rotate the knots internally, sometimes pushing the knot in with tyers or a Sinskey hook.
- Remove ophthalmic viscosurgical device manually.

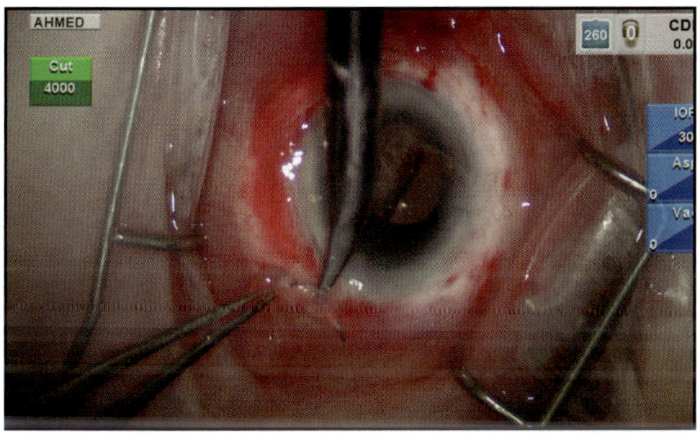

CHAPTER 23

HOW TO IMPLANT A PIGGYBACK INTRAOCULAR LENS

INTRODUCTION

Piggyback intraocular lenses (IOLs) can be placed to correct refractive errors after IOL implantation or to treat negative dysphotopsia. The principles are similar to placing a sulcus IOL.

KEY POINTS

- Do not use this technique in small eyes with minimal sulcus space. Ultrasound biomicroscopy imaging can help determine if there is adequate sulcus. In general, placing piggyback IOLs in axial lengths less than 21 mm should be avoided.
- Ensure that zonules are stable; do not place a piggyback IOL in cases of pseudophacodonesis.
- Capsulorrhexis must be continuous and curvilinear.
- The initial implant should be in the bag; 2 IOLs in the sulcus may increase the risk of iris chafing.
- To reduce the risk of interlenticular opacification, the piggyback IOL should be of a different material than the primary IOL.

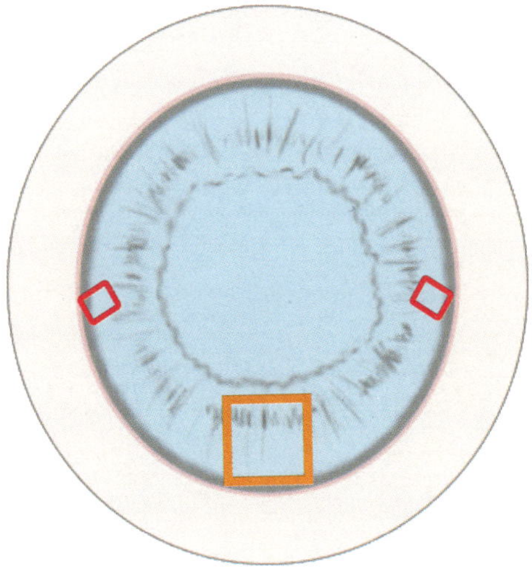

- Standard phaco + knife and fork

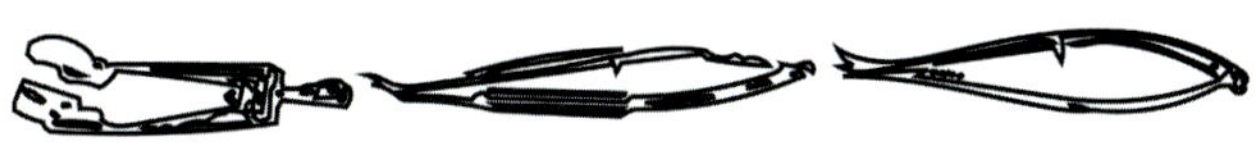

- Kuglen or Sinskey hook
- 3-piece foldable IOL
- Dispersive and cohesive ophthalmic viscosurgical device

Ahmed IK, Campos-Möller X, Shah M, Sheybani A. *Illustrated Advanced Anterior Segment Surgery: A Step-by-Step Guide for Challenging Cases* (pp 173-176).

The sulcus space is filled with cohesive viscoelastic after the previously implanted IOL is determined to be stable.

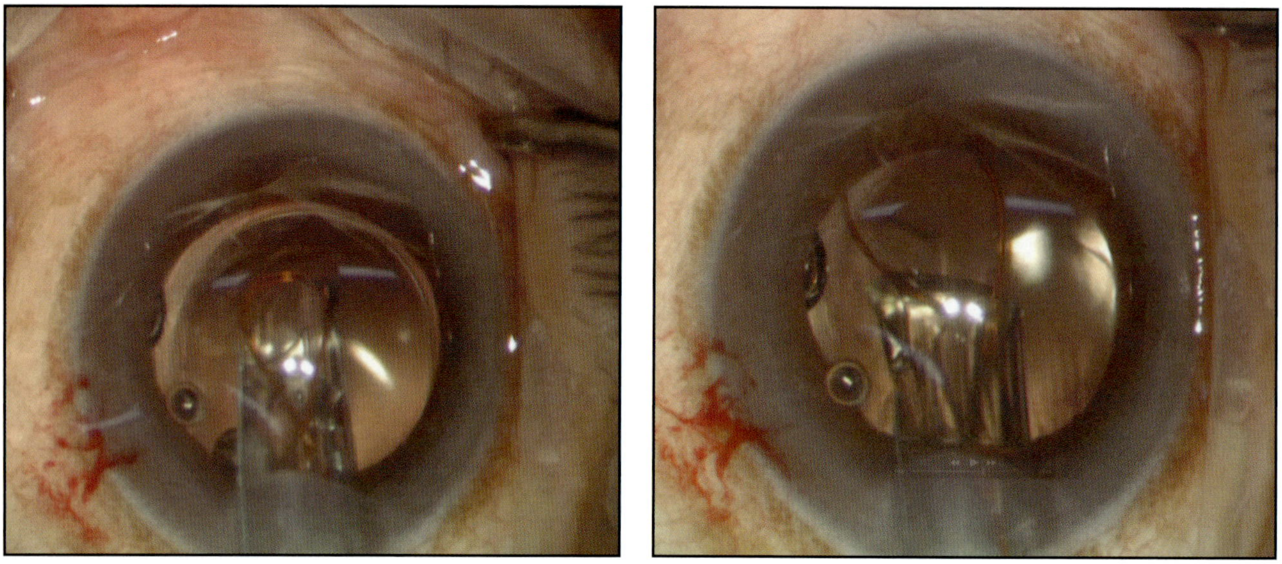

- Intracameral IOL injection, rather than wound-assisted injection, is preferred for more control of haptic delivery into the ciliary sulcus.
- The piggyback IOL is injected into the sulcus space, placing the leading haptic in the correct orientation as the IOL is delivered. Sometimes, this requires rotating the injector during delivery. The leading haptic can be placed under the iris before it unfolds to facilitate the entire haptic's placement into the sulcus.

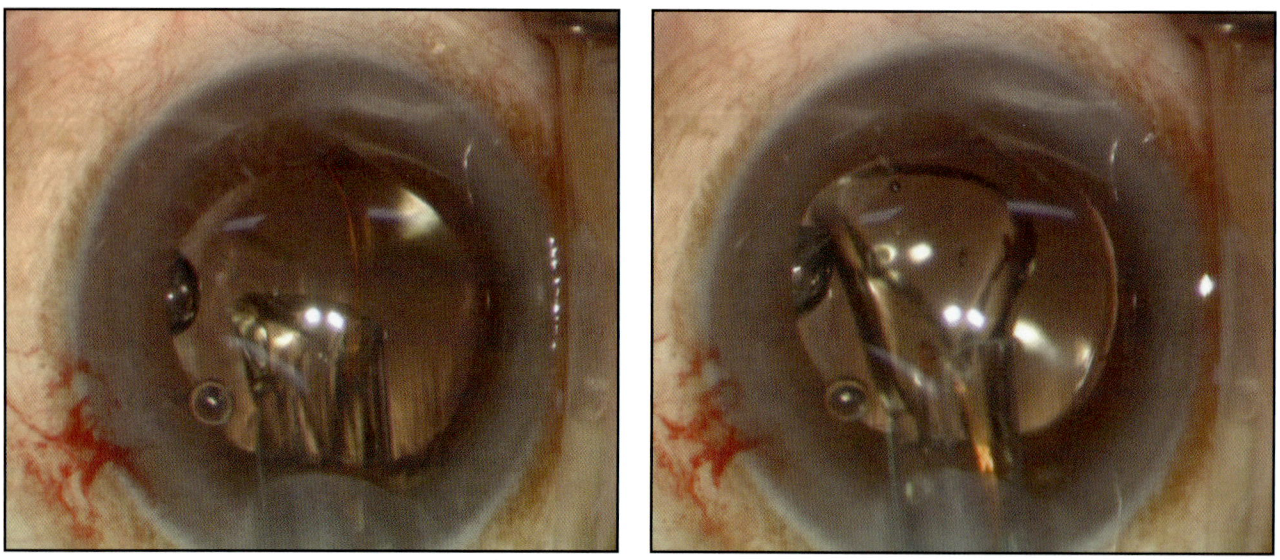

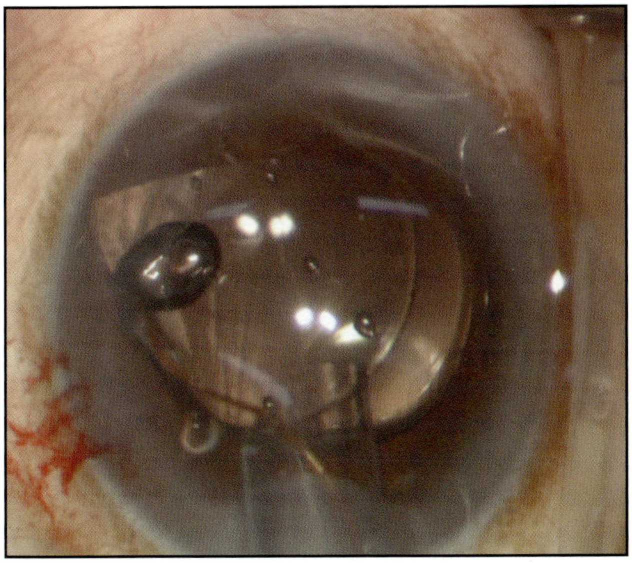

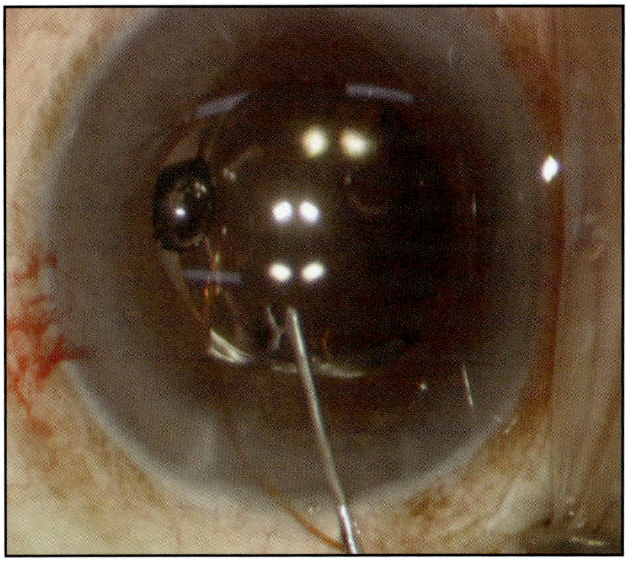

- The trailing haptic is delivered and usually can be left outside the eye.
- The Kuglen hook is used to dial the IOL into the sulcus space by rotating at the haptic-optic junction.
- Once the IOL is in the sulcus space, viscoelastic can be removed in an automated or manual fashion.
- Miochol (acetylcholine) is placed to ensure pupil centration (see also Chapter 14).

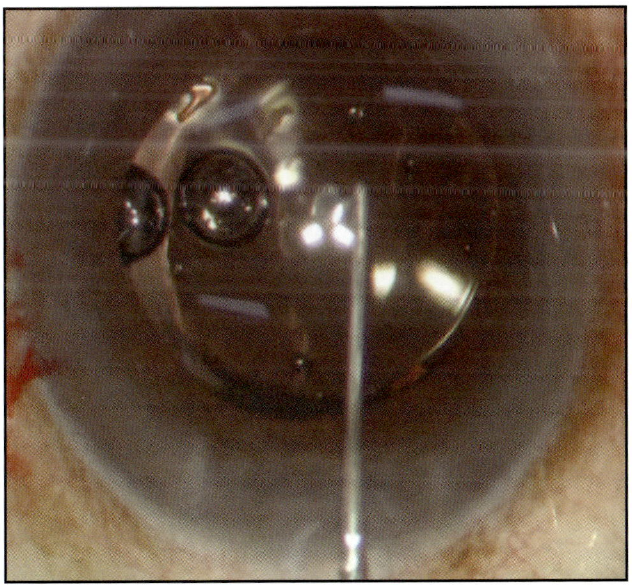

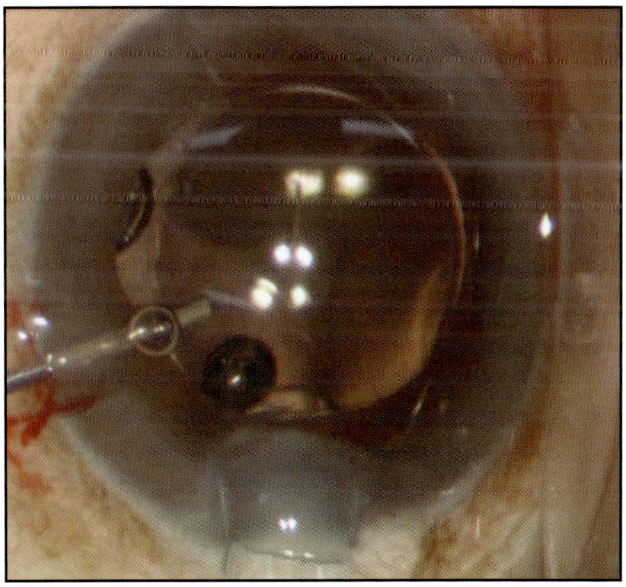

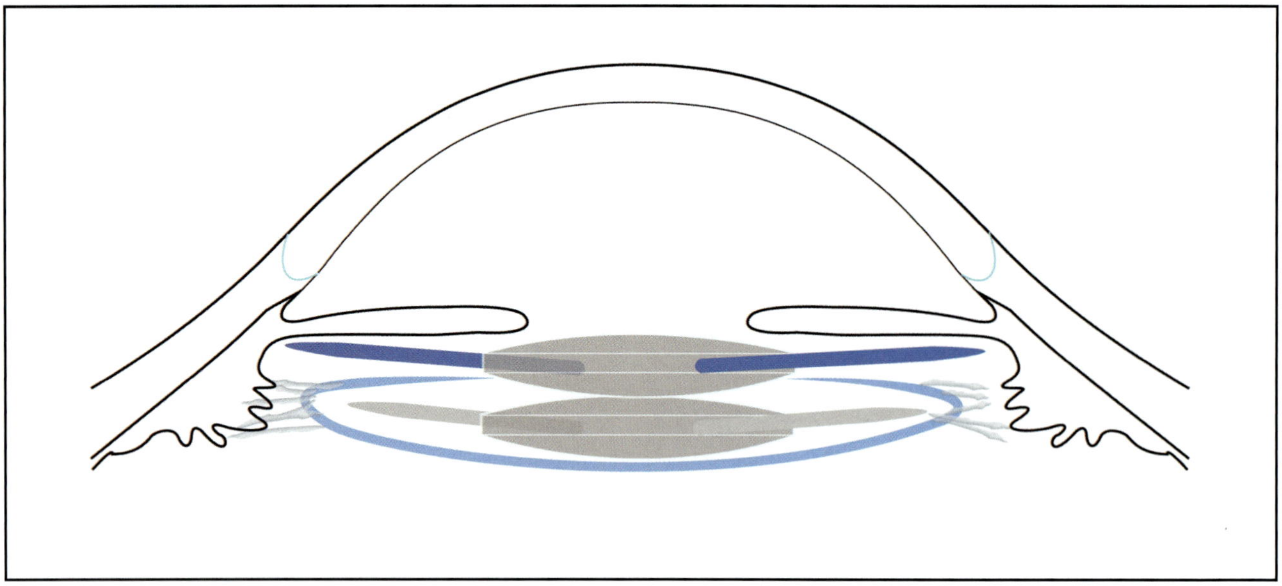

Configuration of a piggyback 3-piece IOL in the ciliary sulcus, anterior to a single-piece IOL in the capsular bag.

CHAPTER 24

HOW TO EXPLANT AN INTRAOCULAR LENS FROM THE CAPSULAR BAG

INTRODUCTION

Intraocular lens (IOL) explantation from the capsular bag may be required for a variety of situations, including refractive surprises, lens opacification, and positive or negative dysphotopsia.

The more time that has elapsed since original IOL implantation, the more adherent the anterior and posterior capsular leaflets can be, particularly when a Soemmering's ring is present.

However, most of the time, one is able to release the haptics easily from the capsular fornix. In case this cannot be performed, one can simply cut the haptics at the optic-haptic junction, explanting the optic only.

KEY POINTS

- Avoid damaging zonules by excessive tugging on the optic or haptics.
- Do not bring the IOL into the anterior chamber until haptics are free and the IOL rotates.
- If the posterior capsule is open, make sure to maintain anterior chamber pressurization with viscoelastic and avoid anterior chamber shallowing. Use dispersive ophthalmic viscosurgical device (OVD) to tamponade vitreous behind the capsular bag.
- Get a good grip on the IOL before attempting to cut to avoid tilting and rotation as the optic is cut.
- Use cohesive OVD under the IOL before cutting to avoid cutting the posterior capsule. Proceed with caution and make sure to have good visualization and focus of the scissors throughout the entire cut.
- During anterior chamber maneuvers, be sure to have a good amount of viscoelastic above and below the optic to protect intraocular structures.

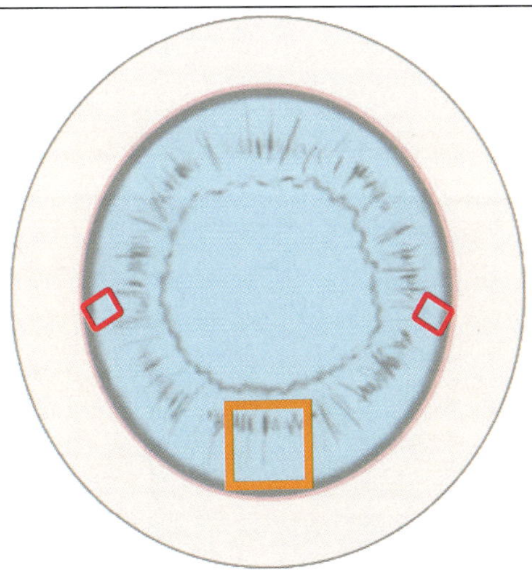

- Knife and fork incision configuration

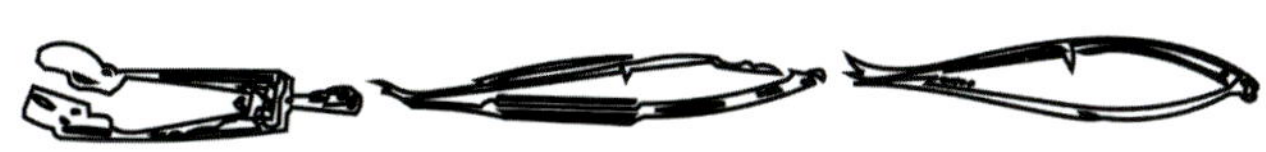

- Keratomes (3-mm main and 1-mm stab)
- Dispersive and cohesive OVD
- Sinskey hook
- Kuglen hook
- Micrograspers (Microsurgical Technology, Inc [MST] 25-g micrograsper shown)
- MST IOL cutting microscissors

Ahmed IK, Campos-Möller X, Shah M, Sheybani A. *Illustrated Advanced Anterior Segment Surgery: A Step-by-Step Guide for Challenging Cases* (pp 177-183).

In this case, we are explanting a toric IOL from an intact bag due to a refractive surprise.

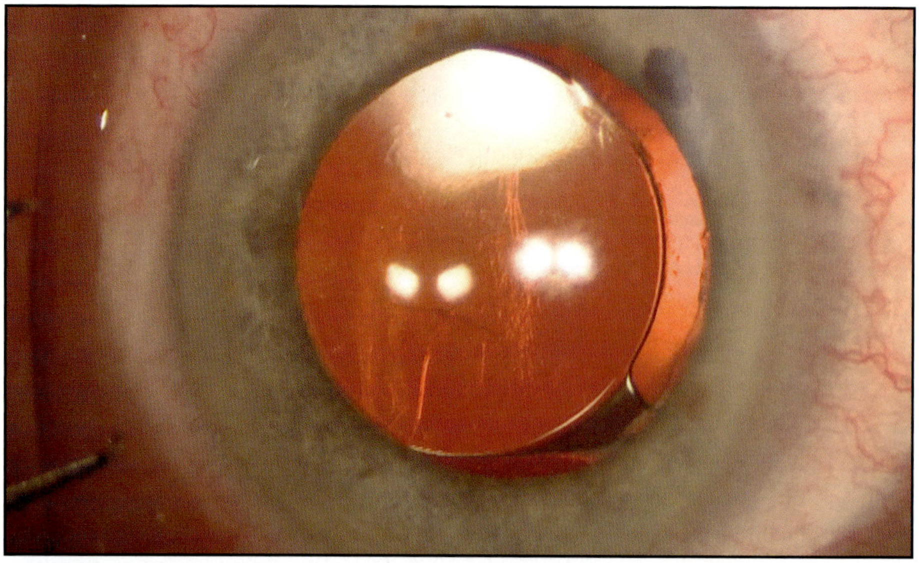

Using a micrograsper, grasp the anterior capsule close to the capsulorrhexis edge, lift and slide a Sinskey hook or OVD cannula to separate the anterior capsule from the IOL optic.

Lightly pushing the optic downward is safer than pulling the rhexis upward to reduce risk of tearing.

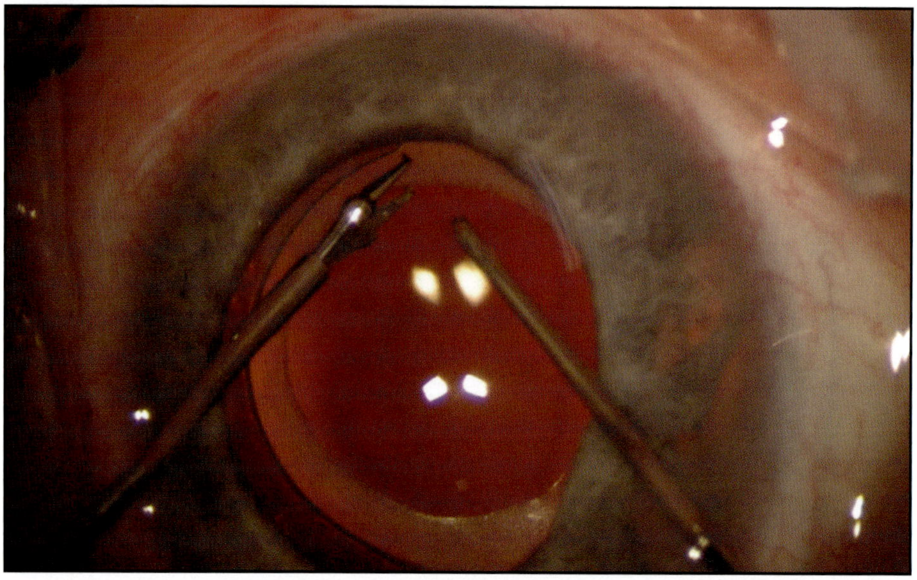

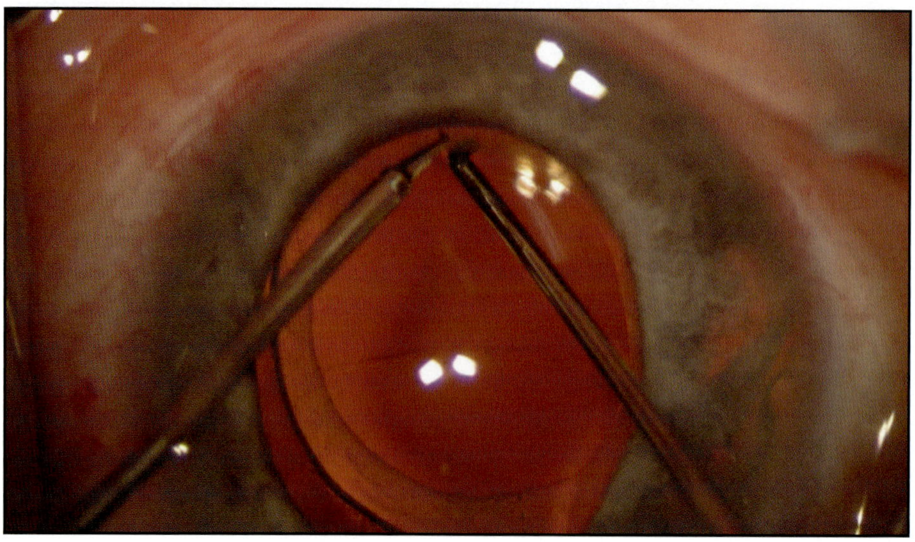

OVD injected to separate haptics from bag. Arrow indicates movement of cannula.

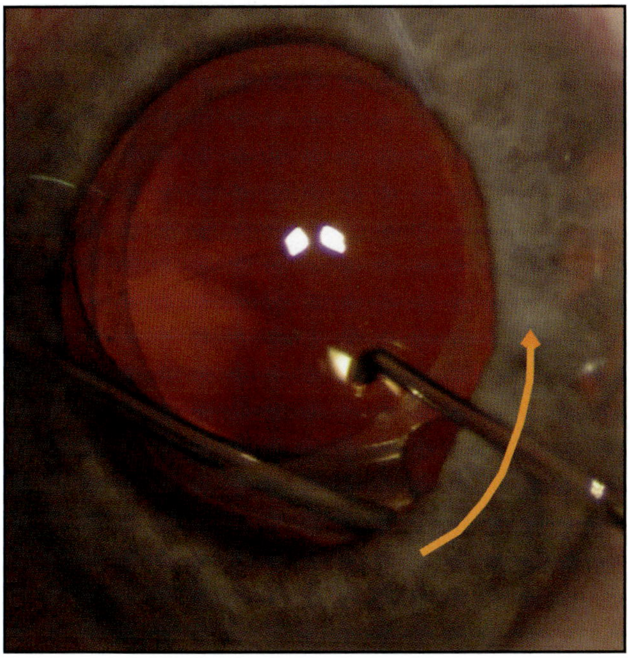

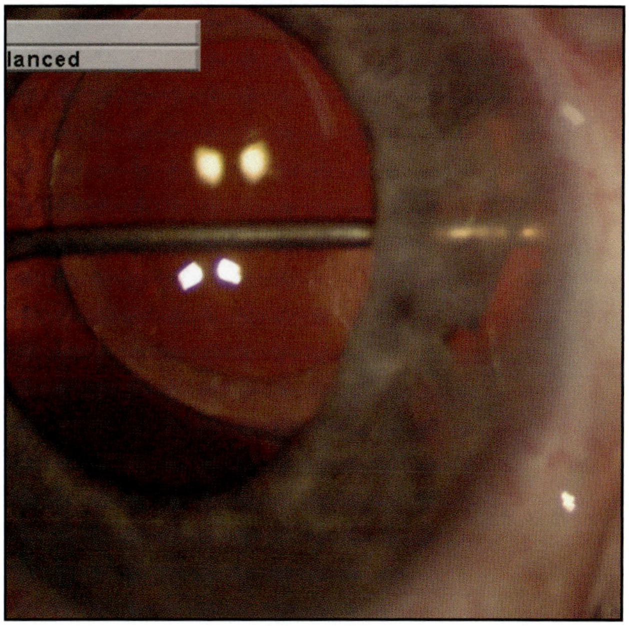

In this patient with pre-existing iris defect, one can observe how the OVD cannula reaches all the way out to the capsular fornix.

Dissect the IOL haptics from the capsular fornix by slowly and moderately injecting cohesive OVD. Make sure to go 360 degrees and all the way out to the capsular fornix, but avoid overfilling the bag. A back and forth "windshield wiper" motion can help release some fibrotic adhesions, but must be used after OVD is injected to prevent capsule rupture. Achieve a 360-degree viscodissection, using alternative incisions as needed. Once the IOL is free, inject more cohesive OVD behind the optic to push the posterior capsule back and allow for manipulation with instruments.

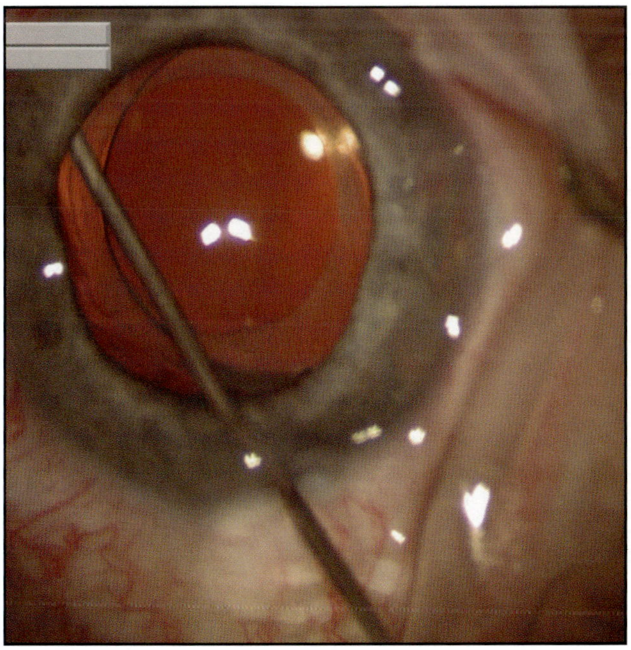

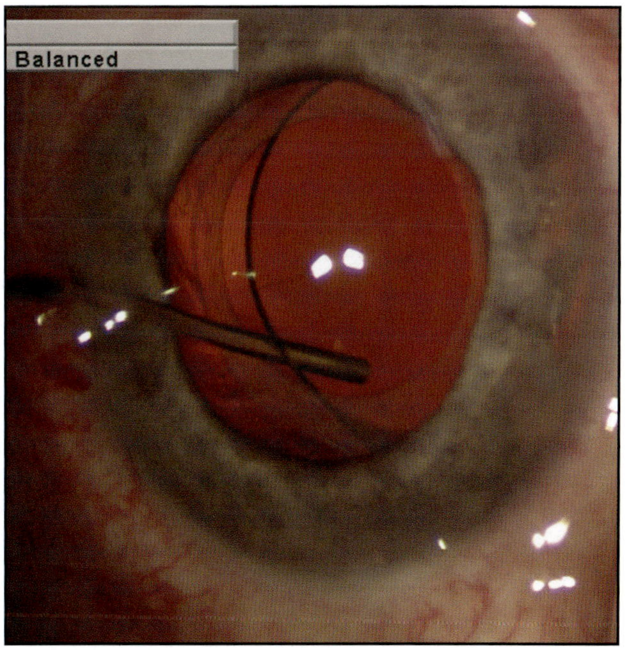

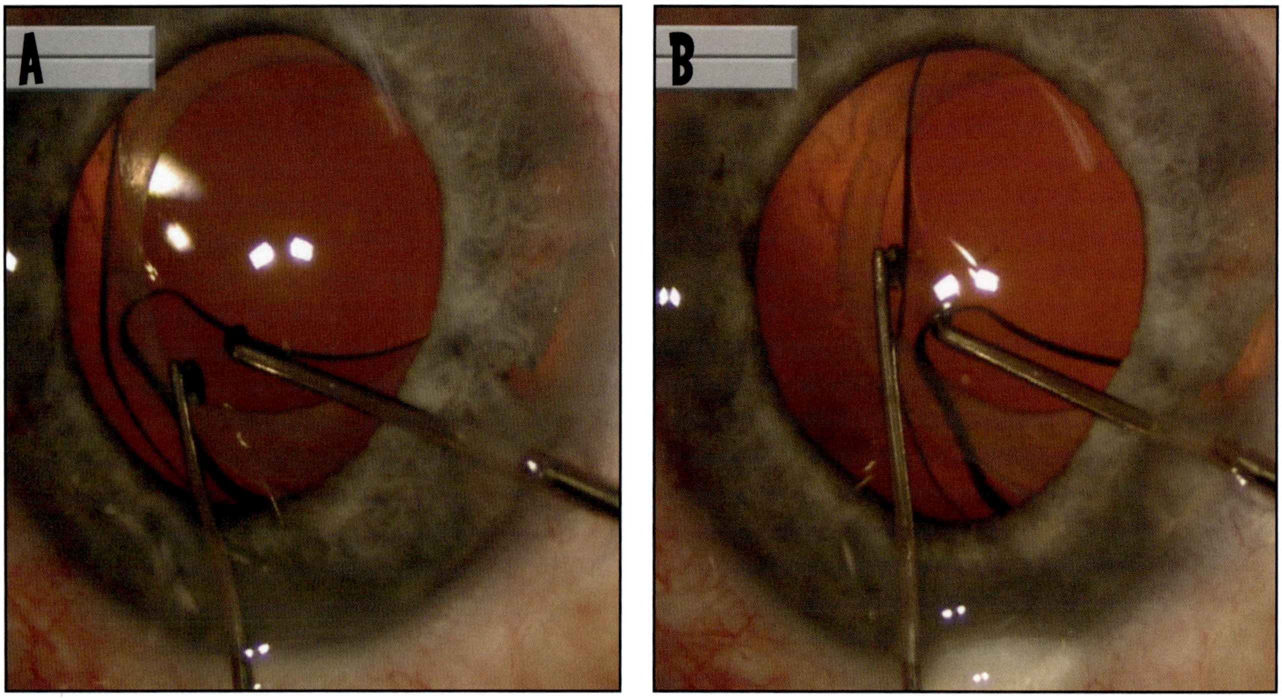

Sinskey and Kuglen hooks are used to manipulate the IOL out of the bag, using a 2-handed "chopstick" maneuver (C). Notice how the Kuglen hook (blunt) is under the optic, while the Sinskey hook (sharp) remains on top. Sinskey hooks can also be used to pull on the optic or haptic edges to position the entire IOL in the anterior chamber in preparation for cutting.

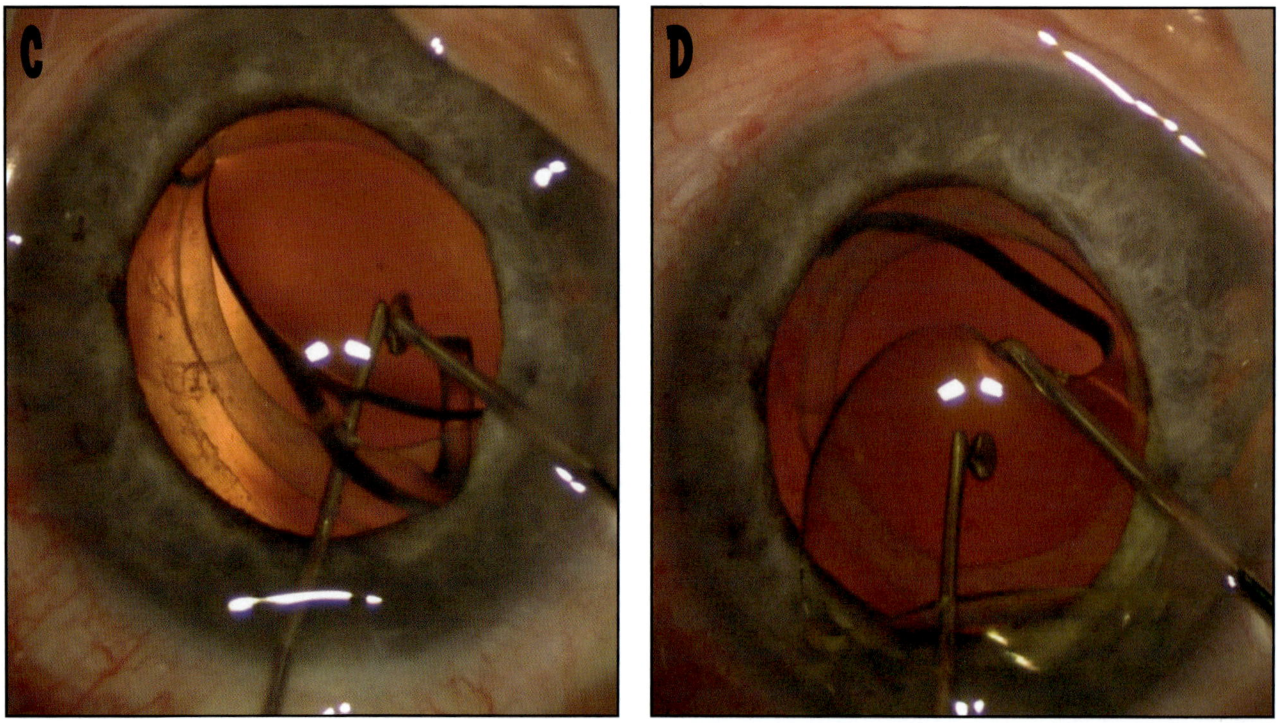

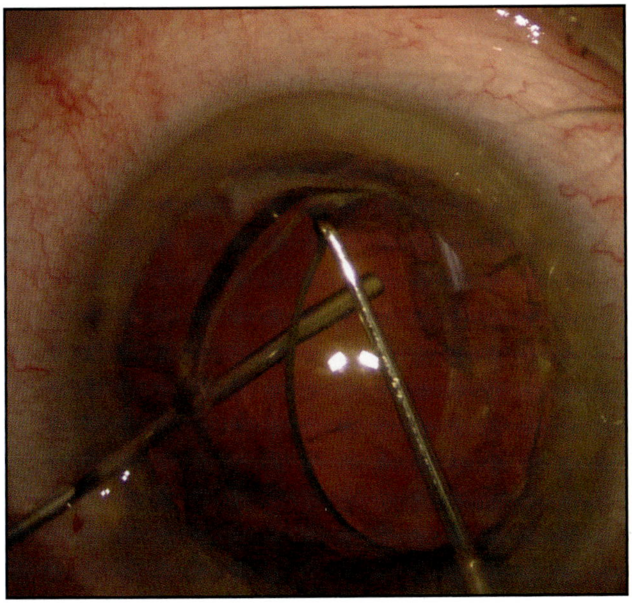

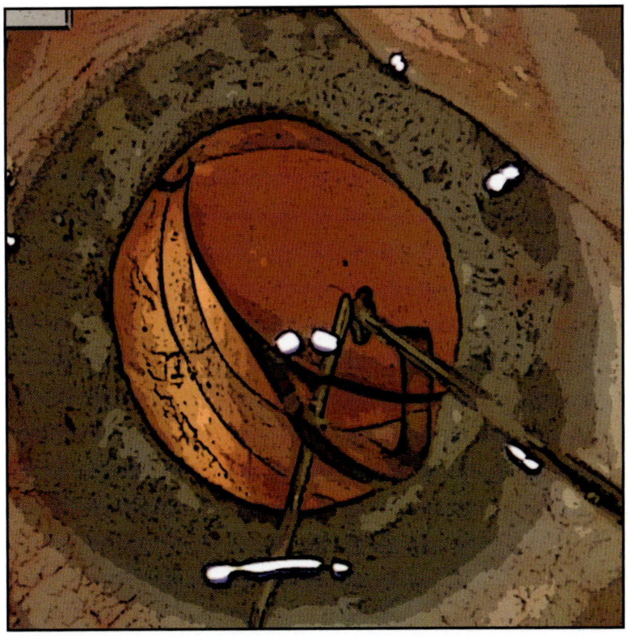

When the posterior capsule is open, make sure to coat the anterior hyaloid with dispersive OVD just beneath the IOL. Overly injecting OVD into the bag can extend posterior capsule defects. Throughout the case, managing the anterior vitreous face by coating with dispersive OVD can prevent vitreous prolapse. Once the IOL is removed, a thorough anterior vitrectomy may be performed.

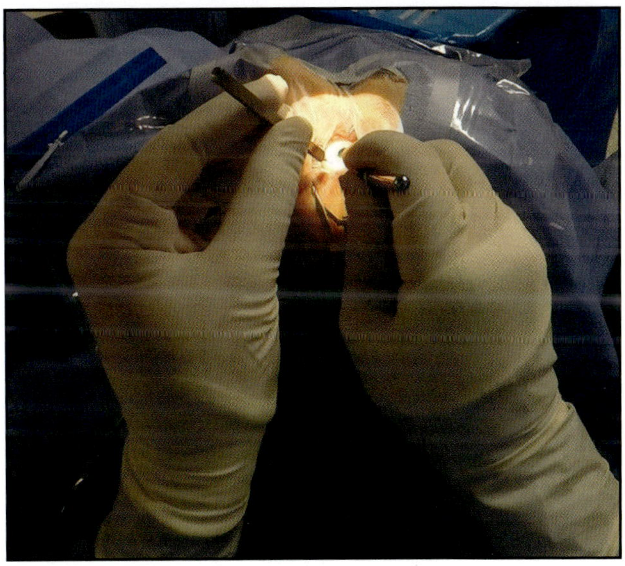

"Chopstick maneuver" to explant IOL from bag once haptics are free.

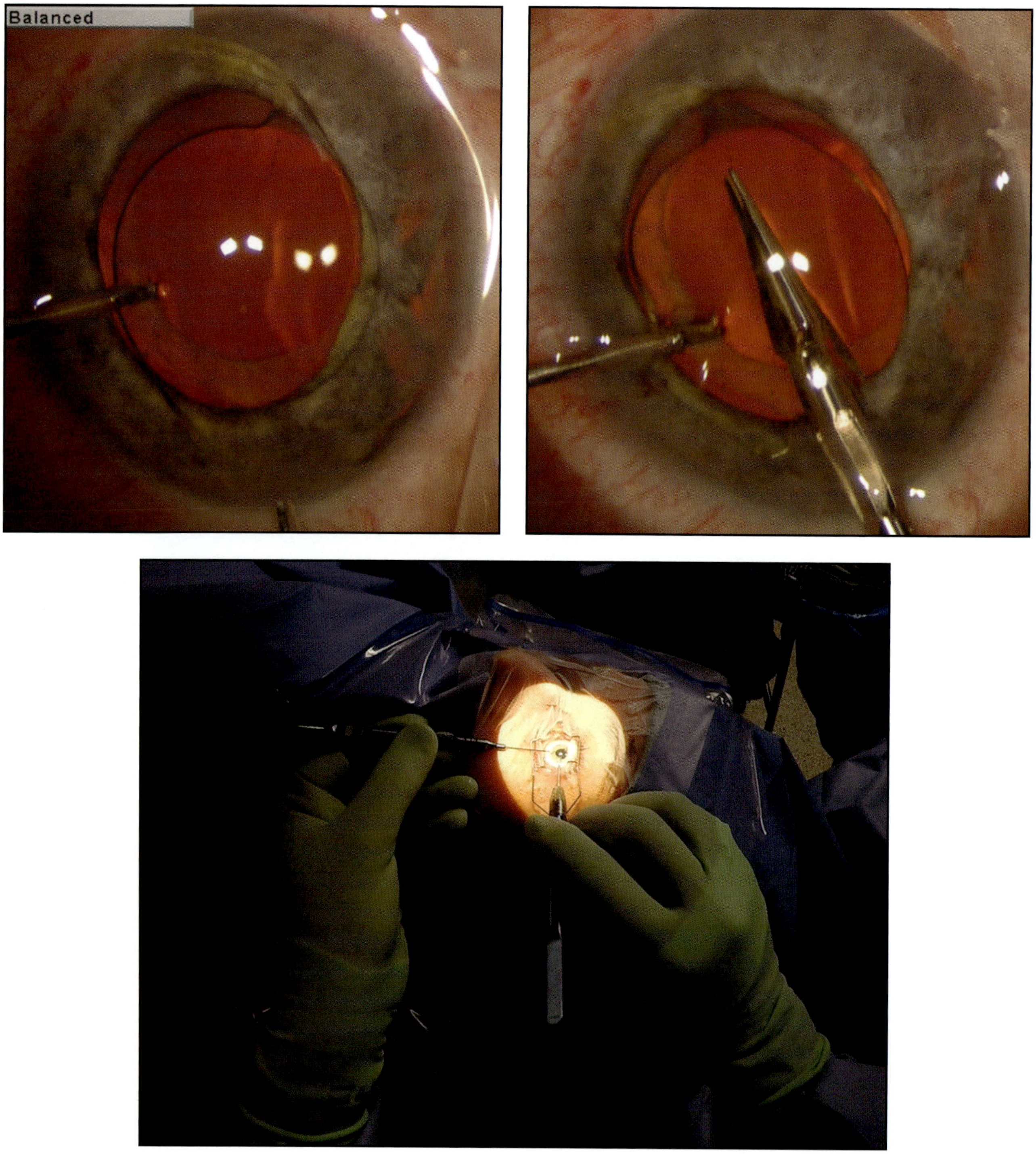

Using a microtyer, get a firm hold on the IOL optic. To prevent IOL tilting, maintain the microtyer shaft parallel to the iris plane at all times. For this, hand position is crucial—stay low. This will help prevent IOL tilting. The best way to ensure that the IOL is being cut into 2 halves of similar size is to cut from proximal to distal optic-haptic junctions. When cutting, expect some torque from the scissors, which will tilt the optic counterclockwise on the scissor shaft axis. This can be counteracted by keeping a low hand position with the opposite instrument, the microtyer.

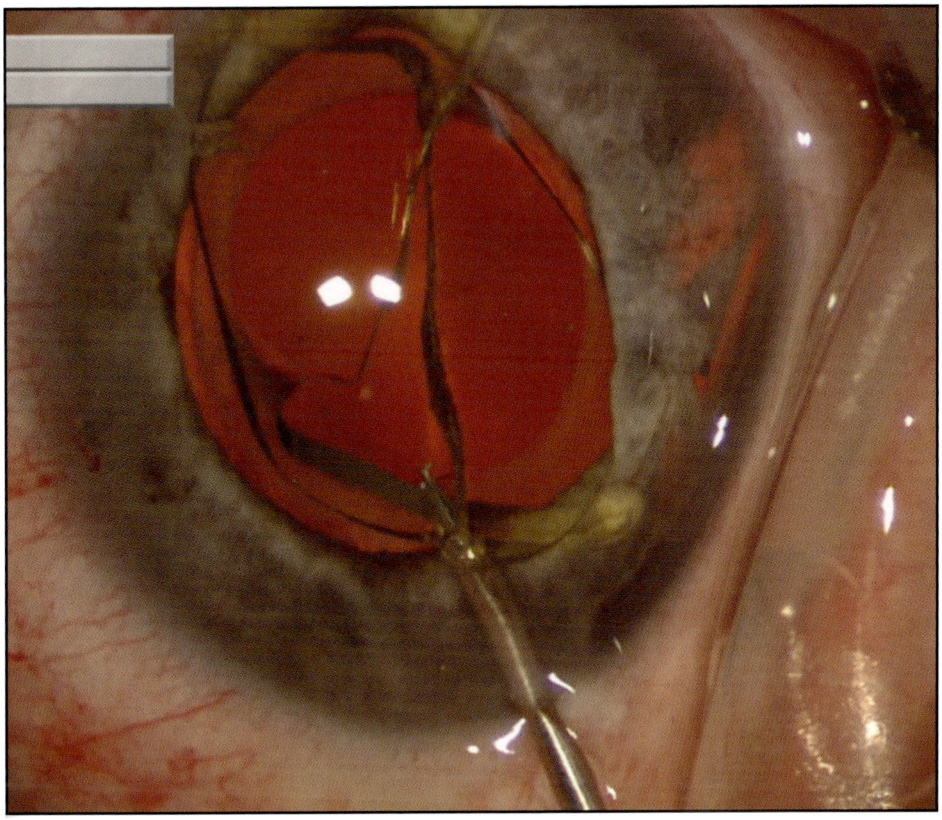

To explant the IOL halves from the anterior chamber, pull on the haptic with a microtyer and then switch to a stronger forceps, such as a Colibri or McPherson, to avoid damaging your microinstruments. For the second half, rotate the piece around such that the second haptic is again oriented toward the temporal corneal incision. It is always easier to explant the halves in this direction

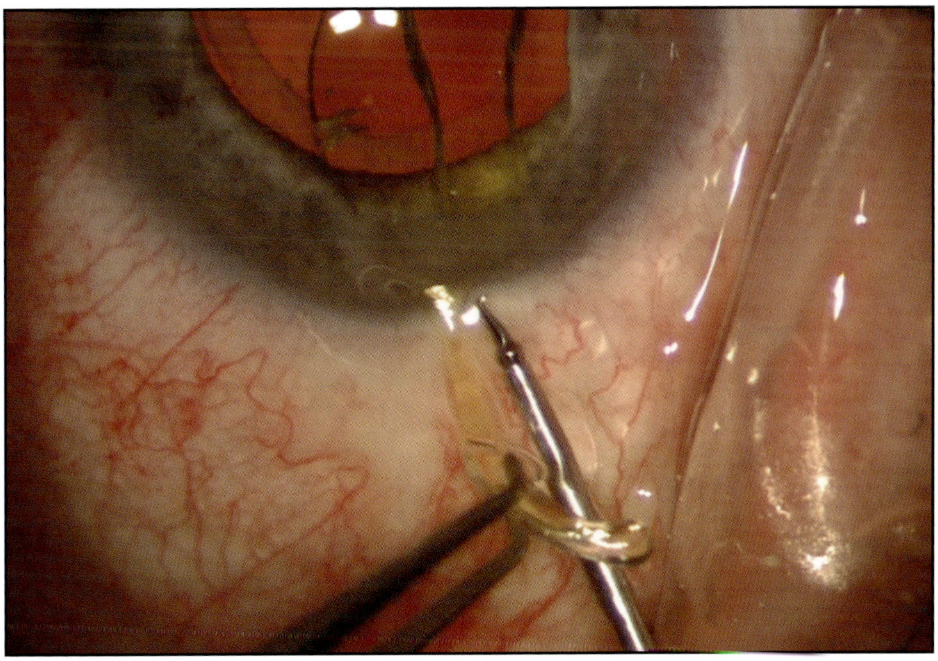

CHAPTER 25

HOW TO REPOSITION AN INTRAOCULAR LENS BY SCLERAL SUTURING

INTRODUCTION

Intraocular lens (IOL) dislocation can occur "in-the-bag" or "out-of-the-bag." This is the single most important distinction. "In-the-bag" IOLs can be suture-loop fixated to sclera, as we will discuss in this chapter. Even single-piece acrylic IOLs can be scleral-fixated this way. Numerous techniques exist to reposition a dislocated IOL. When an IOL is within an intact capsule and the entire IOL-capsule complex has dislocated, repositioning by means of scleral suturing is an option. This technique works for single- or 3-piece IOLs composed of any material.

KEY POINTS

- The fibrotic capsular bag is what holds the suture around the haptics and prevents the suture from sliding off.
- The suture loop should go as close to the optic-haptic junction as possible.
- DO NOT OVERTIGHTEN sutures. This can strip the suture off of the IOL haptic.
- Measuring from scleral spur (where the blue meets the white on the sclera) is key in determining where the IOL will be sutured to the scleral wall. This is the most consistent anatomical landmark. For example, a long eye will have a more posteriorly positioned ciliary body. Measuring from the limbus as the landmark can invariably lead to placing the sutures near or through the ciliary body. This can lead to vitreous hemorrhage and/or uveal chafing.

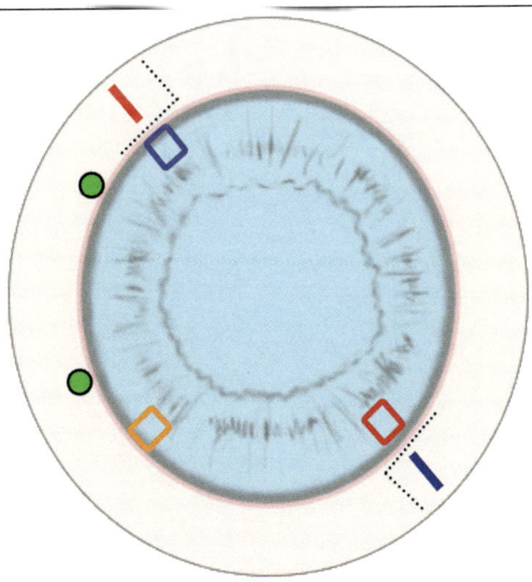

- Knife and fork with additional paracentesis across from the main incision
- L-shaped conjunctival peritomy
- Partial-thickness scleral groove
- Incisions for iris hooks

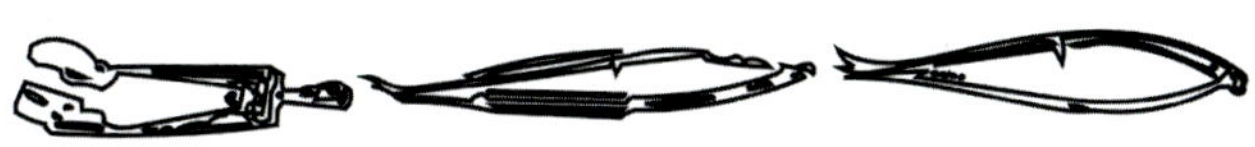

- Microsurgical Technology, Inc microforceps set
- Double-armed Gore-Tex 7-0 suture on CV-8
- 0.5-inch, 25-g hypodermic needle for docking the Gore-Tex suture

  or
- 0.5-inch, 27-g hypodermic needle to dock 9-0 or 10-0 Prolene (Ethicon, Inc) microneedle to dock

Ahmed IK, Campos-Möller X, Shah M, Sheybani A. *Illustrated Advanced Anterior Segment Surgery: A Step-by-Step Guide for Challenging Cases* (pp 185-193).

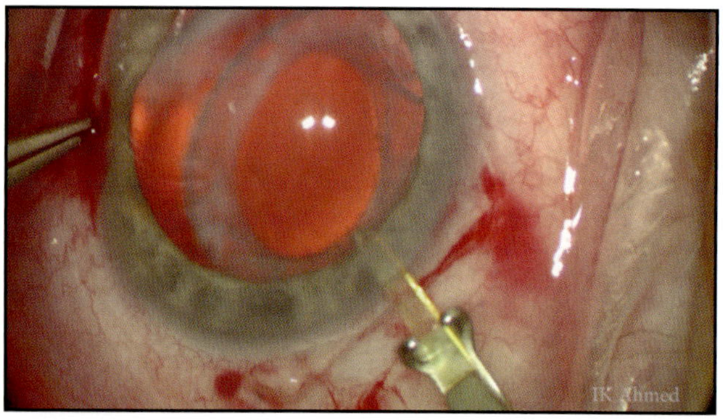

- Use dispersive ophthalmic viscosurgical device to protect the corneal endothelium and to tamponade vitreous in areas of potential prolapse.
- Identify the haptic-optic IOL junctions with a Kuglen hook in order to determine where the scleral suture passes will occur.
- Two conjunctival peritomies are performed 180 degrees apart; location should be adjusted to the clock hour of the IOL optic-haptic junction.

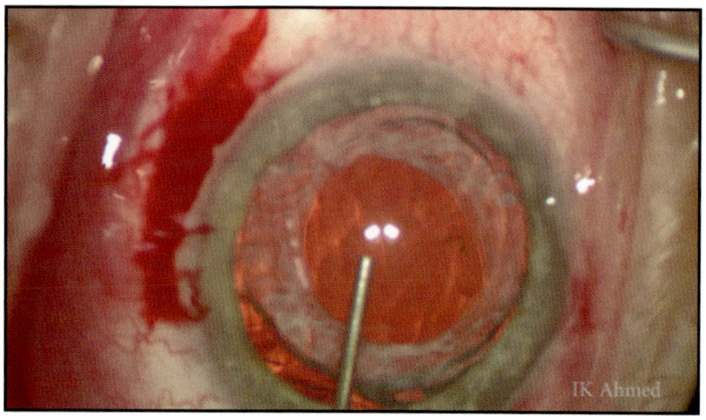

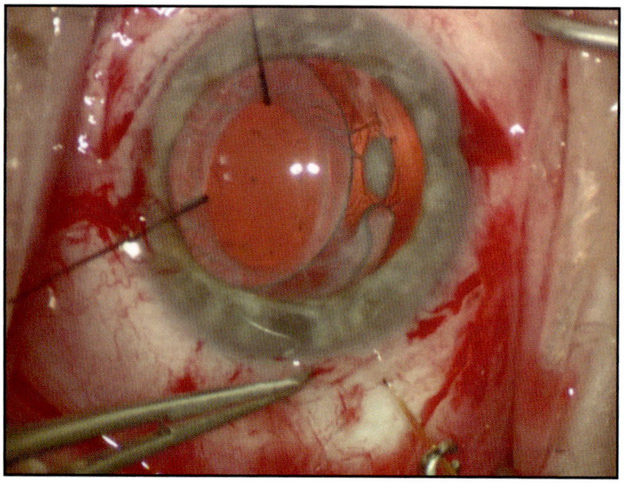

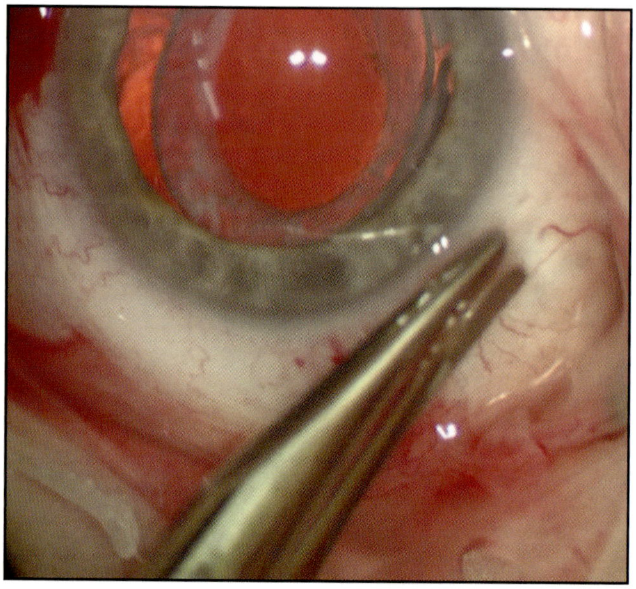

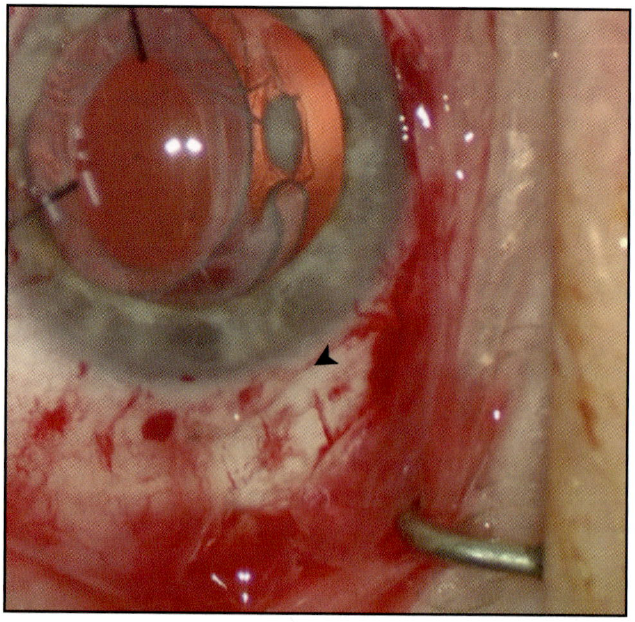

- Create paired radial scleral scratch incisions in line with the intended location for scleral fixation, corresponding to the desired optic-haptic junction positions. The incisions should begin 1 mm posterior to the scleral spur (arrowhead), extend 2.5 mm posteriorly, and be only 10% to 20% thickness.

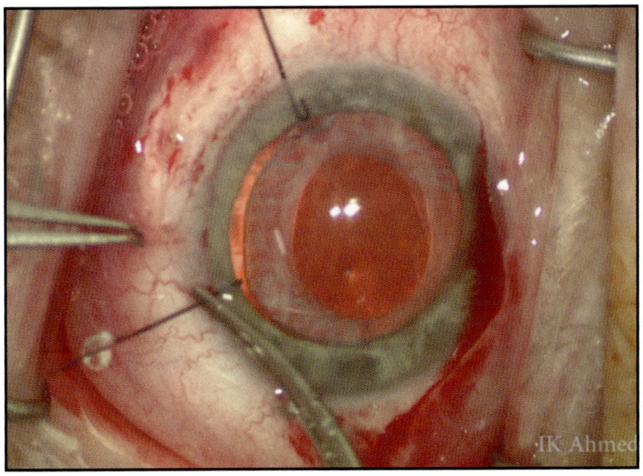

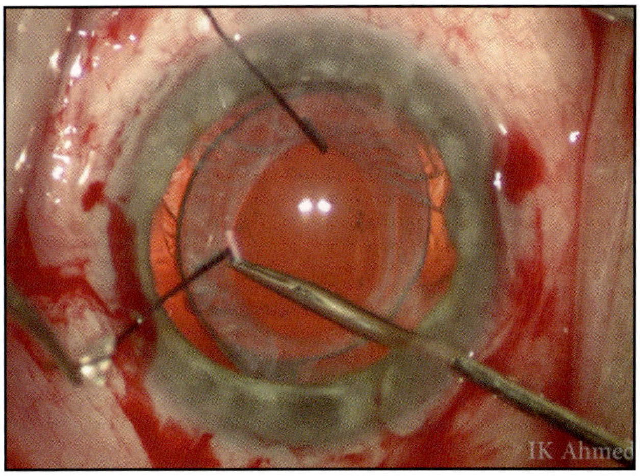

Iris hooks can be placed on the capsulorrhexis edge opposite to the side of planned scleral fixation to stabilize the IOL-bag complex. A micrograsper may be used to facilitate this step by grabbing the capsule and handing it to the iris hook held by the other hand. Do not overtighten these.

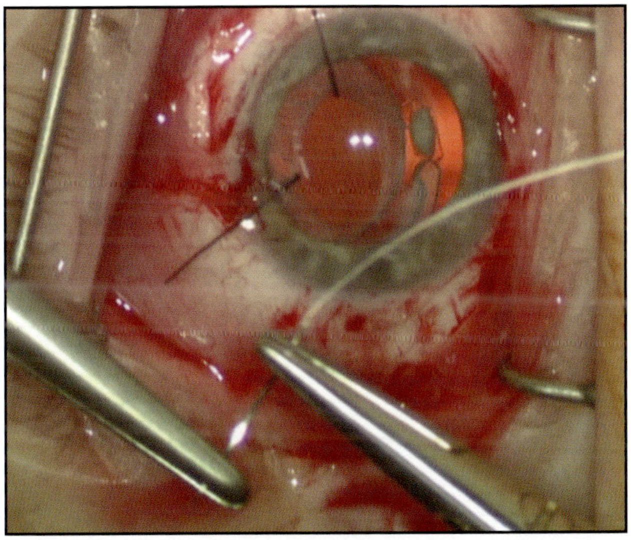

The curved Gore-Tex needle is straightened by 2 heavy needle drivers with a hand-over-hand technique.

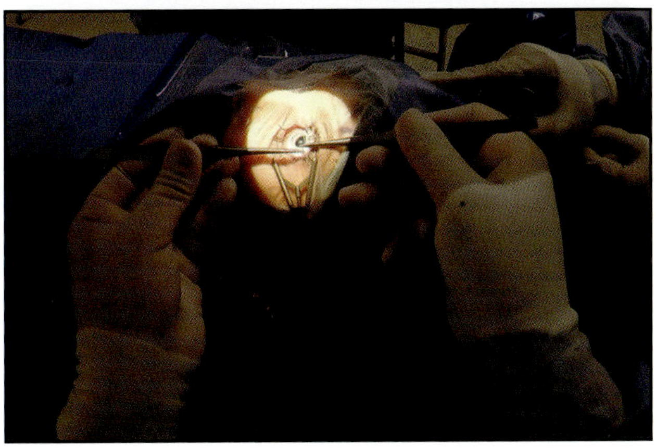

Hand-over-hand technique; notice assistant keeping Gore-Tex suture from falling off the surgical field. The suture is not designed for ophthalmology and is very long.

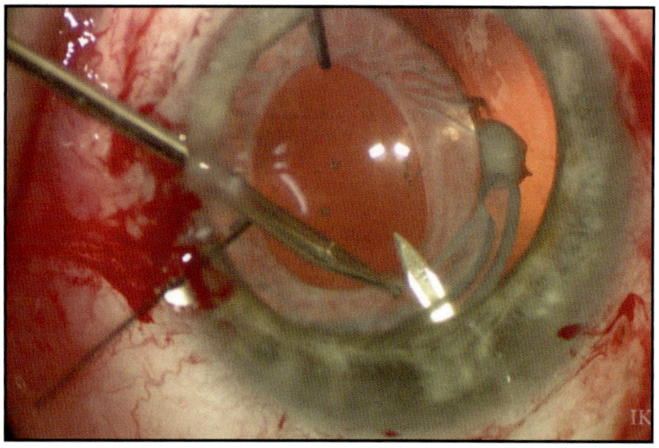

The 25-gauge docking needle is inserted through the posterior portion of the scleral scratch incision (about 3 to 3.5 mm back from the spur). The initial direction of needle entry should be perpendicular to sclera, but upon entry into the eye, the direction should turn to be parallel to the iris plane (Figures 1 and 2 on p 189).

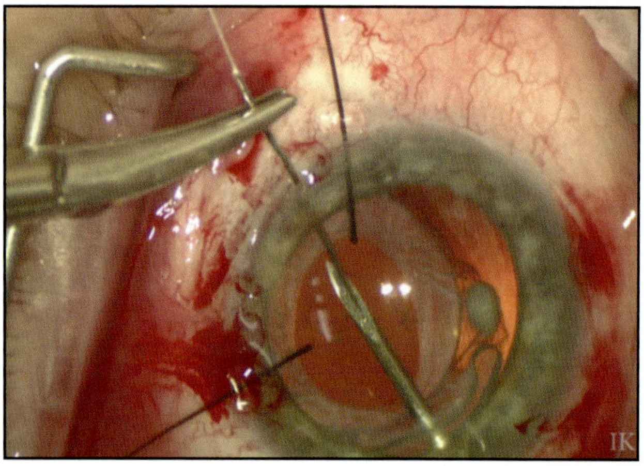

The needle should pass through the fused capsule, right at the "armpit" of the optic-haptic junction. A micrograsper can be useful to help position the needle here. Sometimes it is beneficial to pre-place the Gore-Tex needle into an opposing paracentesis incision in preparation for docking. Be sure not to engage any corneal fibers with suture passage—each needle should pass freely into the anterior chamber through the paracentesis incision. Remove the needle by withdrawing the docking needle carefully as to not torque the needle inside the eye. Avoid any lateral motion as this can tear the capsule and increase the risk of the suture cheese-wiring.

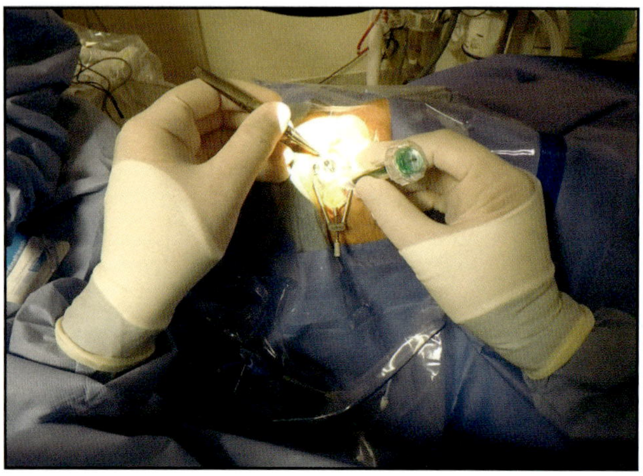

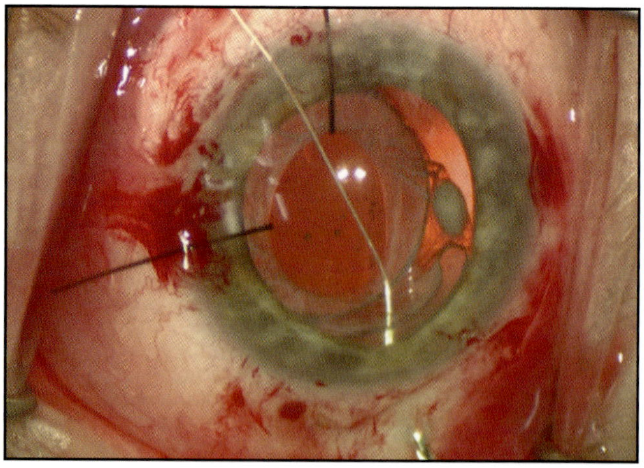

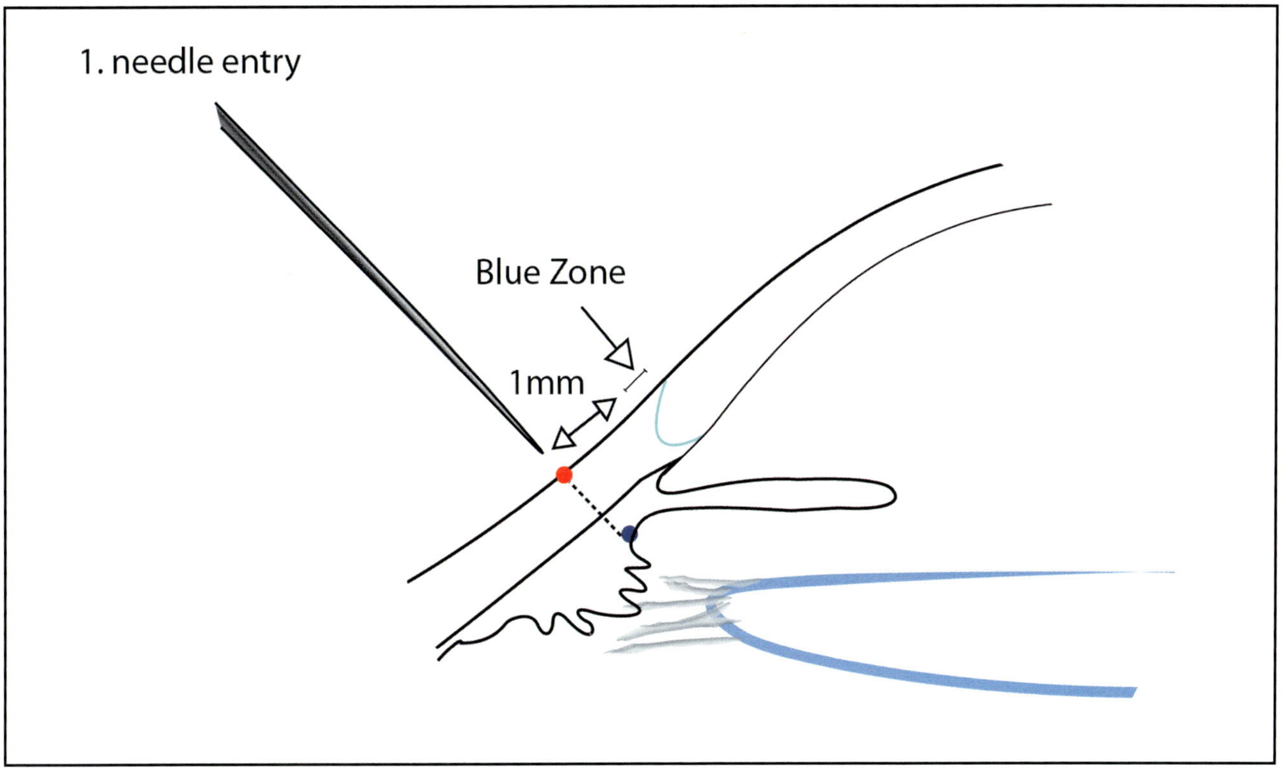

Diagram of needle entry and angle change for sulcus fixation. Needle entry should be done perpendicular to the sclera, 1 mm posterior to the end of the blue zone (corresponding to the corneal wedge). Once the needle has advanced into the scleral thickness, a 45-degree angle change should be carried out in order to enter the ciliary sulcus parallel to the iris plane (dotted arrow).

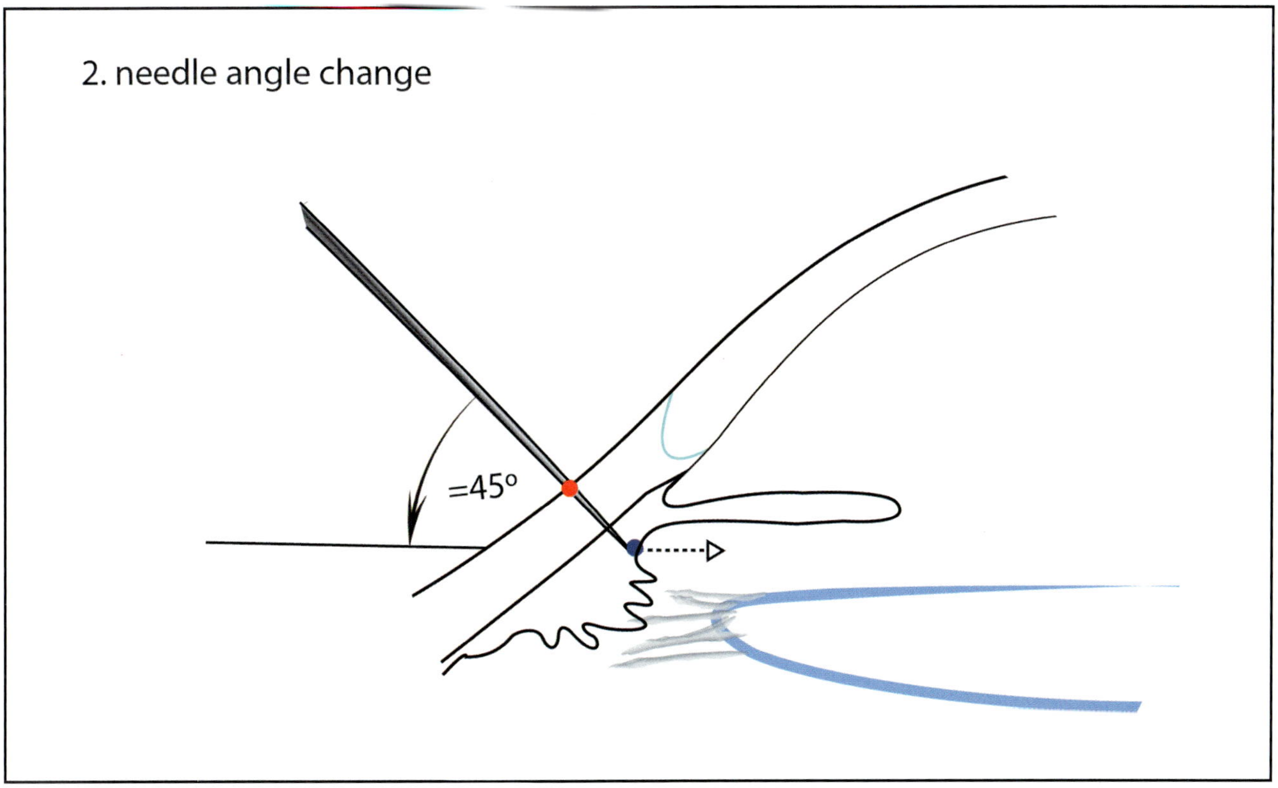

- The second pass of the 25-g needle is made 1 mm posterior to the scleral spur (at the anterior portion of the scleral scratch incision).
- This time, the needle is maneuvered above the IOL/bag complex and under the iris. The change in direction of the 25-g needle is even more pronounced with the second pass.
- Dock the Gore-Tex needle in similar fashion.

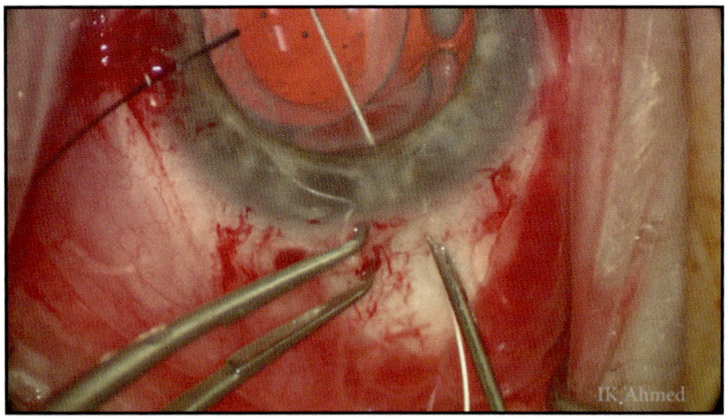

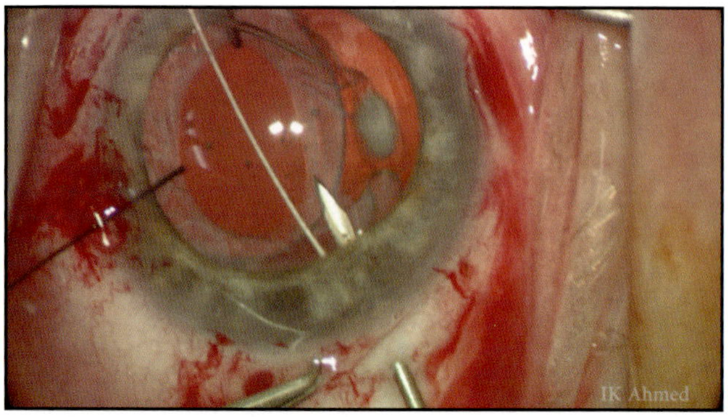

Withdrawing the needle makes a loop of suture around the haptic. Do not overtighten. Wait for the opposite haptic to be looped before centering the IOL. A Kuglen hook can be used to ensure adequate positioning of the loop.

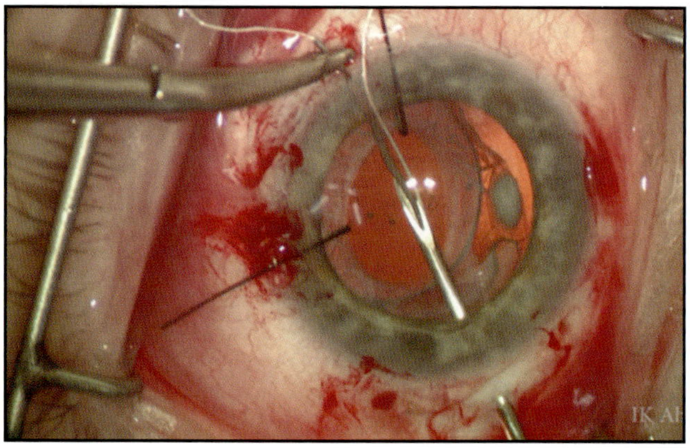

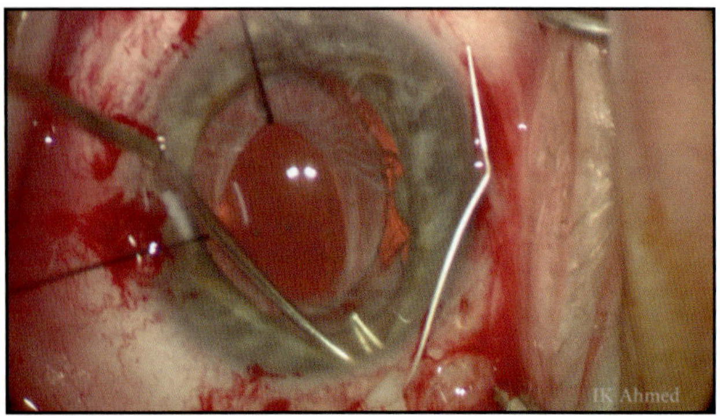

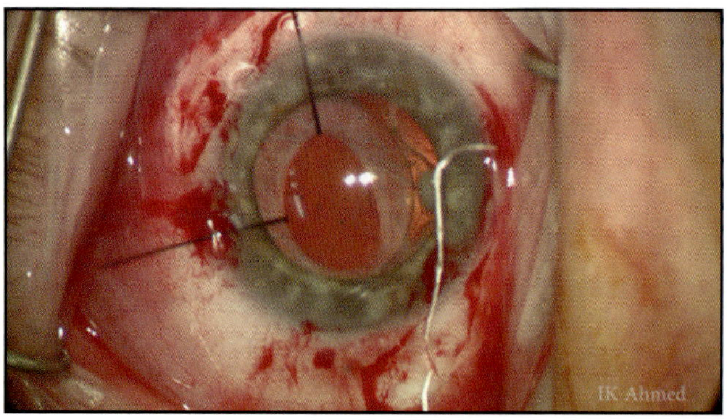

Tie with a slip knot without locking the knot so that final position can be checked after the opposing haptic is secured (see p 76 for slip knot diagram).

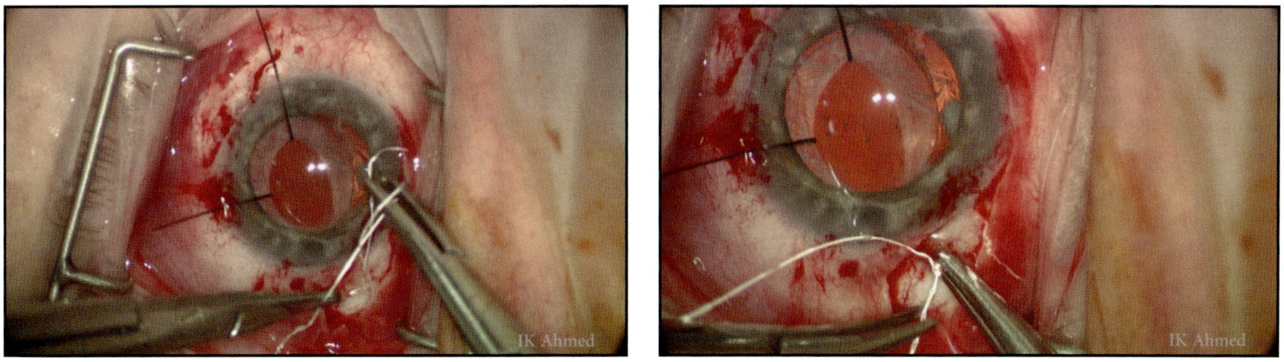

Perform the same scratch incision and suture loop technique 180 degrees apart from the first suture loop. A Kuglen hook can be used to provide countertraction when the capsule is difficult to pierce.

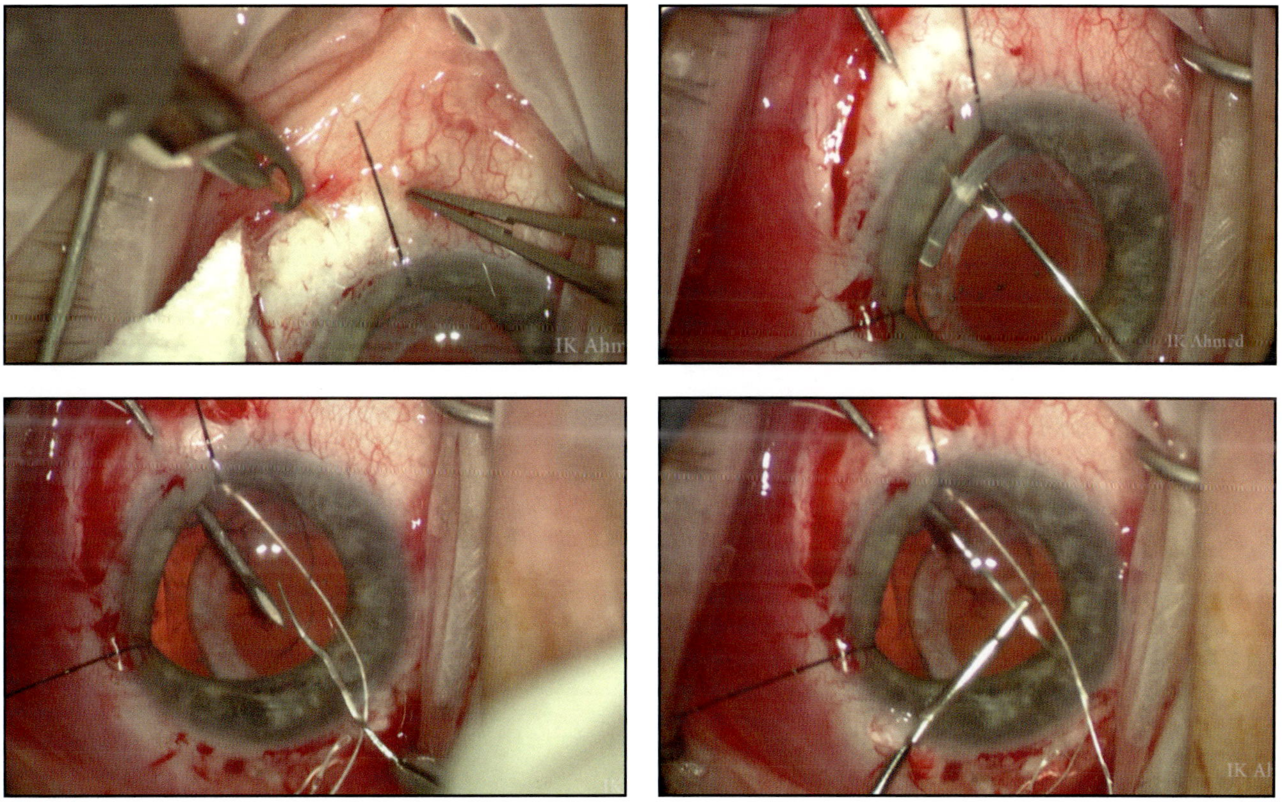

Sometimes a micrograsper can be used through a corneal incision to internally keep the Gore-Tex needle inside the docking needle as it is externalized.

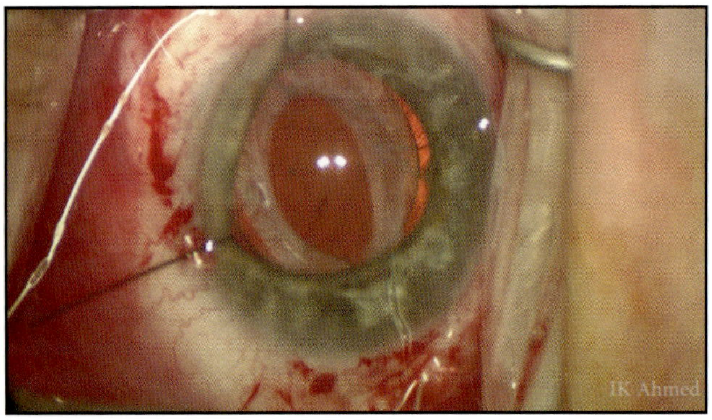

Now is the time to center the IOL by gently adjusting the slip knots on each side. Caution: It is better to go back and forth between knots because an overtightened knot can be very hard to loosen to recenter the IOL.

- Once the knots are locked, cut the tail short and rotate the knot internally. One arm of an open tying forceps can be used to push the knot into the sclerostomy.
- Miochol (acetylcholine) is placed and viscoelastic is removed manually with a 27-g cannula using balanced salt solution. Automated removal can destabilize the IOL or bring vitreous anteriorly.

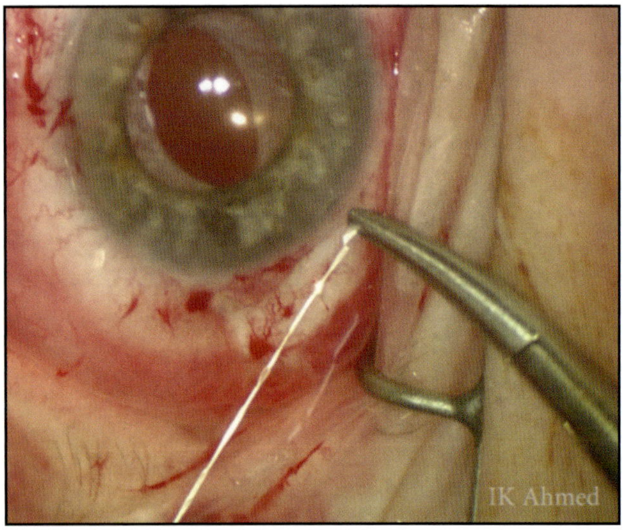

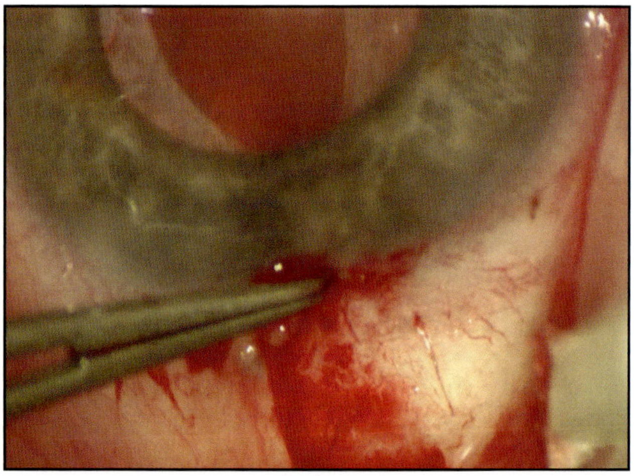

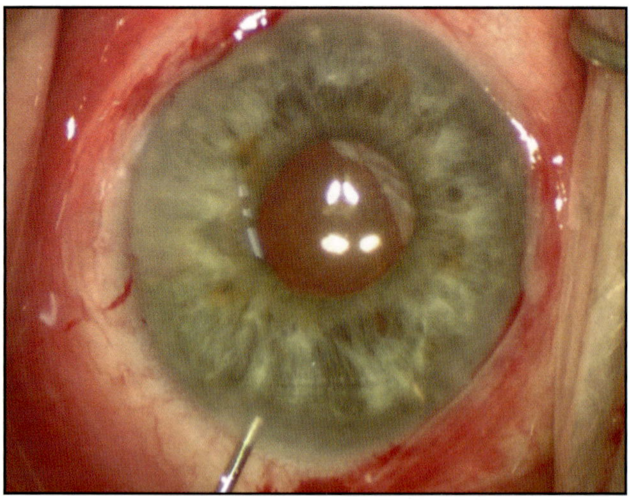

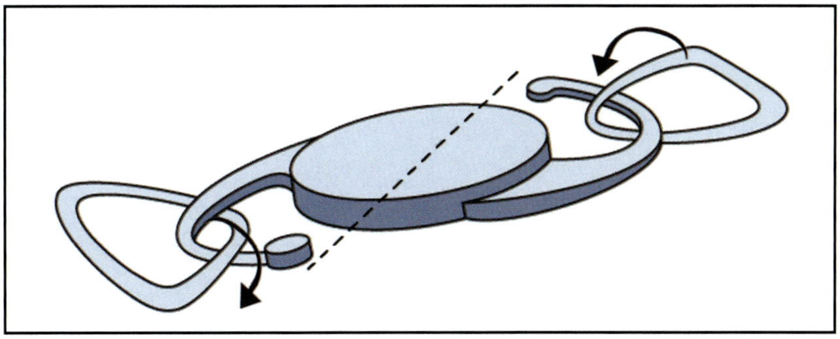

Suture configuration to avoid IOL tilt by balancing the torque generated by the direction of the suture passes.

Opposed direction of suture passes over-under the IOL haptic balances out the torque generated by the sutures and prevents tilt. Dotted line represents axis of rotation, arrows indicate direction of tilt induced by each suture.

A good way to remember this is to always pass the suture closest to the terminal bulb OVER the haptic, and the suture closest to the optic-haptic junction UNDER the haptic.

CHAPTER 26

HOW TO SUTURE IRIS

INTRODUCTION

Repairing iris is performed for several possible reasons. In some cases, it is for cosmesis; in others, it is for function (to improve light sensitivity); and in some cases, it is to create anterior chamber intraocular lens (IOL) support. There are many techniques depending on the situation. We will discuss basic suture and iris cautery principles here. In later chapters, we will discuss the technique in certain situations. The most important assessment occurs at the slit lamp—especially using gonioscopy—to determine the amount and condition of iris preoperatively.

KEY POINTS

- Use Miochol (acetylcholine) after intracameral anesthesia or a block is administered to bring the iris down. Do not start with a dilated pupil.
- Using micrograspers, determine how much iris tissue can be moved. Sometimes, 2 microtyers can be used to simulate what the tissue will look like when sutured by bringing 2 sections of iris together to determine if it will stretch far enough.
- Place a paracentesis 1 clock hour away from the initial place where suture will be passed through iris tissue.
- Do not overpressurize the chamber; it will overly deepen and make suturing difficult. Worse, it can cause the iris to cheese-wire through sutures once they are tied.
- Do not withdraw the docking cannula with the needle inside—it is less controlled and the needle can torque inside the eye. Instead, once the needle is docked, gently push the needle from the opposing corneal wound while the docking cannula is minimally withdrawn. Then disengage the needle from within the cannula and use needle drivers to guide the needle out of the eye.
- Iris cautery can be used to shrink the iris tissue in order to "move" the sphincter or pupillary center toward the area of cautery. It can also be used to focally draw iris toward where one cauterizes to round out sphincter edges for cosmesis.

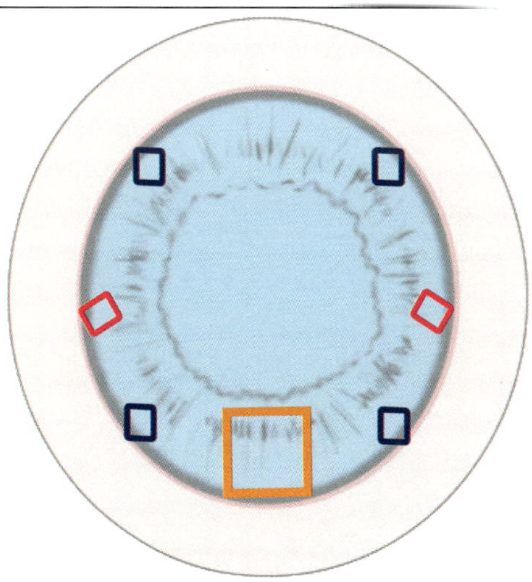

- Knife and fork with additional paracentesis to allow for needle docking

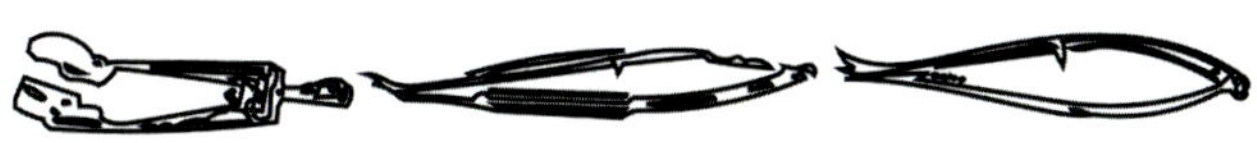

- Microsurgical Technology, Inc micrograsper and microtyer
- Microsurgical Technology, Inc intraocular scissors
- 10-0 polypropylene on a CIF-4 or PC-7 needle
- Fine bipolar cautery (pencil-tip)
- 27-g cannula

Ahmed IK, Campos-Möller X, Shah M, Sheybani A. *Illustrated Advanced Anterior Segment Surgery: A Step-by-Step Guide for Challenging Cases* (pp 195-205).

THE SIEPSER SLIDING KNOT

The Siepser sliding knot offers the advantage of laying a knot on iris tissue without disturbing the tissue (having to draw it to a paracentesis like in McCannel suturing), yet does not require microinstrumentation. It is more time consuming than the other techniques described and has a steeper learning curve (see http://www.ncbi.nlm.nih.gov/pubmed/7944159).

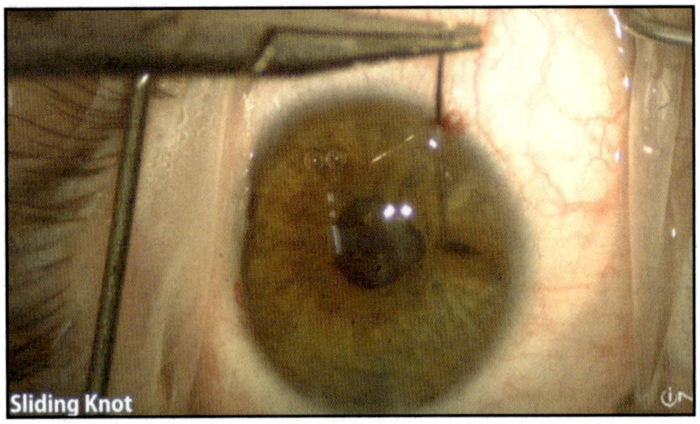

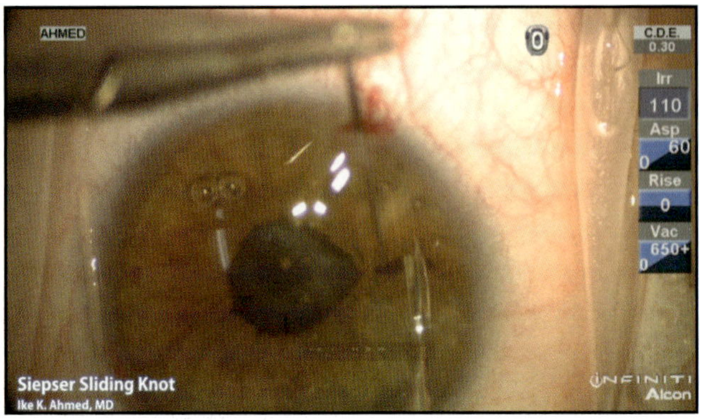

Two opposing paracenteses are created for the needle passes. An imaginary line from one incision to the other should be approximately at 90 degrees from the defect and bisect it in half. Sometimes, these paracenteses will be more peripheral than others, and this will depend on the localization and extent of the defect. The 10-0 polypropylene suture needle is inserted into the distal paracentesis by "wiggling" it back and forth to avoid catching stromal fibers. A micrograsper is used to hold the iris, through which the needle will pass. Once the second pass is made, a 27-g cannula is inserted through the opposing paracentesis and used to dock the needle. To guide the needle out of the eye, a combination of "push and pull" is done with the needle driver and the 27-g cannula. Do not only pull, as the needle may come out of the cannula. Do not only push, as this will create excessive downward force on the cornea, iris, and possibly lens.

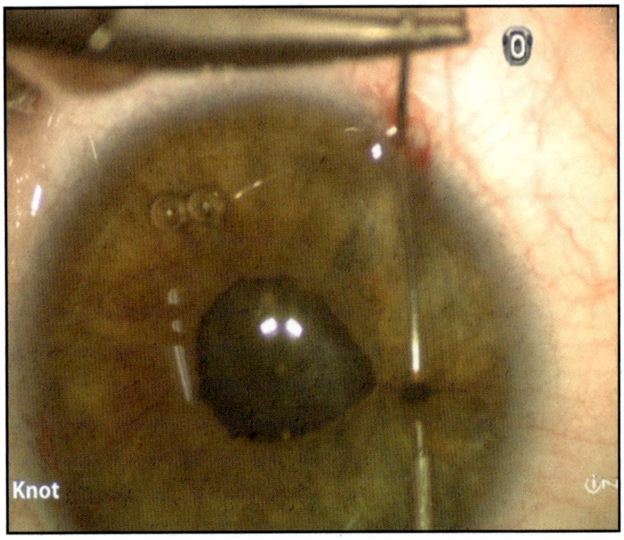

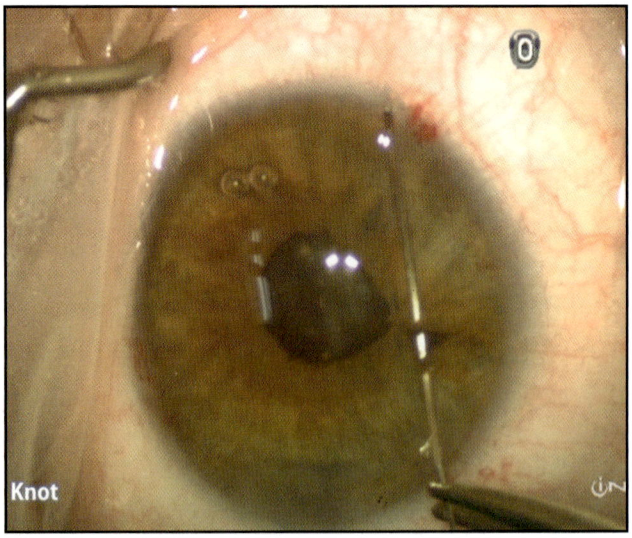

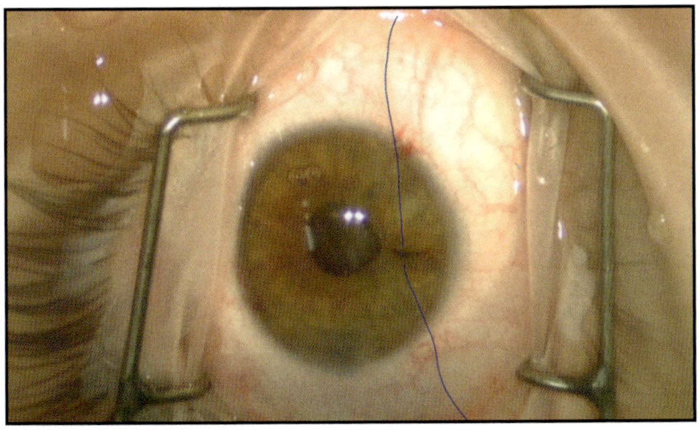

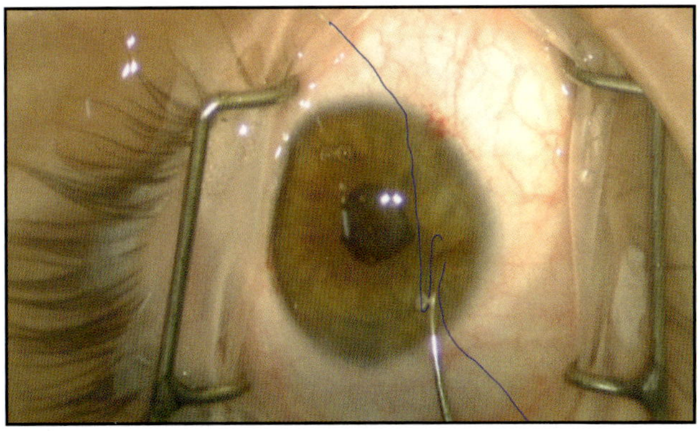

There is a proximal and distal strand. A Kuglen hook is used through the proximal paracentesis, hooking around the suture near the distal paracentesis. The suture is pulled out of the eye through the proximal paracentesis, creating a loop of suture. The loop has one side that is going through iris, and another that is going through the distal paracentesis. Tugging on the 2 sides of the loop will help identify them. It is key to have them properly identified before starting any suturing maneuver.

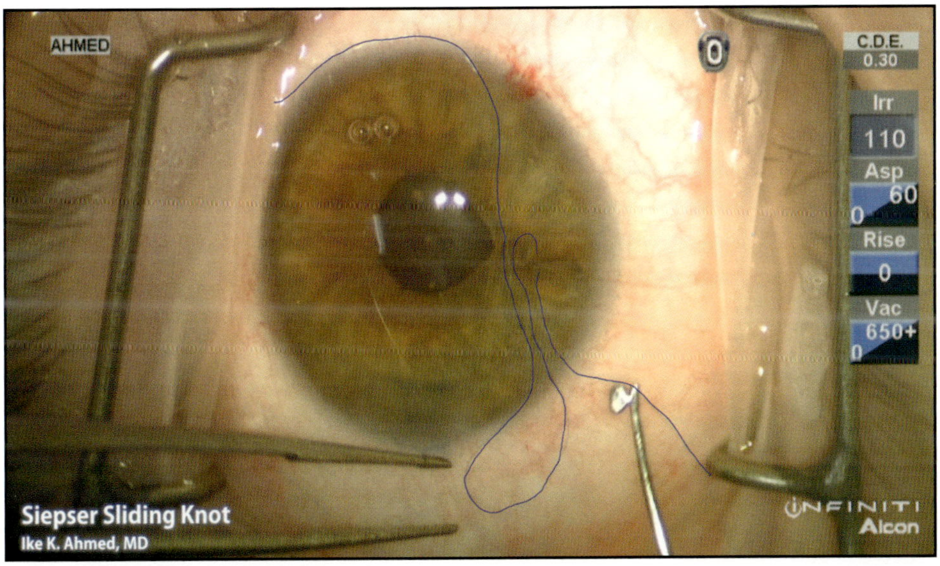

Cut the proximal strand short. Use tying forceps to triple throw distal strand 1 around another pair of tyers.

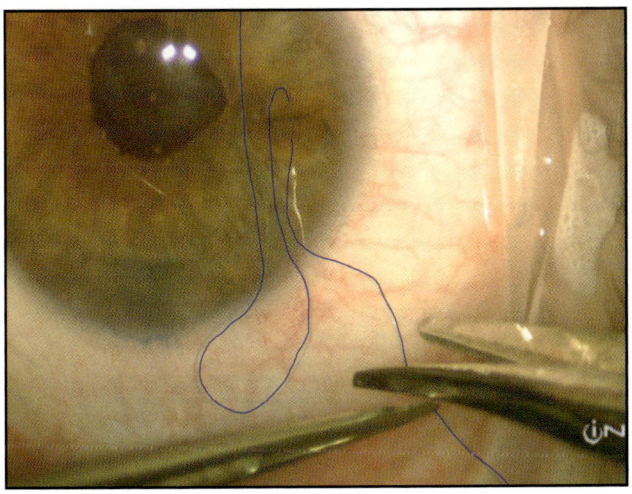

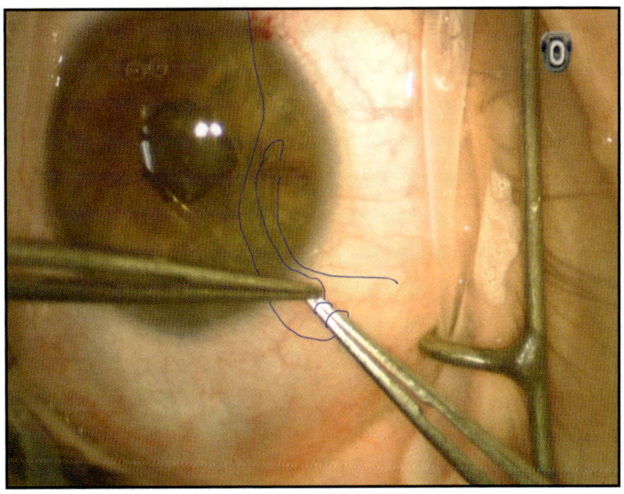

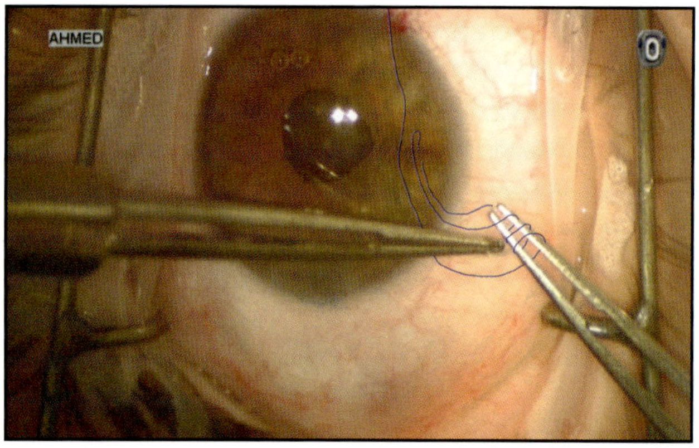

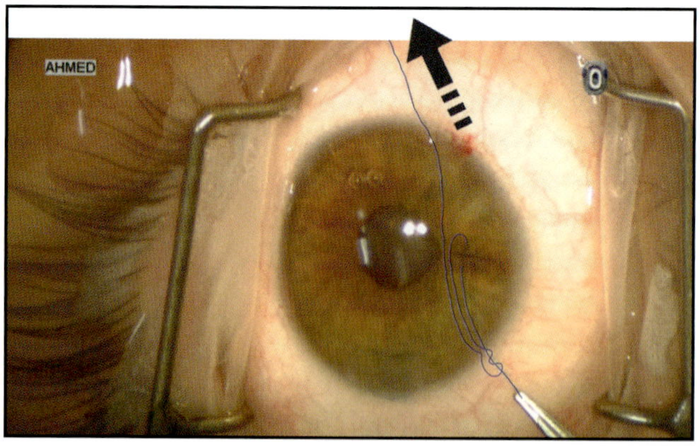

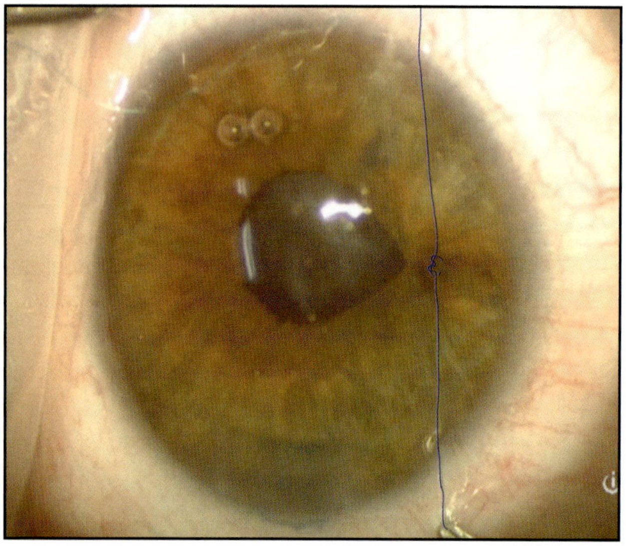

Then grab the proximal strand (strand #3) with the tyers that have the triple throw around them.

With the other pair of tyers (left hand in image), grab the distal strand close to the distal paracentesis and pull to slide the knot into the eye. DO NOT PULL ON THE PROXIMAL END as this can air-lock the knot.

Repeat creating a loop, using a single throw but looping the suture in the opposite direction as the first triple throw to lock the knot. A third time around, a single throw in the same direction as the first triple throw will finish locking the suture. Cut the suture with intraocular scissors just above the knot. If microscissors are not available, a 25-g needle can be used to cut the sutures as well.

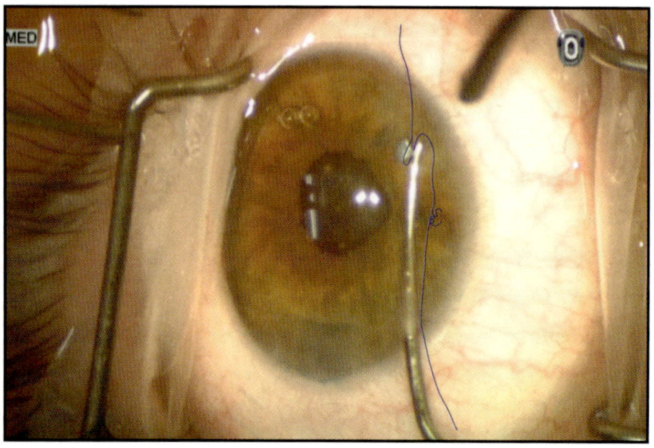

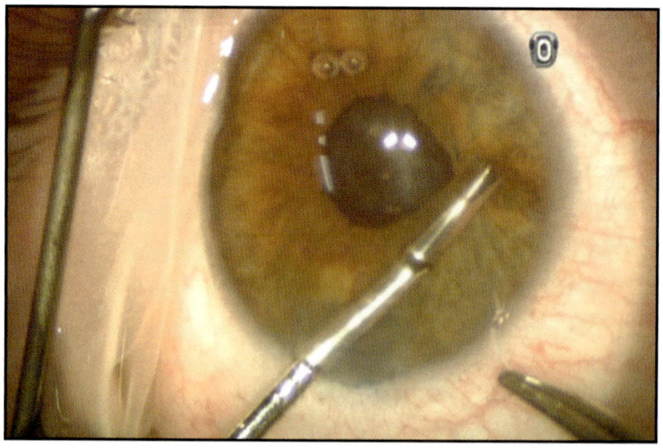

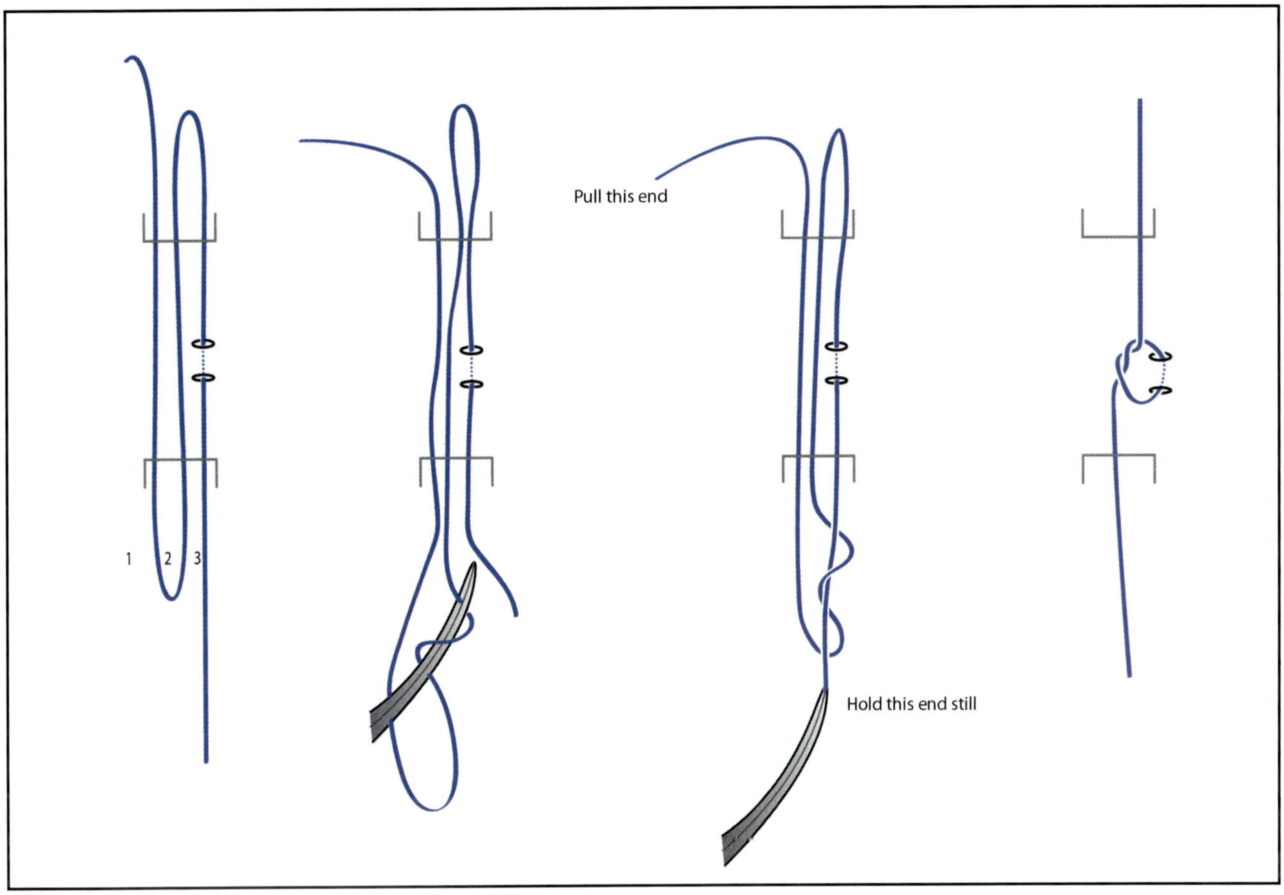
Pull this end
1
2
3
Hold this end still

THE AHMED KNOT OR MODIFIED MCCANNEL KNOT

This technique is a modification of the technique described by McCannel in (see http://www.ncbi.nlm.nih.gov/pubmed/778720). This requires microtying instruments to draw the knot over iris tissue. It is conceptually simpler than the Siepser sliding knot and does not disturb iris tissue. This is our preferred way to suture iris tissue.

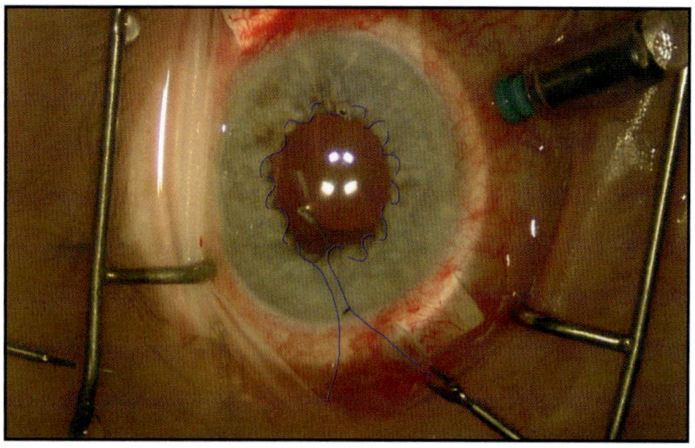

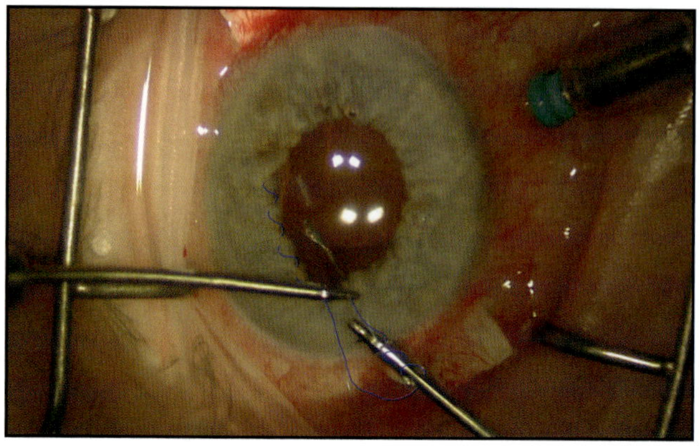

After suture passes through iris are made (in this case, a pupil cerclage, but the technique can be used for a simple iris defect repair as well) as above, both ends of the suture are withdrawn through the same wound using a Kuglen hook. A tyer (or microtyer in this case) in the nondominant hand is used to throw 2 or 3 loops around a curved microtyer.

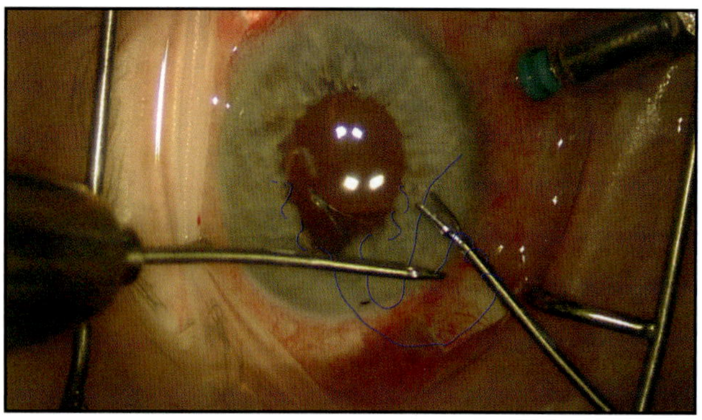

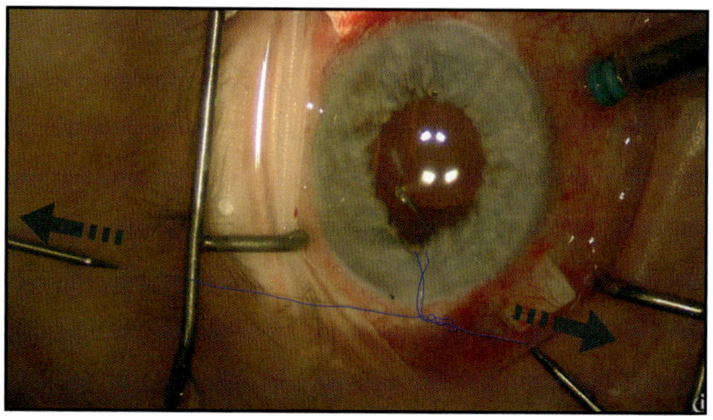

One suture end is held outside the eye with a tying forceps, while the other is introduced into the eye with a microtyer. This way, the pupil is not overly traumatized as in a traditional McCannel suture as the iris remains in place and the knot is brought over the area of suture pass.

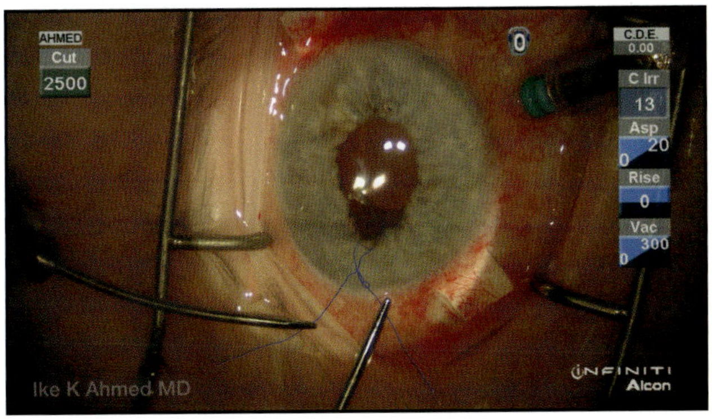

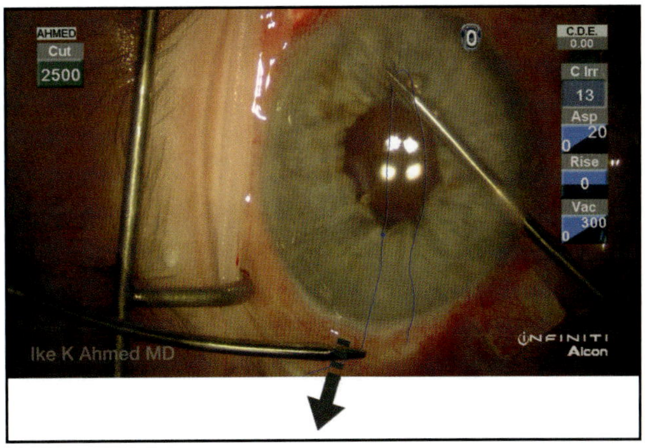

These steps are repeated for 2 more single throws, performing the loop in the opposite direction each time, to end up with a 3-1-1 knot configuration. Finally, the suture is cut with the aid of microscissors.

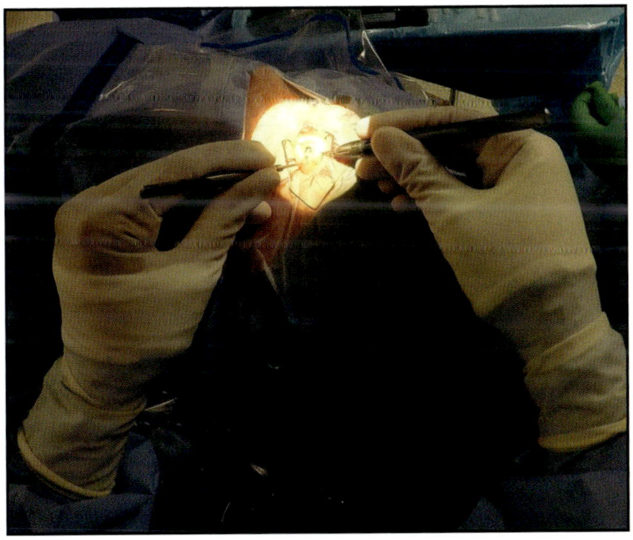

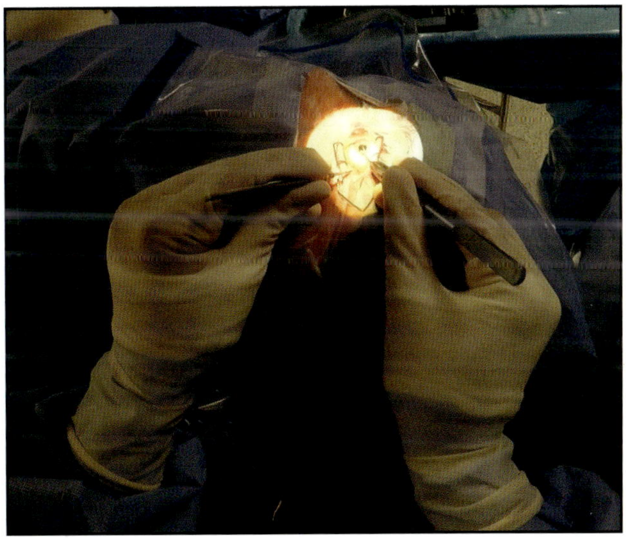

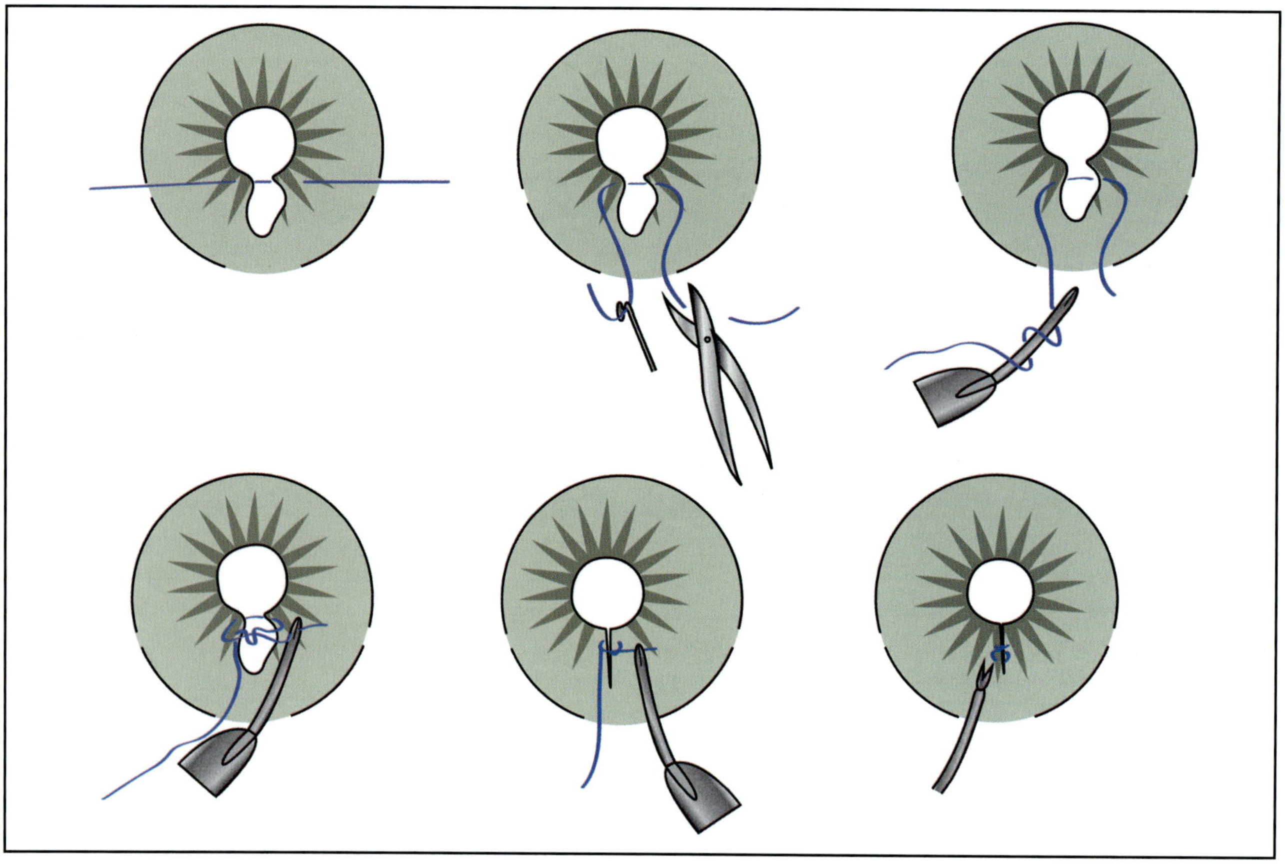

INTRAOCULAR KNOT TECHNIQUE

Intraocular tying seems challenging; however, with 2 microtying instruments, it can be performed without much difficulty. The key is to create paracentesis incisions that are wide enough to allow for proper movement of the instruments (approximately 2 mm). The long arm of the suture should remain outside the eye while the short arm should be 3 to 5 mm internally; otherwise, there will be too much suture in the anterior chamber. Ensure a clear view by using dispersive viscoelastic to sweep liberated iris pigment out of the surgeon's view.

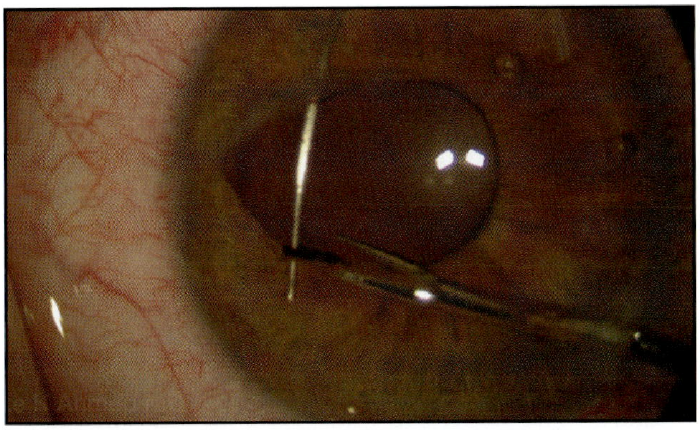

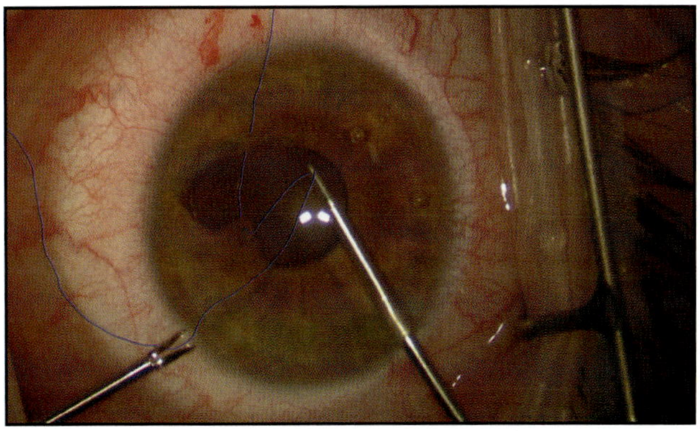

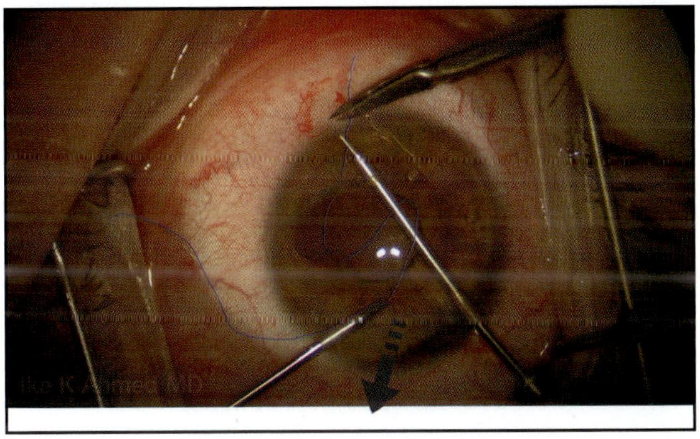

Once the suture is placed through iris tissue, the surgeon should plan on having a long arm and short arm of suture. Leaving the long arm near the nondominant hand can make tying the knot easier. The long arm will remain external to the eye through the paracentesis through which the suture was originally passed. Otherwise, a Sinskey hook can be used to retrieve the long arm through an incision closer to the surgeon's nondominant hand. TAKE CARE NOT TO PULL THE OPPOSING SUTURE OUT OF THE IRIS AS THE LONG ARM IS MANIPULATED. To create the short arm, cut the end opposite the long arm outside the eye near a paracentesis with Westcott scissors. Slowly draw the short arm into the eye by pulling on the long arm of the suture external to the eye.

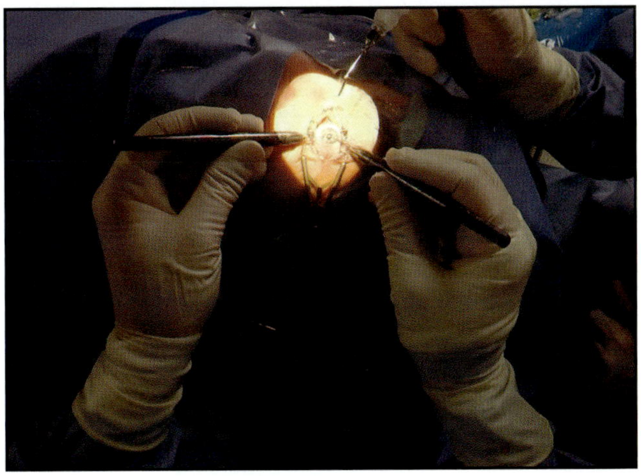

Two microtying forceps are placed through 2 opposing paracentesis incisions—knife and fork configuration is optimal. Arranging the short arm of the suture 90 degrees apart from the long arm, pointing up, can make grabbing this suture tail easier once the loops of the knot are created. This can be done with the microtyers or a Kuglen hook. The cohesive viscoelastic helps maintain this configuration. The nondominant hand loops the long arm of the suture around the microtyer in the dominant hand.

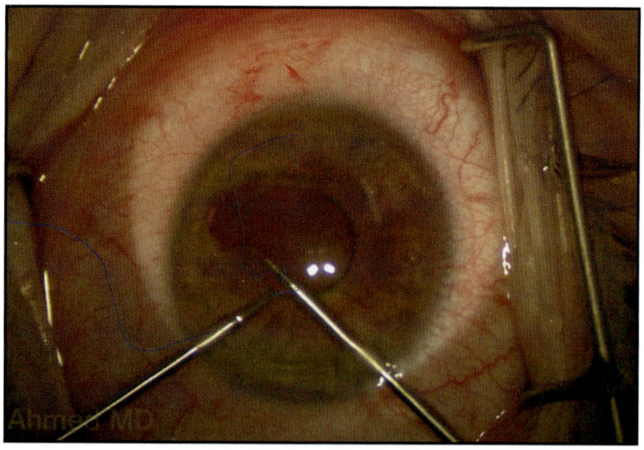

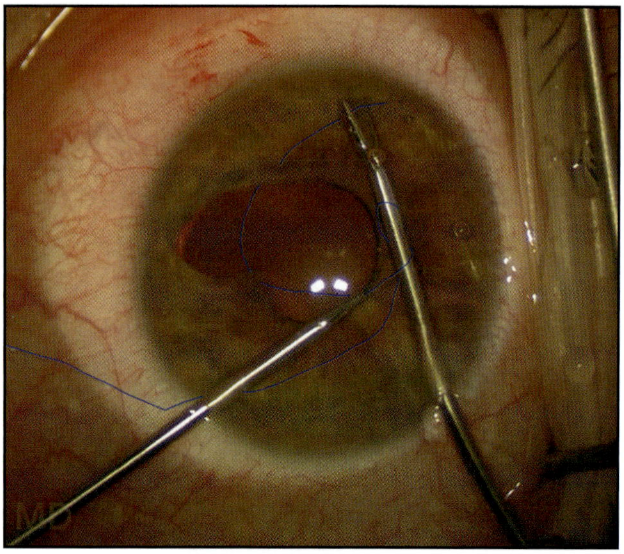

The dominant hand then grasps the short arm of the suture. Pull the long arm microtyers outward through the paracentesis incisions until the loop of the suture is laid down over the tissue. Pulling the long arm by grabbing the externalized portion of this suture while HOLDING the short arm STATIONARY allows for minimal tissue disruption. The short arm can also be returned to its position, as was previously described in preparation for the locking throws. The loop is then recreated and laid over the knot by repeating the steps above. The knot is then cut with intraocular scissors. Make sure the short arm is retrieved, holding it with microtying forceps while it is cut to facilitate retrieval.

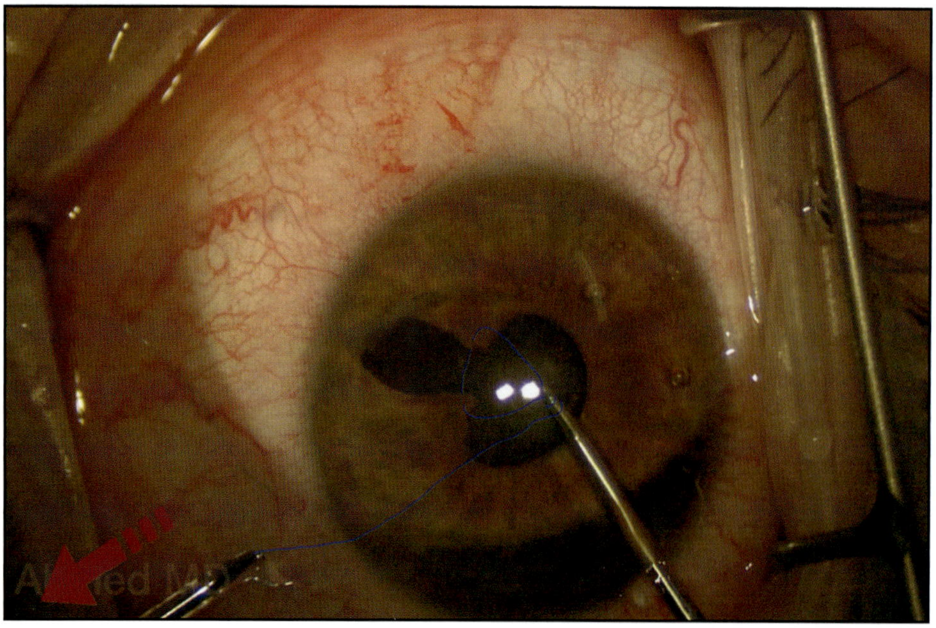

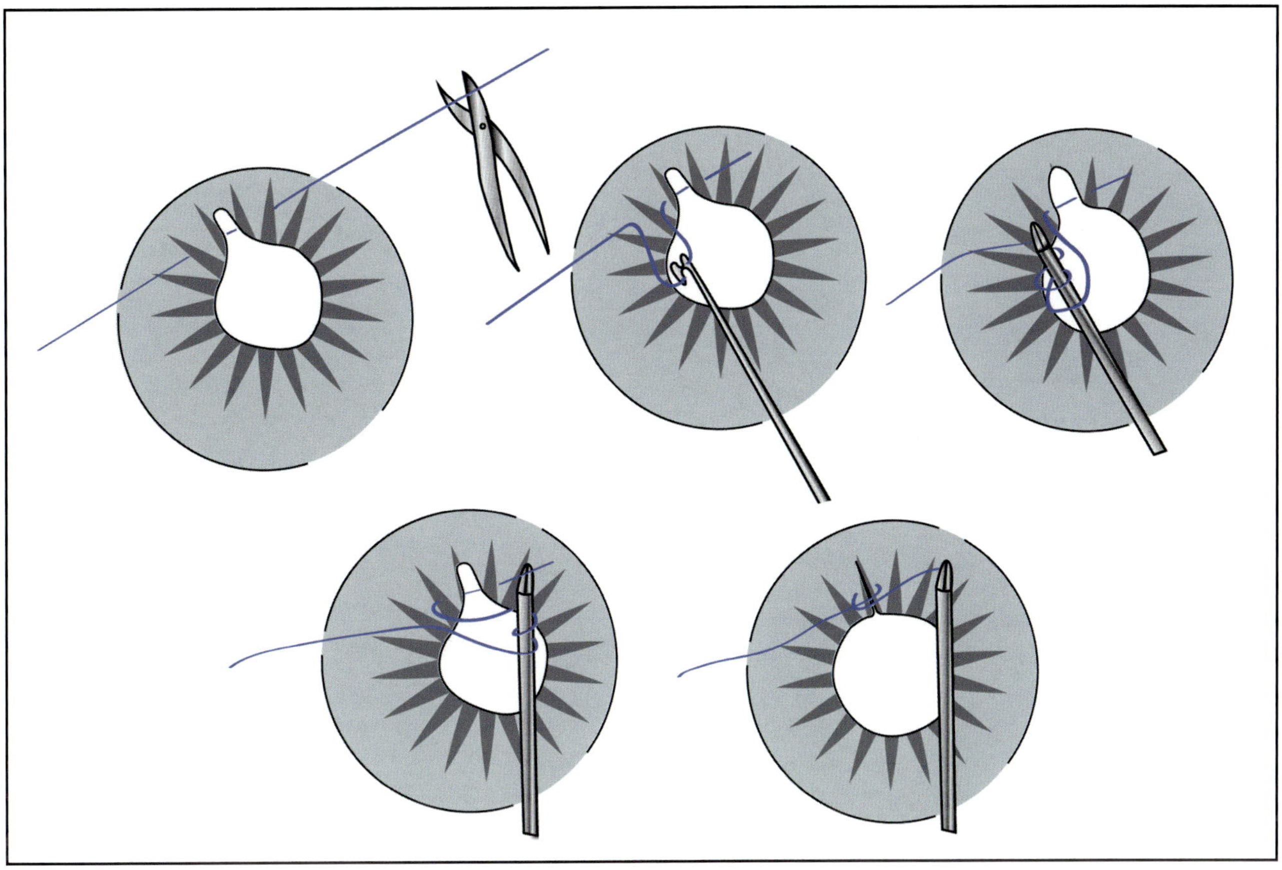

CHAPTER 27

HOW TO PERFORM GONIOSYNECHIALYSIS

INTRODUCTION

This technique gently separates peripheral anterior synechiae from the angle. It can be used to improve outflow through the trabecular meshwork, or it can be used to free iris tissue when iris repairs are performed. Advantages of the technique described here stem from angle visualization during the procedure. This can limit hemorrhage and help the surgeon ensure that iris tissue is minimally traumatized as the peripheral and not central iris is manipulated.

KEY POINTS

- A single-mirror gonioscopy mirror, preferably with a curved recessed space beneath the mirror, is used to view the angle. The image through the mirror is flipped and reversed. The curved recessed space allows for manipulation of instruments beneath the lens.
- Be wary of the fact that the view through the gonioscopy mirror is reversed; it is very easy to get turned around and traumatize the corneal endothelium!

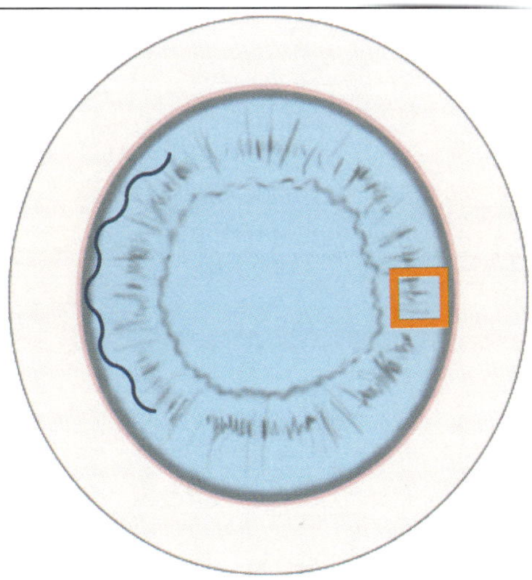

- 2.0-mm incision opposite to the area of anterior synechiae to be released

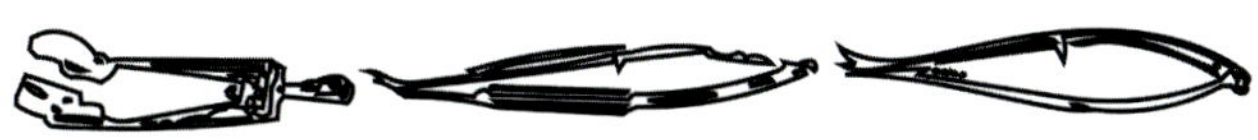

- Microsurgical Technology, Inc micrograsping forceps
- Single-mirror gonioscopy lens (ocular "Ahmed" lens used here)
- Intracameral acetylcholine
- Cohesive viscoelastic

Ahmed IK, Campos-Möller X, Shah M, Sheybani A. *Illustrated Advanced Anterior Segment Surgery: A Step-by-Step Guide for Challenging Cases* (pp 207-210).

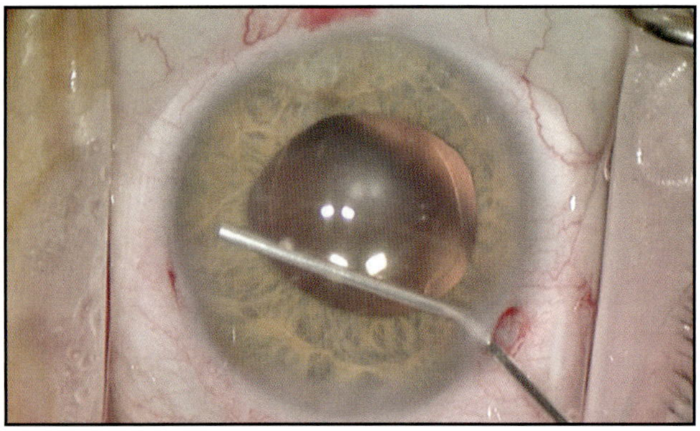

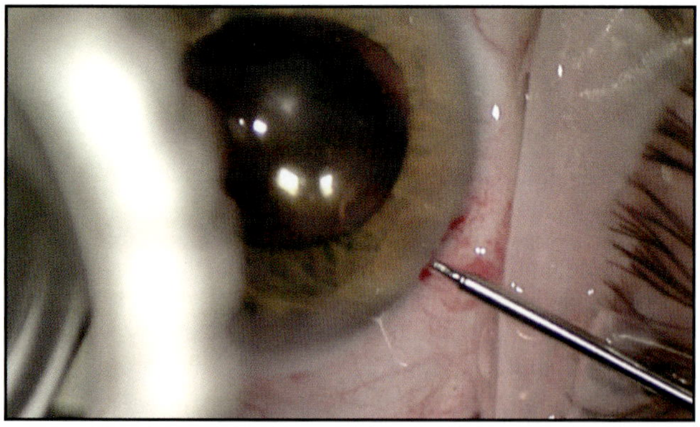

- An intracameral miotic should be used, especially if the goniosynechialysis is to be performed after another intraocular procedure that required dilation. Cohesive viscoelastic is used in the anterior chamber angle to push the iris posteriorly. Do not overfill.
- A 1.5- to 2-mm incision is created approximately 180 degrees from the area with the peripheral anterior synechiae.

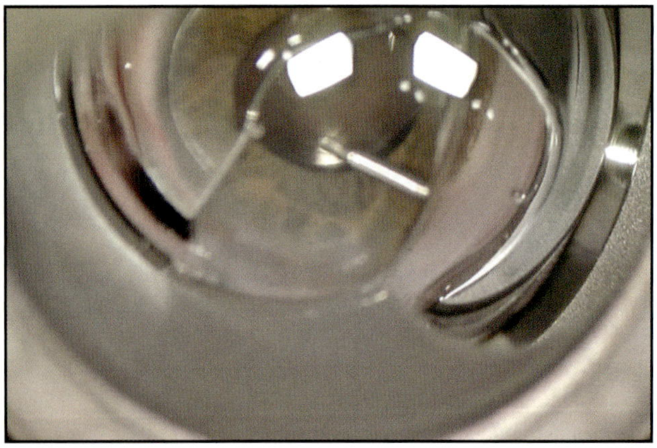

- A coupling agent such as cohesive viscoelastic or methylcellulose is placed on the cornea to improve the gonioscopic view.

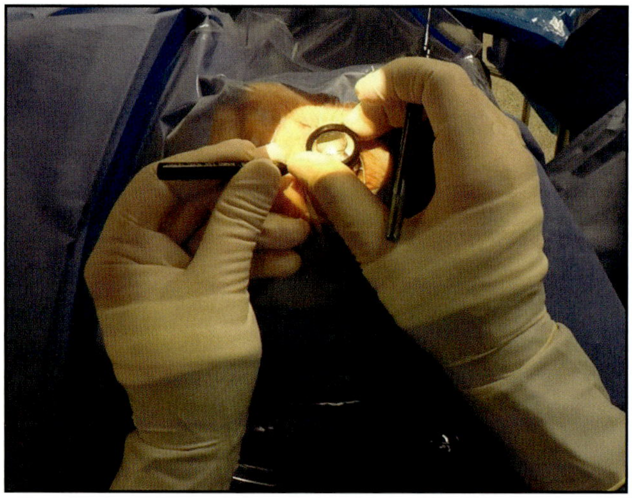

- The gonioscopy mirror is held in the nondominant hand.
- Avoid exerting downward pressure on the eye as this will generate corneal striae, which will obstruct the view. The lens should "float" on the coupling agent without making direct contact with the cornea. This can be evidenced when a meniscus between the lens and coupling agent just barely forms.

- If using a single-mirror lens, the mirror should be oriented 180 degrees from the area to be treated, which usually corresponds to the incision site.

- A Microsurgical Technology, Inc micrograsper is placed through the paracentesis directly across from the desired area of synechialysis.
- The recessed portion of the lens allows for instrument manipulation beneath the mirror without the instrument being limited in movement by the gonioscope.

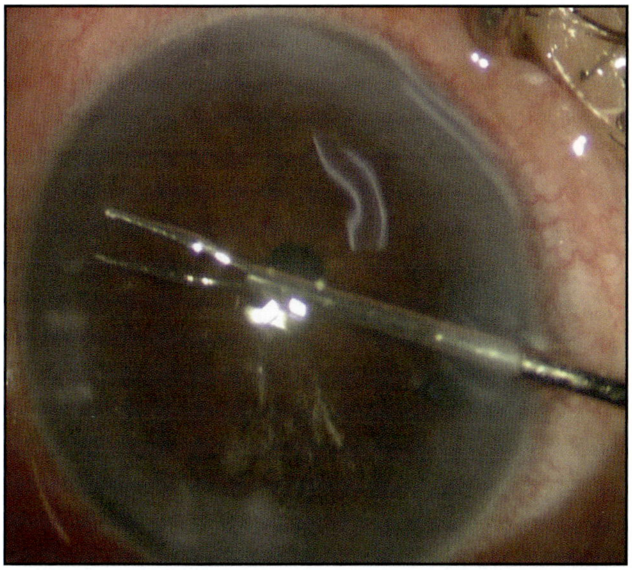

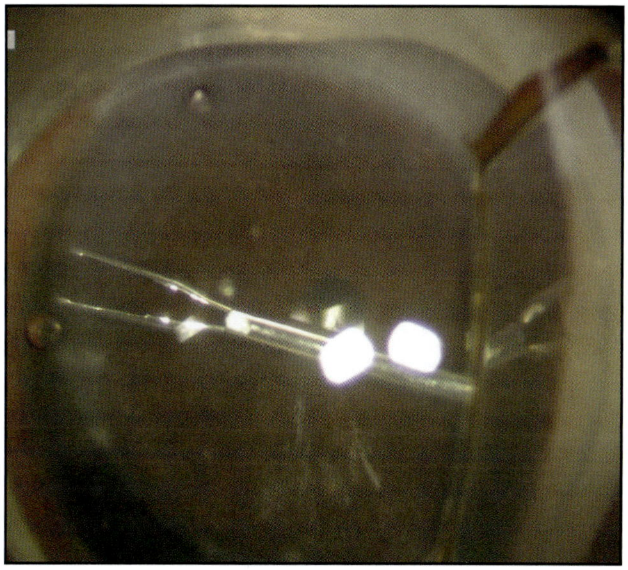

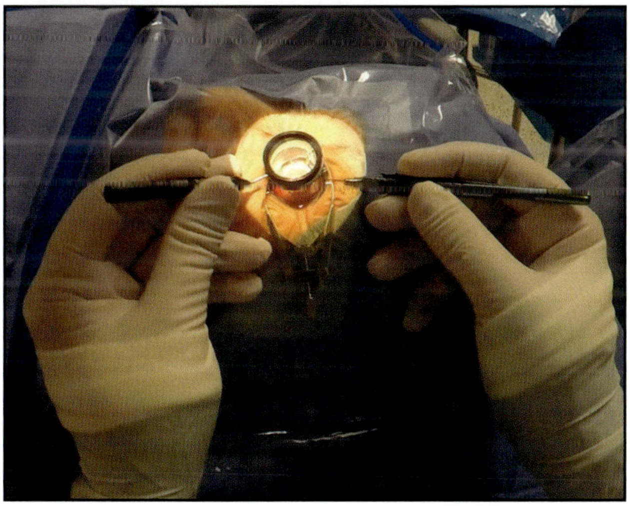

The forceps can be directed into the angle by directly viewing it through the center of the gonioscope (not looking through the mirror). Once the instrument is in the peripheral angle, looking through the mirror will show the surgeon the opposing angle view. Anteroposterior (vertical) adjustments can easily be made while viewing through the mirror, whereas horizontal adjustments are easier to achieve looking straight through the center.

Adequate visualization through the mirror will require focusing down, relative to the central direct view.

Iris is grasped peripherally by gently pushing down on iris with open jaws, grasping iris, then gently pulling centrally (away form the angle).

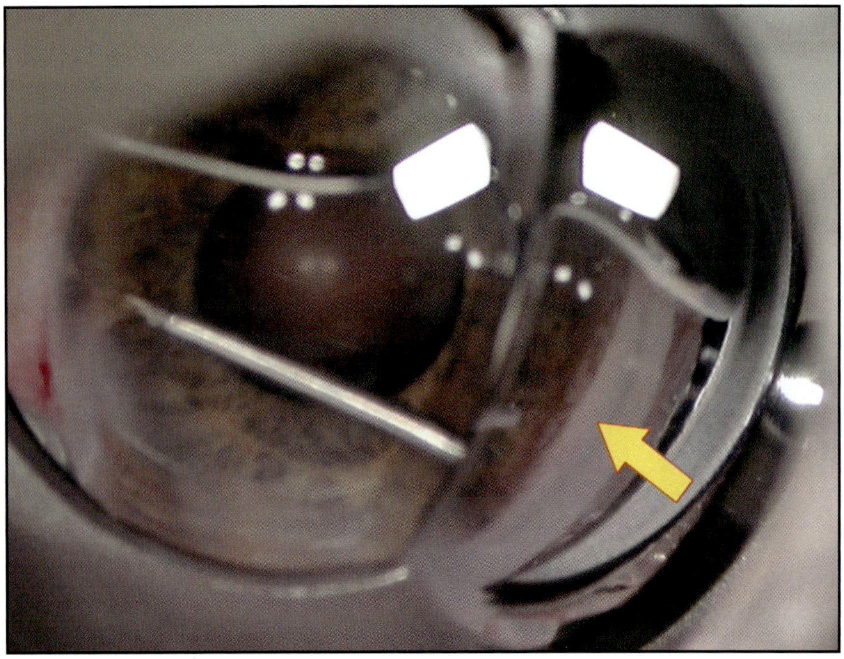

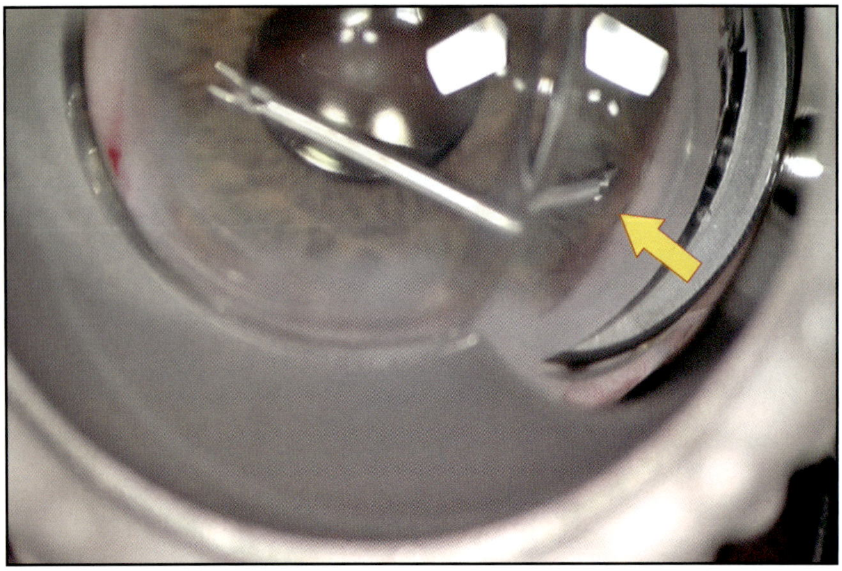

- When the jaws are closed, make sure not to pull back at the same time, but remain in the same location.
- If there is significant angle hemorrhage, viscoelastic can be injected into the eye to pressurize and tamponade the blood. Doing this with a direct view is preferable, taking care not to push the blood onto the endothelium or into the plane of visualization as this can obstruct the view.
- Synechialysis is performed by repeatedly grabbing peripheral iris and pulling centrally, moving along the angle usually a single clock hour at a time.
- An alternative to using micrograspers is to use the irrigation/aspiration handpiece of a phacoemulsification platform.
- The irrigation/aspiration is taken to the peripheral angle with the aspiration port facing down, then vacuum is engaged and a very slight downward motion is made with the cannula, similar to what was done in this chapter with a micrograsper.

CHAPTER 28

HOW TO PERFORM PUPILLOPLASTY IN CORECTOPIA

INTRODUCTION

Corectopia presents unique problems in iris repair cases. Shifting the pupil center while closing the resultant defect can be challenging. Using a combination of techniques is required. In some cases, iris cautery and partial cerclage techniques are needed. In others, relaxing incisions are required to help deliver tissue to areas that are lacking. Here, we describe a combination of techniques used to repair corectopia in a congenital case.

KEY POINTS

- Iris cautery should be performed before suturing to ensure the pupil can be drawn over.
- Interrupted sutures are preferred as less tissue is incorporated in a single pass as compared to partial cerclage techniques, especially if relaxing incisions are made.

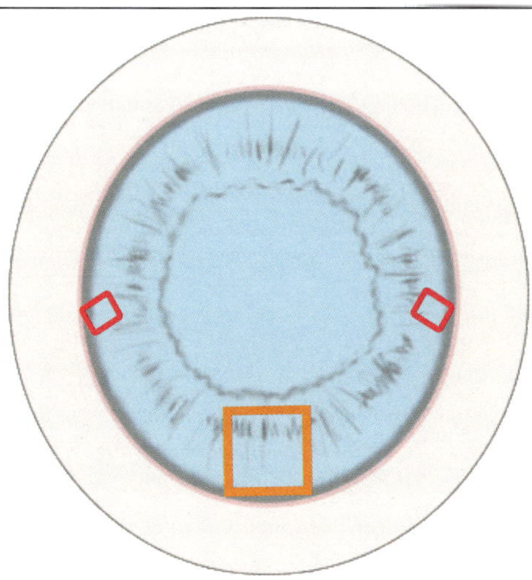

- Knife and fork with additional paracentesis close to the intended suture passes and docking.

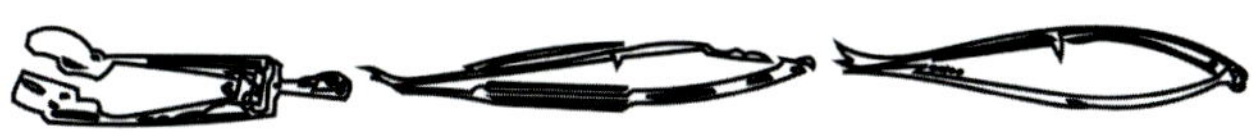

- Microsurgical Technology, Inc micrograsper and microtyer
- Microsurgical Technology, Inc intraocular scissors
- 10-0 polypropylene on a CIF-4 or PC-7 needle
- Fine bipolar cautery (pencil-tip)
- 27-g cannula

Ahmed IK, Campos-Möller X, Shah M, Sheybani A. *Illustrated Advanced Anterior Segment Surgery: A Step-by-Step Guide for Challenging Cases* (pp 211-215).

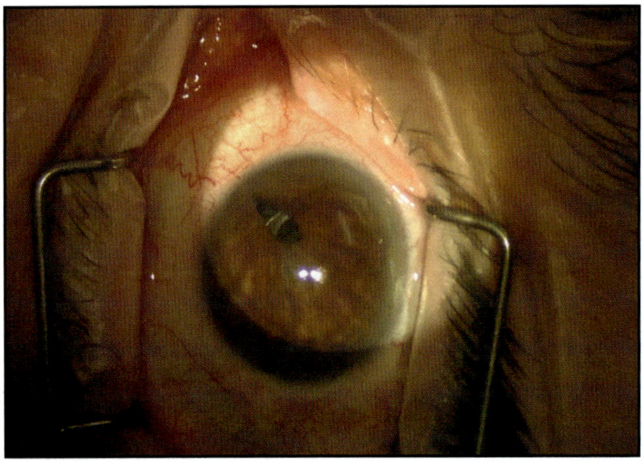

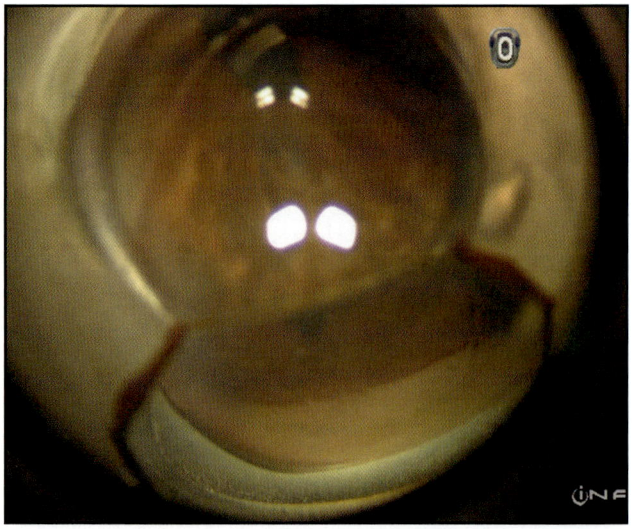

Gonioscopy can identify the extent of remaining iris tissue; if present, relaxing incisions will be helpful to mobilize iris. Goniosynechialysis can be performed as needed to mobilize peripheral iris that may be scarred into the angle (see Chapter 27).

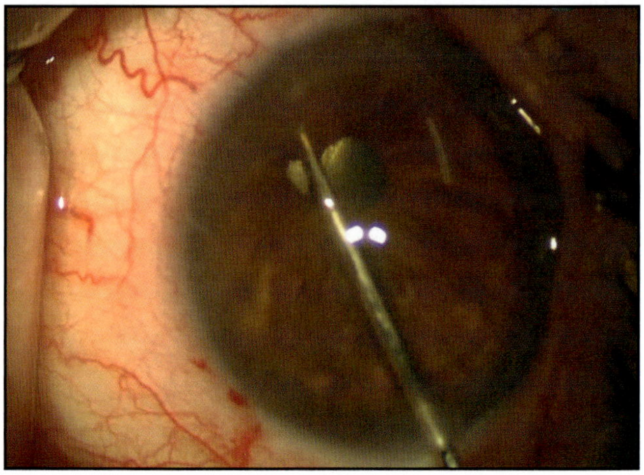

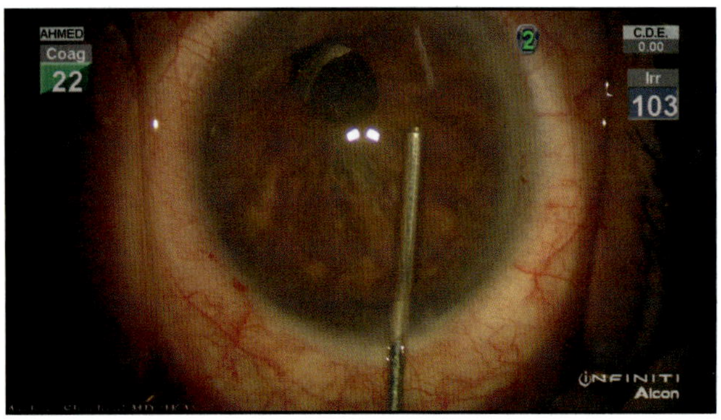

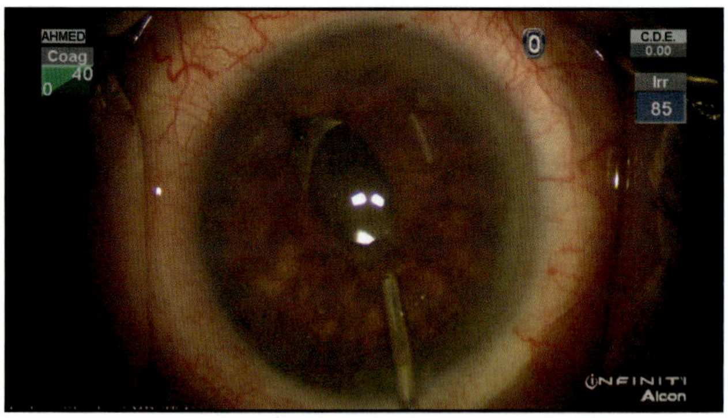

Iris cautery can be used to shrink the iris tissue in order to relocate the pupil. Cautery should be used in linear mode. Typically, very light cautery is needed. It can also be used to focally draw iris toward where one cauterizes to round out sphincter edges for cosmesis. Tissue will contract at the site where the cautery is being applied. Multiple applications at different sites may be required. It is best to go slowly at first because contracted tissue cannot be relaxed, so the defect can be worsened if care is not taken. A greater effect on the pupil will be observed when cautery is applied near the pupil margin, so exercise caution.

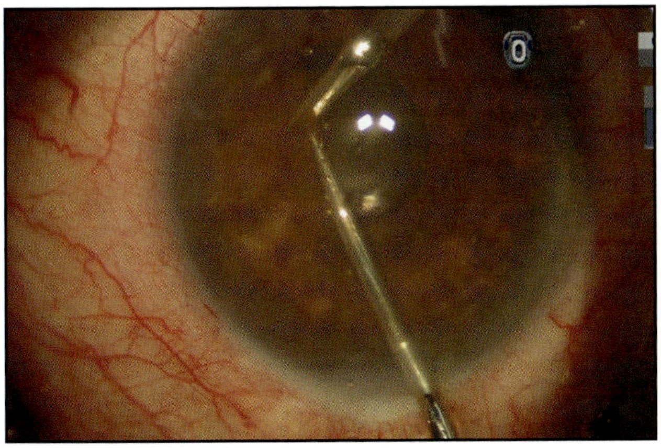

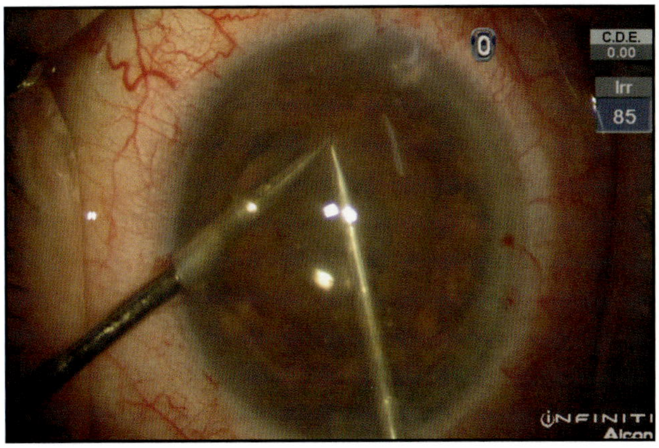

Relaxing incisions are made using micrograspers and microscissors. They are made PERPENDICULAR to the iris—make these cuts small.

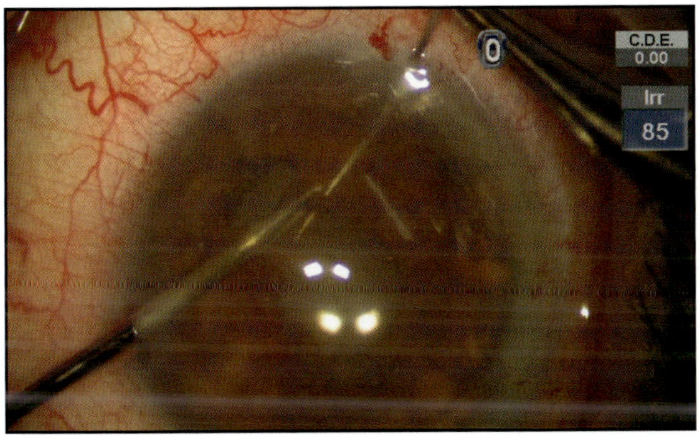

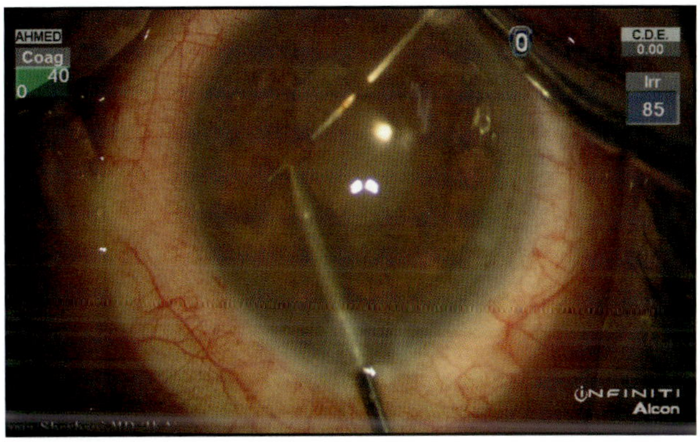

Interrupted suture passes are performed, connecting the innermost leaflets of the relaxing incisions. This way, there is less tension drawing the iris peripherally. Without relaxing incisions, the pupil would not achieve optimal centration. Micrograspers are used to hold the iris leaflet while the CIF-4 needle of the 10-0 Prolene (Ethicon, Inc) suture is inserted through a paracentesis. Avoid lateral motion of the needle. It is often easier to keep the needle stationary while using the micrograspers to deliver the iris tissue to the needle. A 27-g cannula inserted through an opposing paracentesis is used to dock the needle, which is then externalized. Iris suturing techniques are described in Chapter 26.

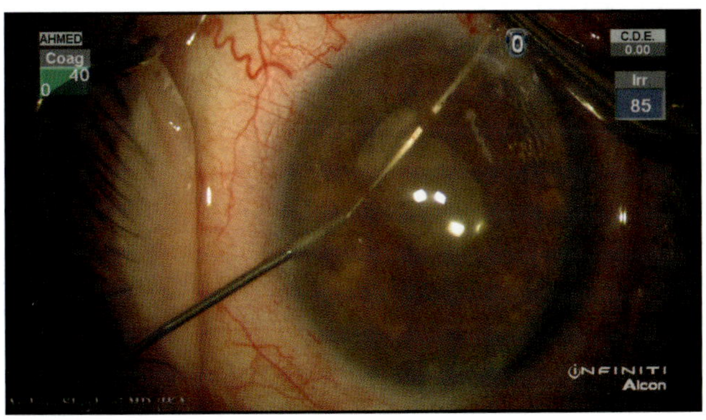

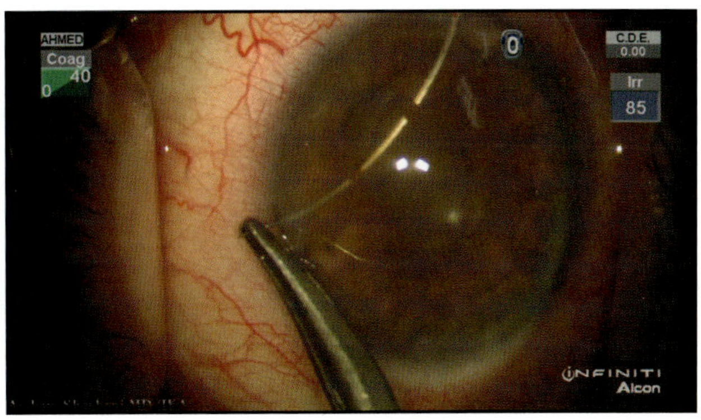

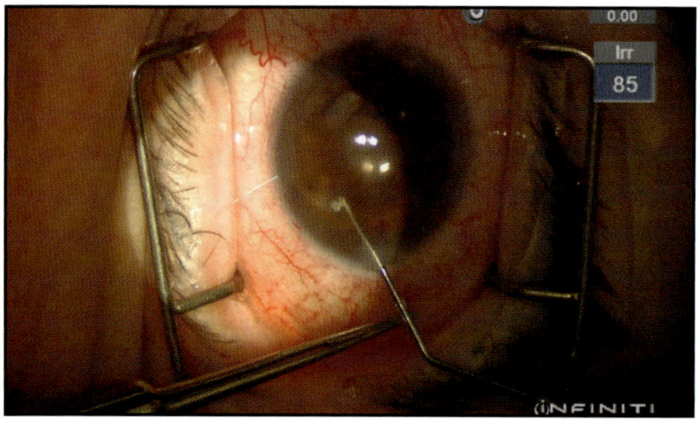

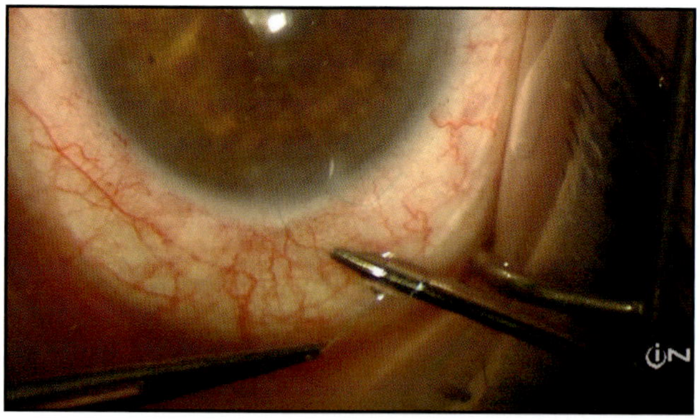

In this case, we used 2 interrupted Ahmed (modified McCannel) sutures to close the defect. See illustration at the end of this chapter for an explanation of the knot.

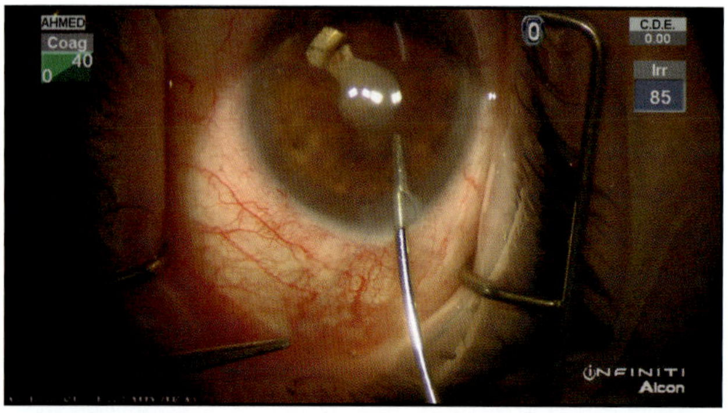

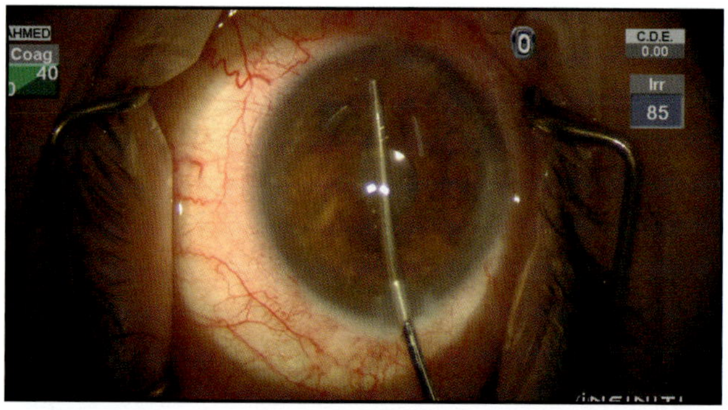

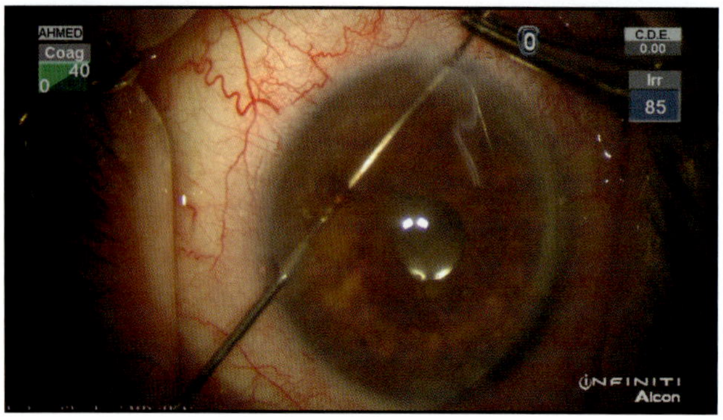

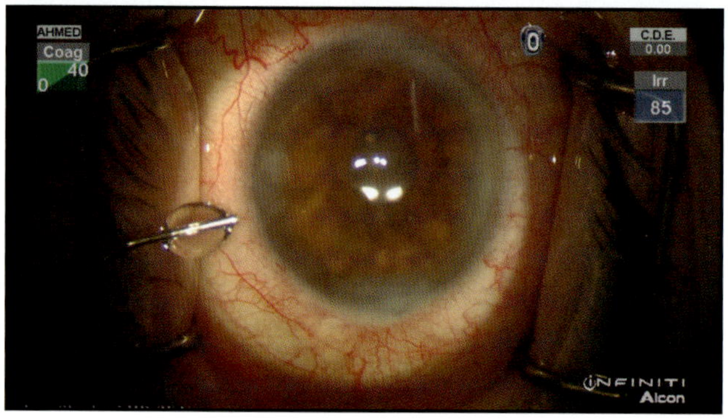

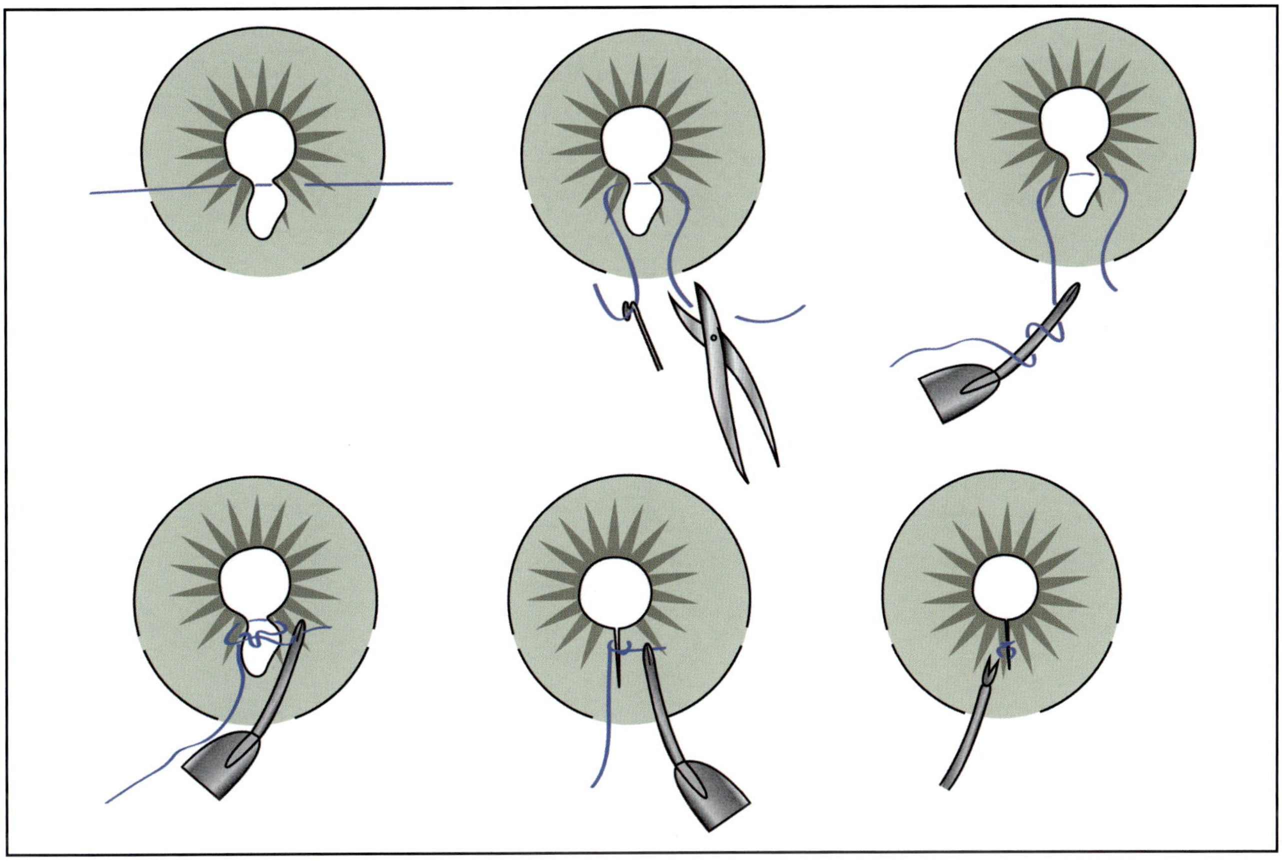

CHAPTER 29

HOW TO PERFORM AN IRIS CERCLAGE

INTRODUCTION

An atonic, mydriatic pupil can be a source of significant photophobia. Furthermore, when considering lens extraction in these cases, the potential for dysphotopsia due to light coming around the intraocular lens (IOL) edge warrants surgical management of this condition. The iris cerclage technique offers an elegant solution to this problem, and creates a rounded pupil margin at a titratable pupillary diameter.

KEY POINTS

- Coordinating the passage of a long suture needle with small manipulation of iris tissue can be difficult; it is often easier to think of the motion of the 2 hands as separate steps instead of moving the 2 simultaneously.
- The more bites you take, the more smooth and rounded the pupil margin will appear.
- Take advantage of strategically placed multiple incisions.
- Refer to Chapter 26 for pearls on iris suturing.
- As it has been mentioned numerous times, be prepared to use your dominant and nondominant hands equally!

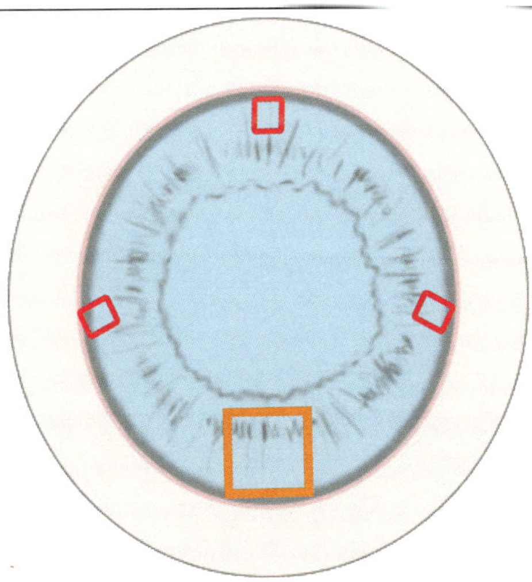

- Knife, fork, temporal incision, and a nasal incision

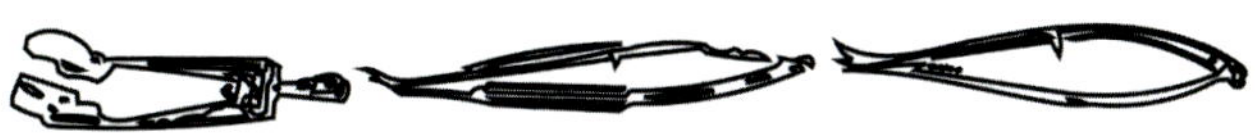

- Iris micrograspers
- Microtying forceps
- Intraocular scissors
- 10-0 Prolene (Ethicon, Inc) on CIF-4 needle (keep this suture double armed)
- Needle driver
- Cohesive viscoelastic

Ahmed IK, Campos-Möller X, Shah M, Sheybani A. *Illustrated Advanced Anterior Segment Surgery: A Step-by-Step Guide for Challenging Cases* (pp 217-224).

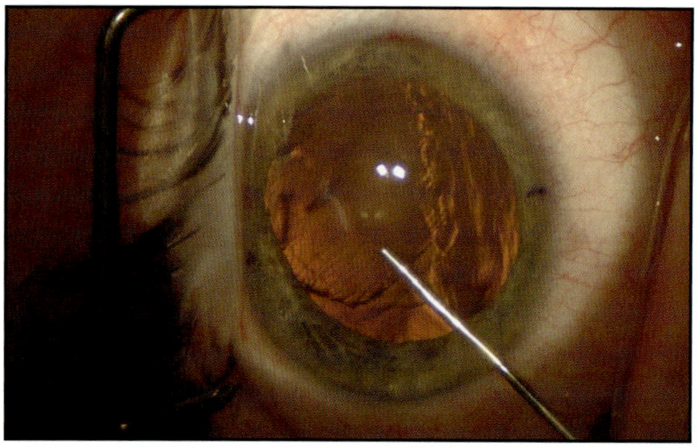

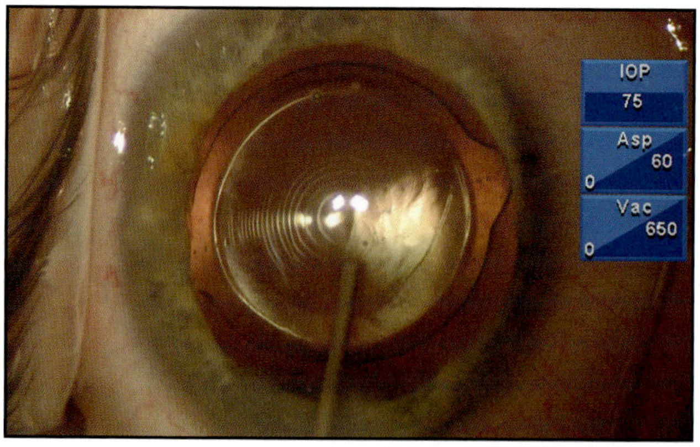

- Instill acetylcholine intracamerally to maximize pupillary constriction.
- Ensure adequate cohesive viscoelastic is present in the anterior chamber.
- Use iris micrograspers to gently assist in constricting the pupil, pulling on the pupil margin toward the center.
- This provides an initial sense of what the iris consistency will be like as you begin to suture.

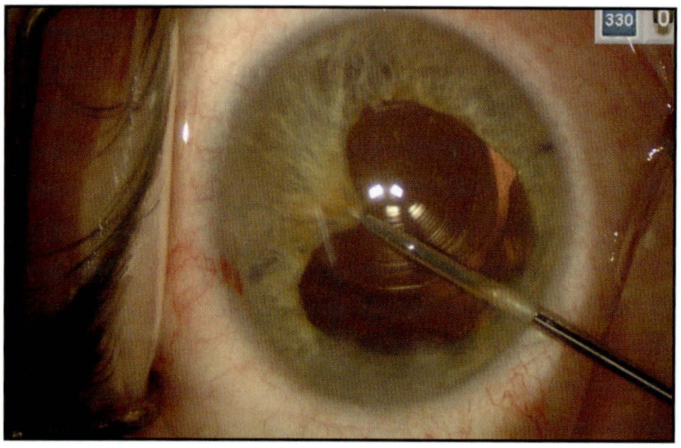

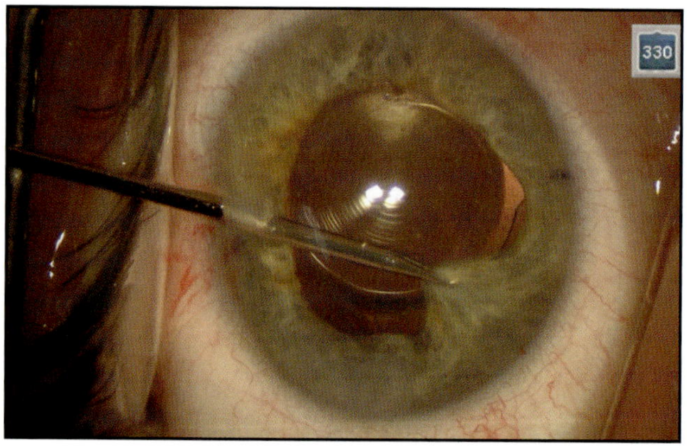

- Insert one arm of the 10-0 suture through the nasal paracentesis.
- Using the iris micrograspers in your other hand, pass the needle through the iris approximately 0.5 mm away from the pupil margin with the needle pointing toward the center off the pupil.
- Once you have successfully made your first bite, rotate the needle approximately 45 degrees.
- Begin taking small bites of iris stroma, remaining approximately 0.5 mm inside the pupillary margin and spacing bites about 1 mm apart.

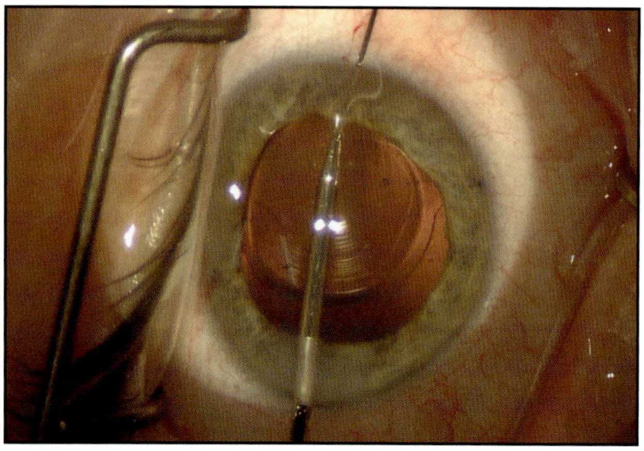

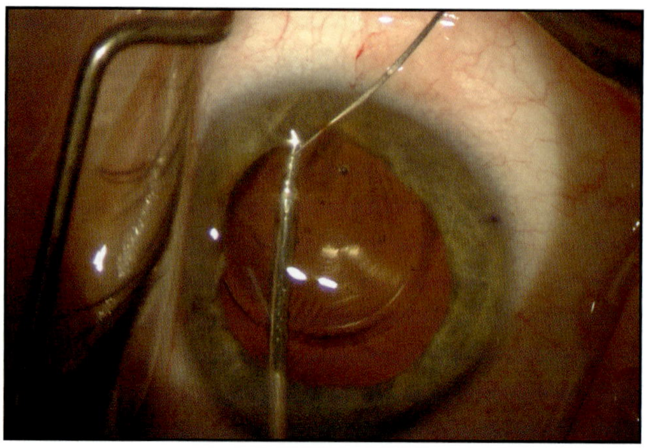

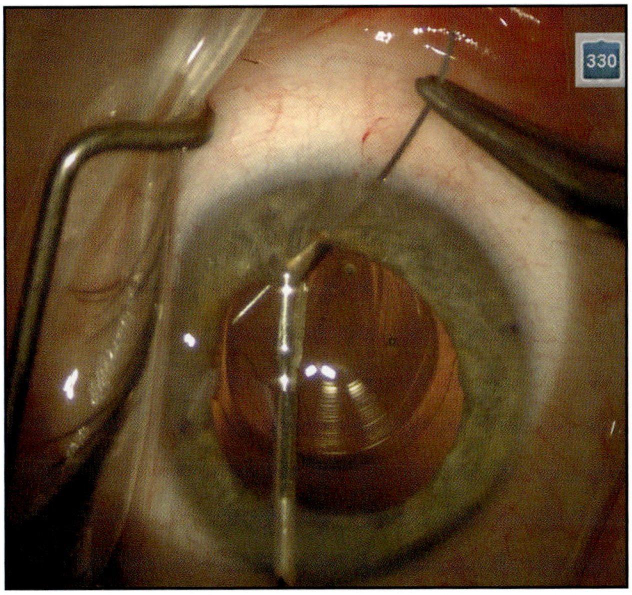

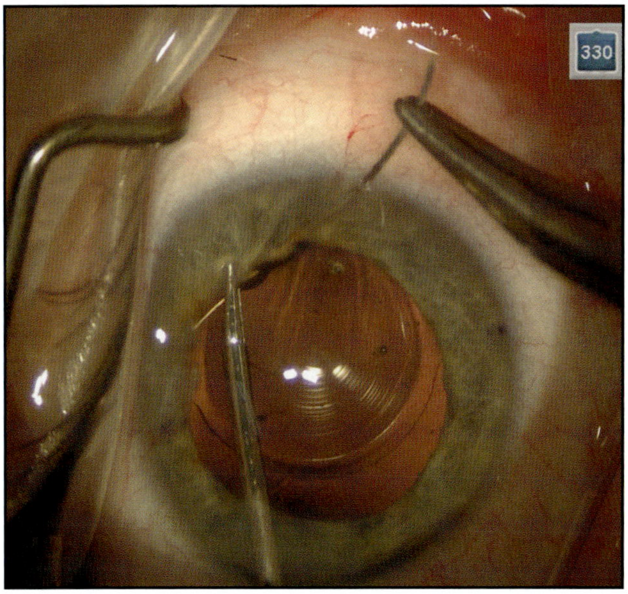

- When taking bites, rely on your iris micrograspers to do the bulk of the work The needle stays stationary and advances slowly as the micrograsper lays iris onto the needle. The needle is large, unwieldy, and, as a result, should largely remain still.
- The micrograspers should follow a running, almost circular path as they bring iris tissue to the needle and drive the collected tissue back along the long arm of the needle before going back for another bite of tissue.
- Do not take too small a bite, as you risk cheese-wiring!

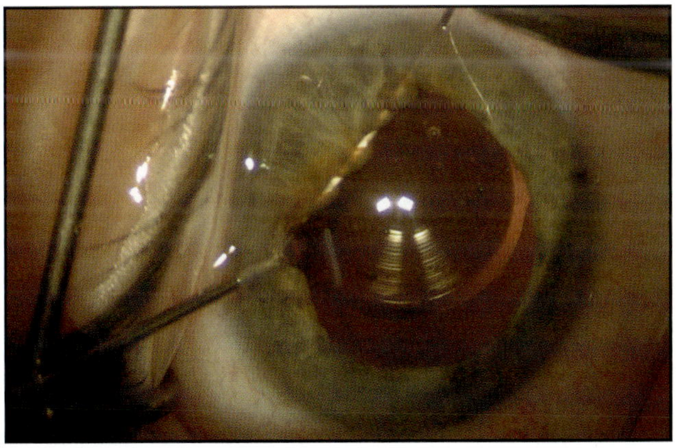

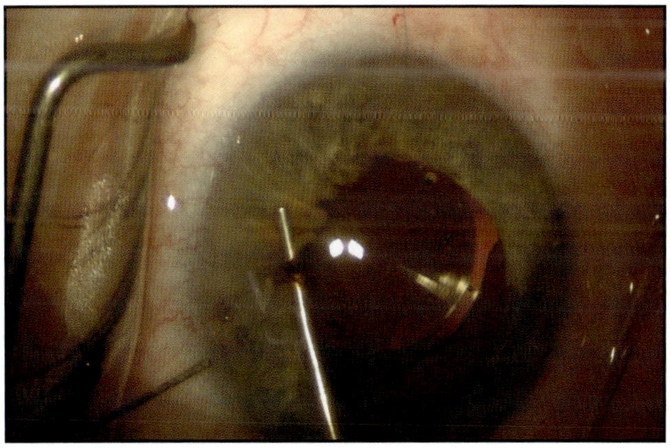

- When you are close to one of the superior or inferior paracentesis incisions, withdraw the iris micrograspers and instead introduce the viscoelastic cannula through the paracentesis you are approaching.
- Dock the needle in the cannula to allow the needle and suture to leave the eye without engaging corneal fibers.
- Gently pull out the needle and allow the suture to advance.
- Move slowly, as rapid motion can result in an iridodialysis or bleeding from the angle.
- As you are withdrawing, consider using the blunt viscoelastic cannula to provide countertraction on the iris to prevent it from being pulled along with the suture toward the paracentesis.

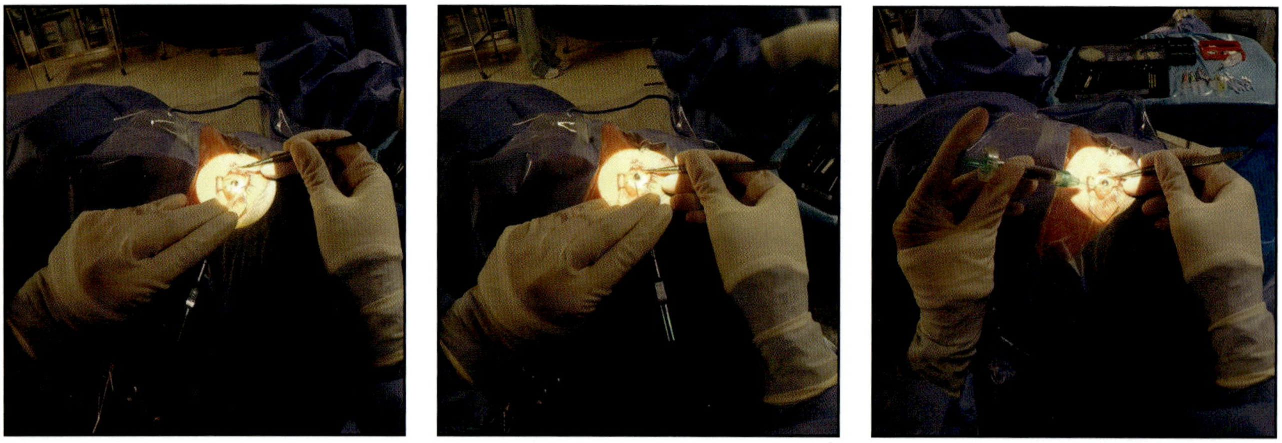

First suture passes are done inferonasally, holding the needle driver hand relatively still, while the left hand holds a micrograsper and does most of the movements. Later, a 27-g cannula is used to dock and retrieve the needle.

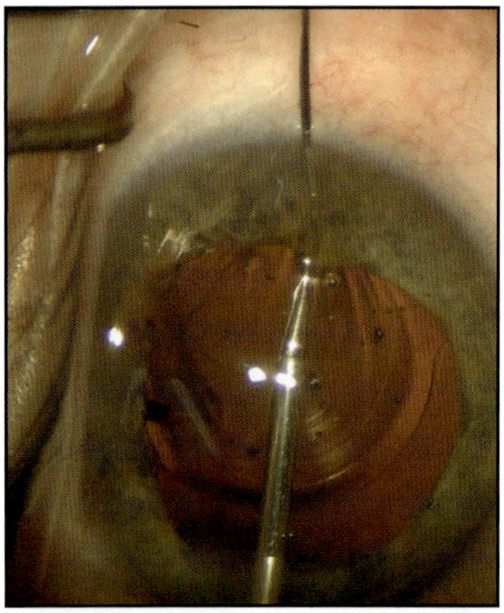

- For the superonasal quadrant, repeat the same steps as described above using the opposite hands for the needle driver and iris micrograspers as you proceed from the nasal to the other paracentesis.
- When introducing the second arm of the suture, make sure the first bite is relatively close to the initial bite of the first arm. Spacing this too far can result in a focal defect in the pupil contour.

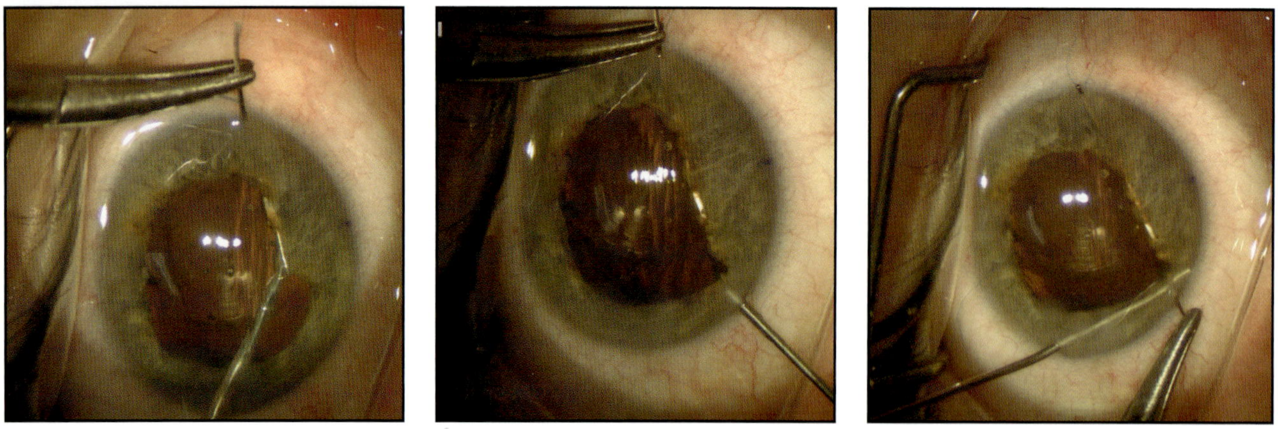

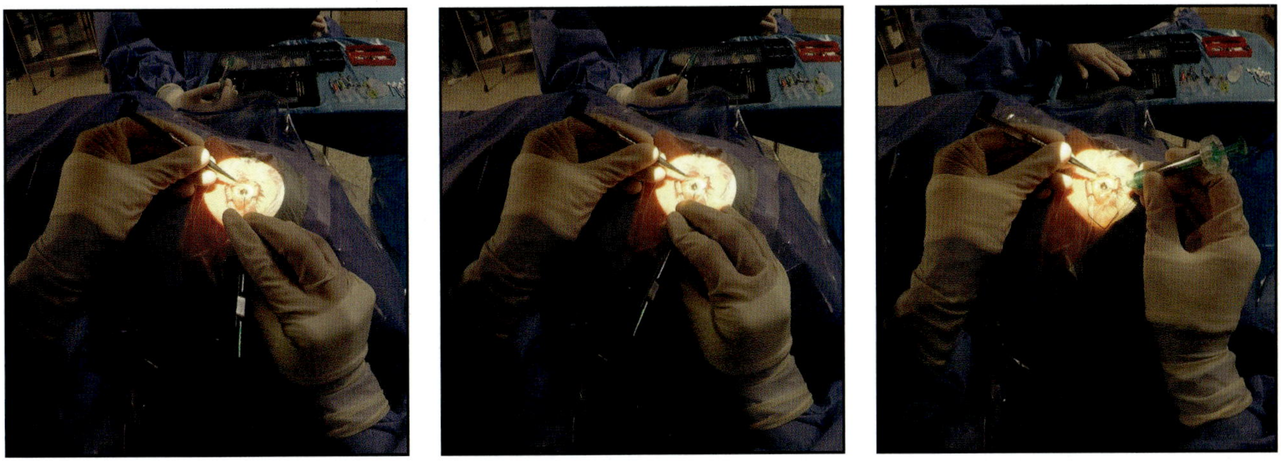

Instruments switch hands for the superonasal quadrant. Again, the micrograsper hand does most of the movements.

- After completing this, you will repeat the same suturing technique by reintroducing each needle through the paracentesis incision it had previously exited from.
- Take care not to entrap any corneal fibers during needle entry.
- This time, both needles are retrieved through the temporal incision, using the docking technique as described above. The 27-g cannula can be used to sweep the iris and keep it from coming out of the incisions when the suture is being pulled.

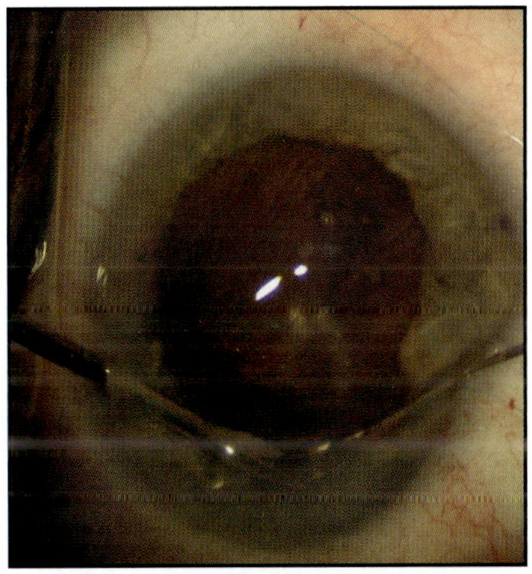

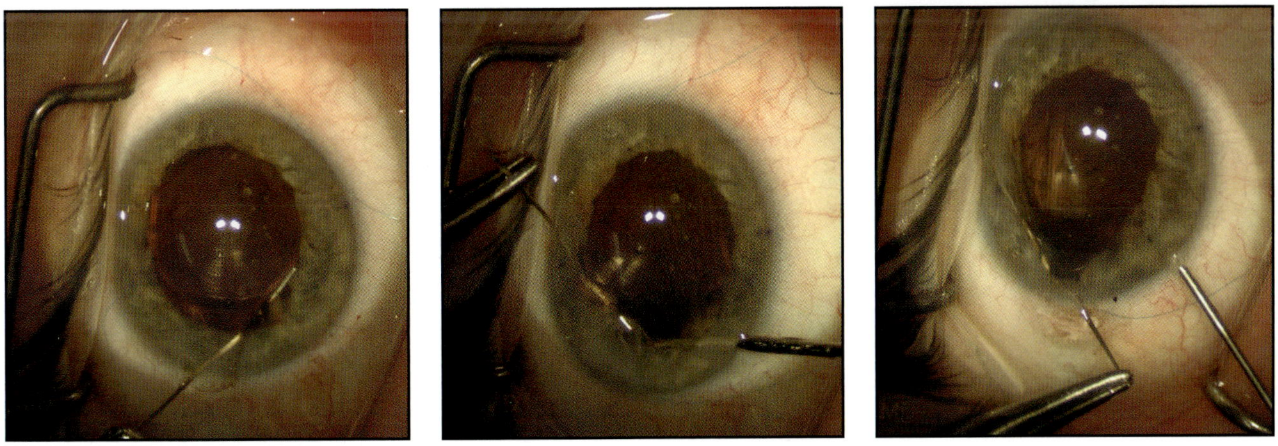

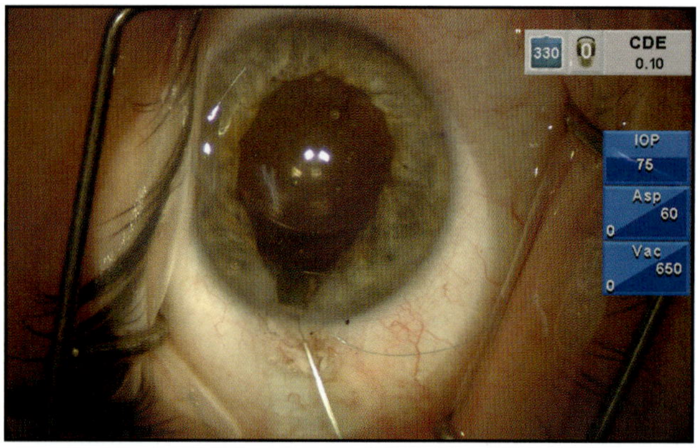

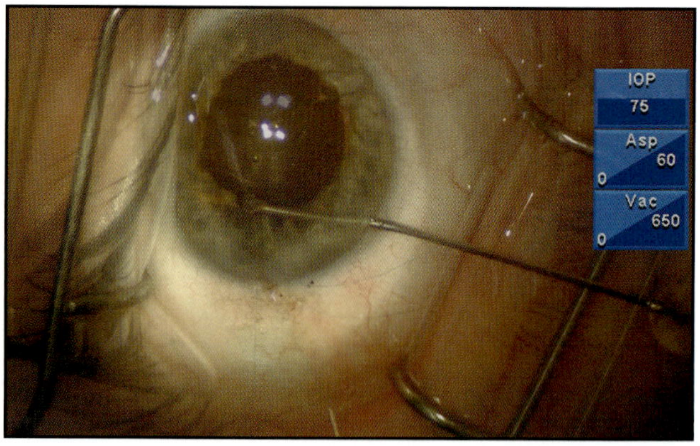

- Provide gentle tension in order to achieve a pupil diameter that is symmetrical to the fellow eye; typically, around 3 to 3.5 mm is adequate in minimizing photophobia and allowing an adequate examination of the posterior segment.
- Refer to the diagram at the end of this chapter for the Ahmed (modified McCannel) suturing technique, using straight tyers and microtying forceps.
- After the knot has been tied and suture ends have been trimmed, use a Kuglen hook to gently move iris tissue around the running suture to smooth out the pupillary margin.

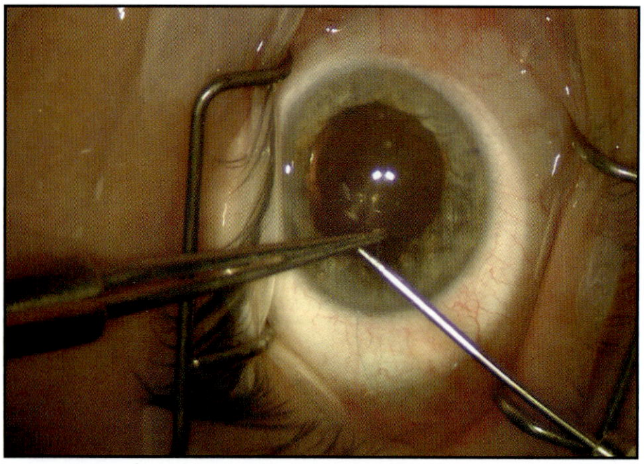

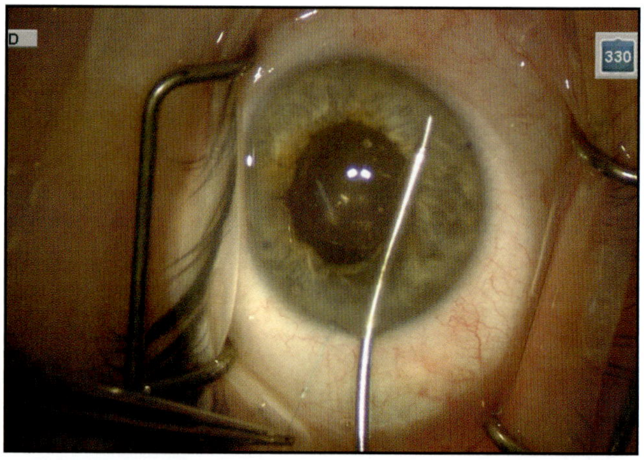

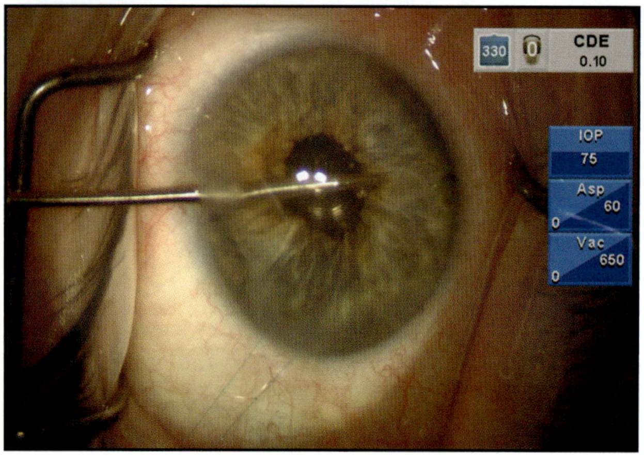

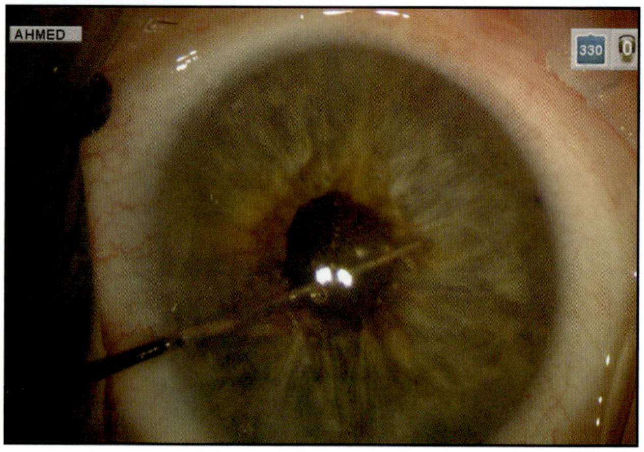

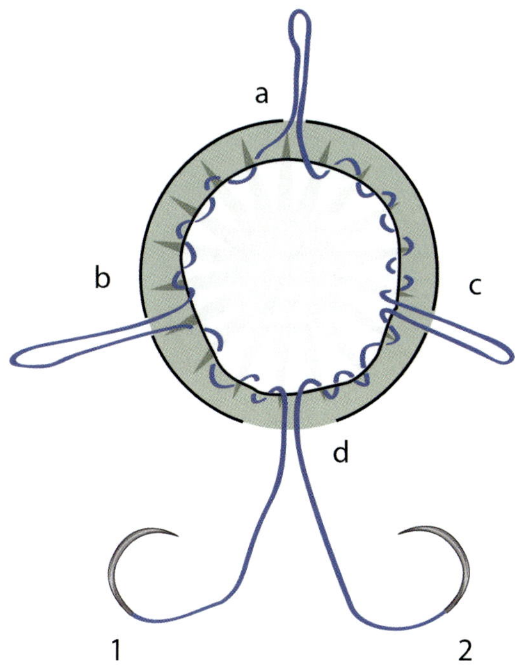

This diagram illustrates the path of the suture before it is tightened. Needle 1 goes through nasal incision, takes bites until it comes out through incision (b), does a 180-degree turn and goes back in through incision (b), taking more bites on the temporal iris until it comes out of the temporal incision (d). The needle on the other end of the suture (2) goes in through the nasal incision, takes bites on the other half of the nasal iris until it comes out of incision (c), does a 180-degree turn and goes back in through incision (c), taking more bites until it comes out of the temporal incision (d). Note: The temporal, superior, and nasal loops should be shorter than shown, as this is only for schematic purposes.

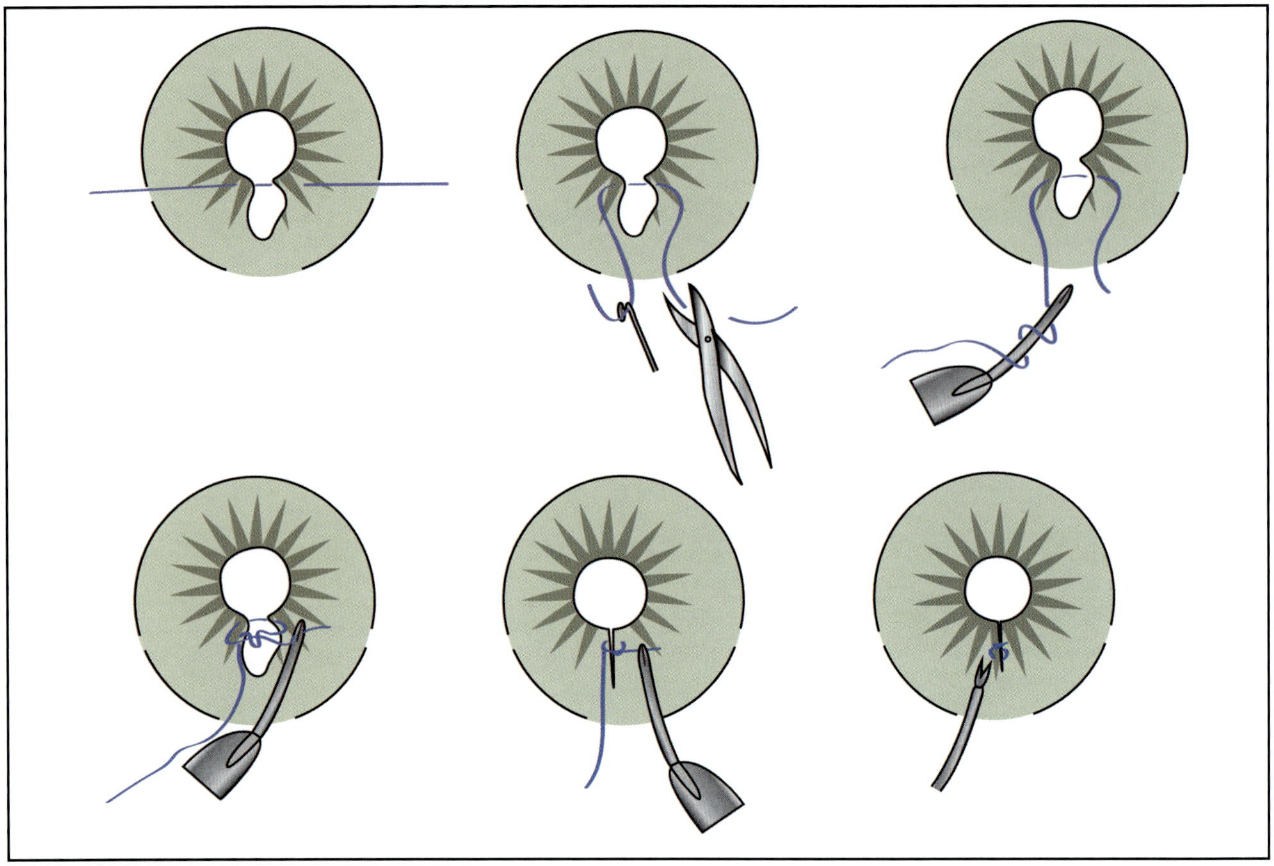

CHAPTER 30

HOW TO INSERT ANIRIDIA IMPLANTS

INTRODUCTION

In the setting of small iris defects, one can consider in-the-bag partial aniridia implants. An intact capsule is required for implantation, so the majority are placed at the time of cataract extraction. Theoretically, an implant can be placed after intraocular lens (IOL) implantation has occurred so long as the capsule can be atraumatically expanded fully. In the setting of total aniridia, iris prosthesis implants are required. In the setting of an intact capsular bag, an in-the-bag iris prosthesis can be implanted. For partial sectorial aniridia, we prefer the Morcher 96 range, with or without iridoplasty. For total or near total aniridia, we prefer the HumanOptics artificial iris (intracapsular without tissue) or the Morcher 50E implants. The former is the most cosmetically appealing but is custom-made and usually has a higher cost. All of these implants have similar results in terms of visual rehabilitation resolution of photophobia.

KEY POINTS

Morcher 96/50 series:

- Implanting these devices is similar to implanting capsular tension rings without an injector in that the bag must be completely inflated with cohesive viscoelastic.
- The fin should be placed first; do not place the fin as the trailing end, otherwise it is more difficult to manipulate.
- Ideal placement of aniridia segments occurs before the IOL has been placed.
- Sometimes a combination of partial aniridia ring and sutured pupilloplasty may be performed.

HumanOptics artificial iris:

- Ideal placement of the HumanOptics implant occurs after the IOL has been placed.
- Size the HumanOptics implant to 9 mm for normal eyes, adjusting for smaller or larger eyes.
- For in-the-bag implantation, the fiberless model must be used.

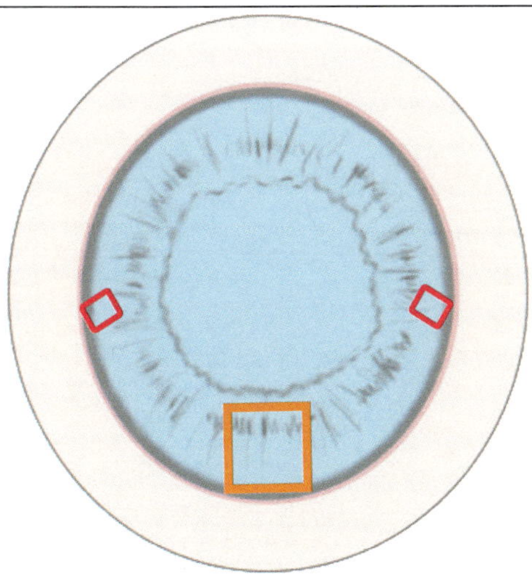

- Standard phaco 3.25 mm with knife and fork

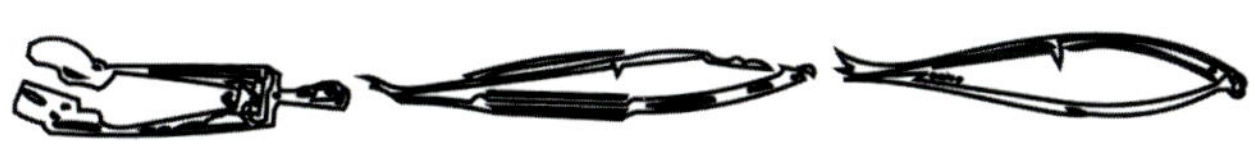

- Kuglen and Sinskey hooks
- Micrograspers
- Corneal trephine for HumanOptics
- Choice of iris prosthesis implant: Morcher 96 or 50 series, HumanOptics artificial iris

Ahmed IK, Campos-Möller X, Shah M, Sheybani A. *Illustrated Advanced Anterior Segment Surgery: A Step-by-Step Guide for Challenging Cases* (pp 225-236).

In this case, we are implanting a Morcher 96E partial aniridia implant for treating glare and photophobia in a patient with a partial iris defect. The IOL was also exchanged in this case, but we will begin this chapter after IOL explantation (see Chapter 24). Dispersive ophthalmic viscosurgical device (OVD) is used to coat the cornea and cohesive OVD to fully fill the capsular bag.

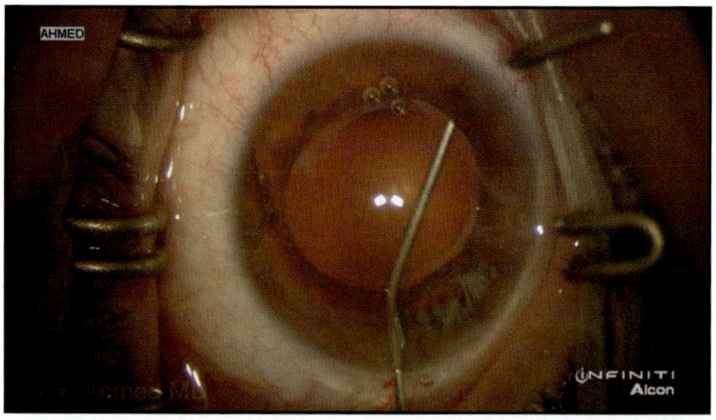

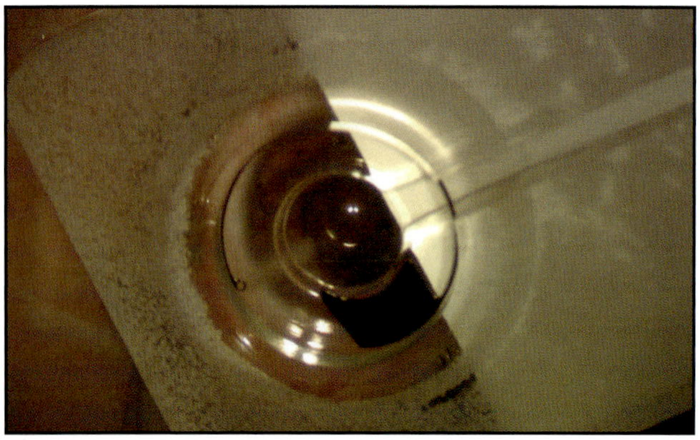

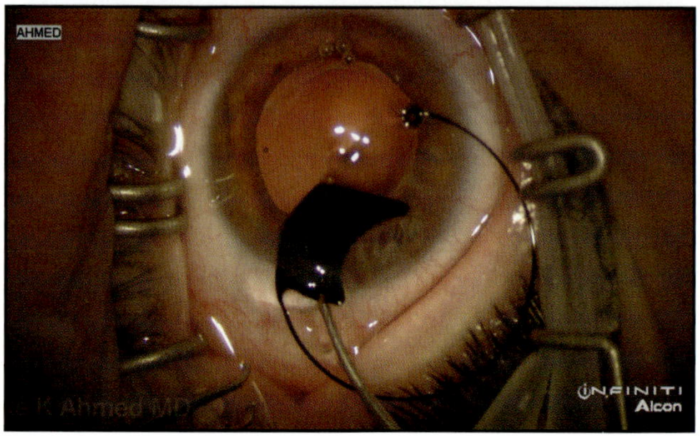

Care must be taken to not flip the implant over as it is easier to rotate it clockwise. Using a toothless tyer, the partial aniridia ring is placed "fin-first" through a 3-mm, clear corneal incision, and then rotated by the "armpit" into the capsular bag with a Sinskey or Kuglen hook.

Often, the temporal clear corneal incision will have to be enlarged to accommodate the fin of the aniridia implant. Refer to the manufacturer's guidelines, as different sized segments require different wound sizes.

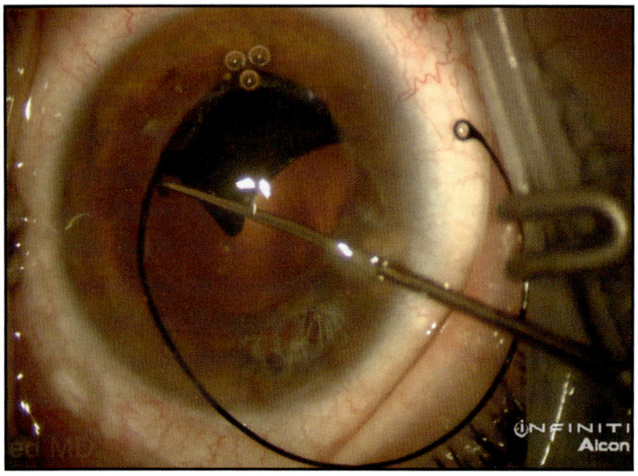

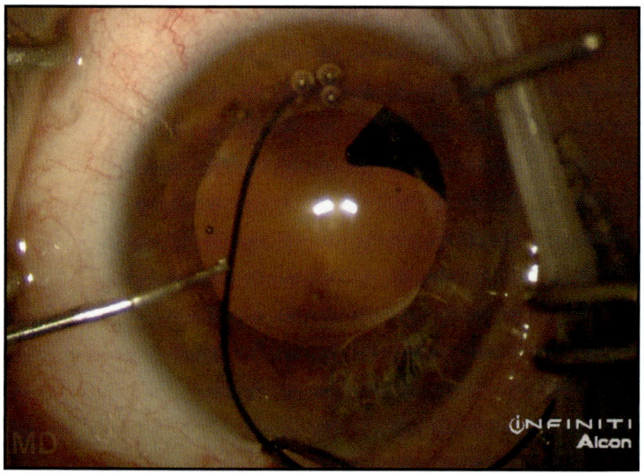

A bimanual maneuver with Sinskey and Kuglen hooks can help guide the ring into the bag in a similar way as a capsular tension ring. Using the Sinskey in the trailing eyelet and the tip of the Kuglen as a guide, the ring can be atraumatically inserted into the bag.

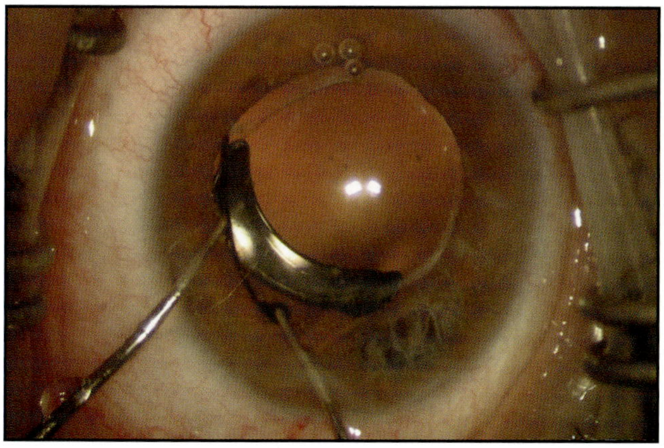

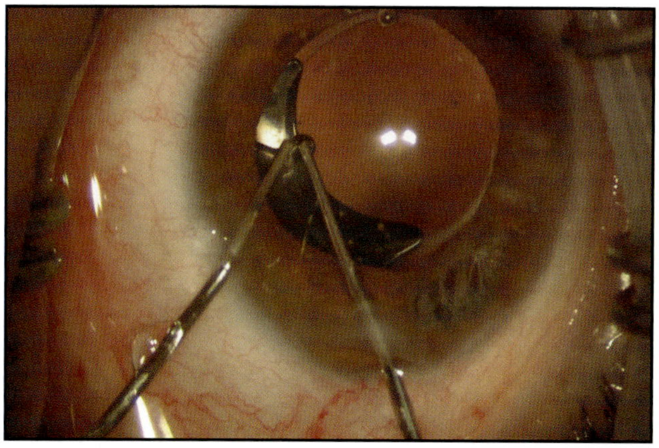

Avoid excessive flexion of the ring, as it can break. The ring can be rotated clockwise or counterclockwise, but it is best to manipulate the edge of the fin instead of the eyelet. For IOL placement, we prefer inserting the cartridge into the anterior chamber instead of a wound-assisted technique, as this minimizes the possibility of rotating the aniridia ring out of position. The IOL must be placed under the aniridia implant to avoid IOL tilt. Consider refilling the capsular bag with cohesive viscoelastic to ensure there is ample space posterior to the aniridia implant. Viscoelastic is removed after the IOL has been implanted.

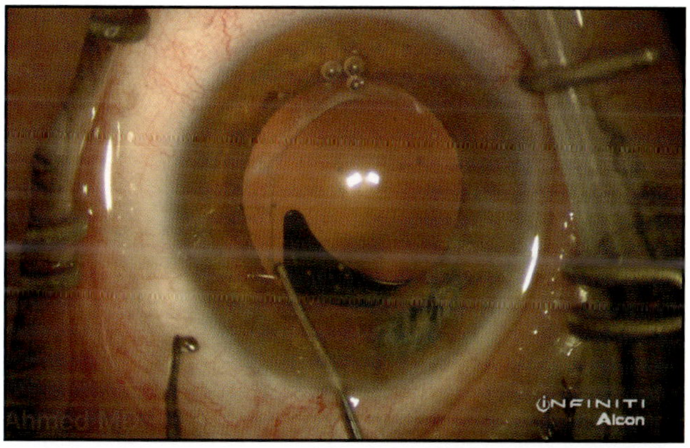

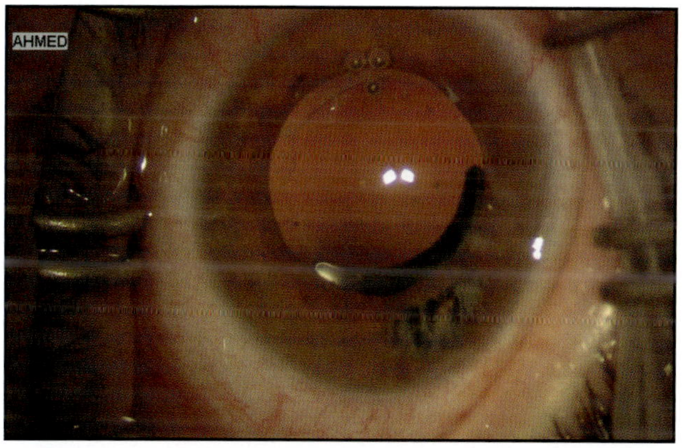

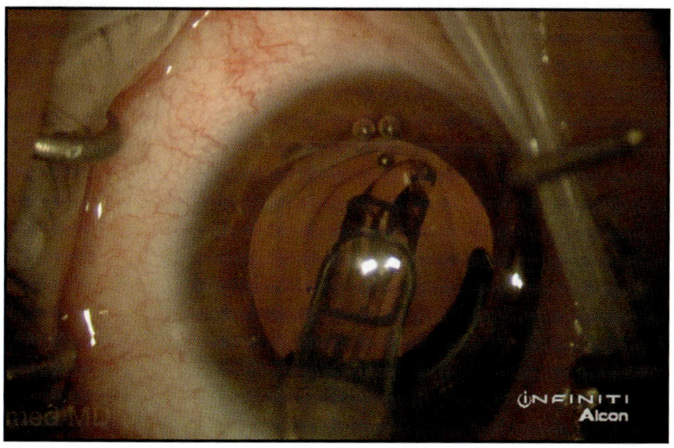

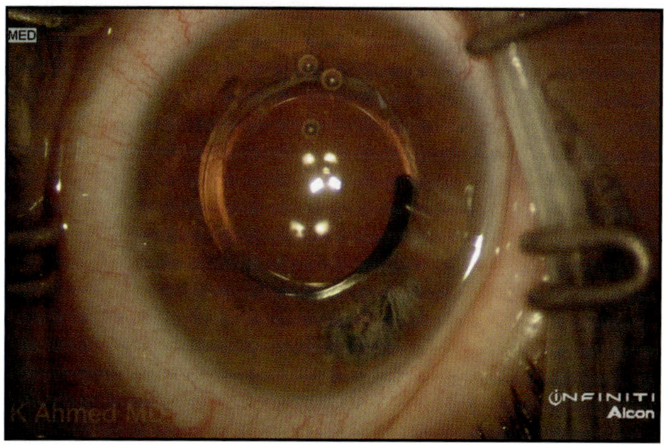

HOW TO IMPLANT MORCHER 50F/50E TOTAL ANIRIDIA RINGS

Key points:

- Two Morcher 50E or 50F devices are needed for full overlap.
- The 50E is easier to place than the 50F as the fins of the 50E are narrower and do not lock together as easily in the bag.
- The IOL should be placed after both rings are placed in the bag. Place the first ring in the bag and elevate it anteriorly in the bag on a bed of cohesive OVD before placing the second ring.
- Do not place these implants in a bag with an anterior capsule tear. Use caution if there is a posterior capsule tear as these devices will stretch the bag similar to a capsular tension ring and can cause splitting of the bag.

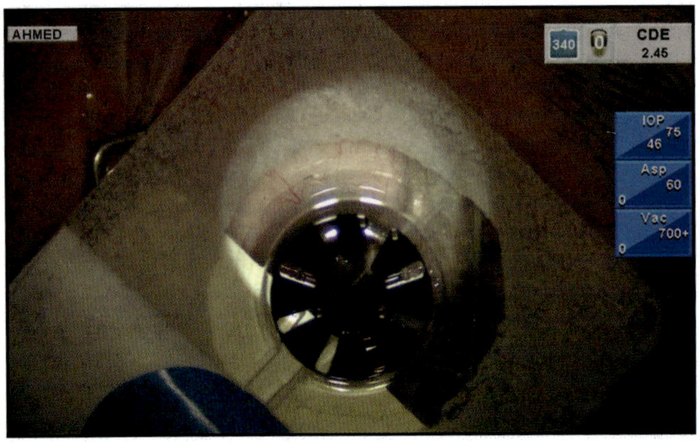

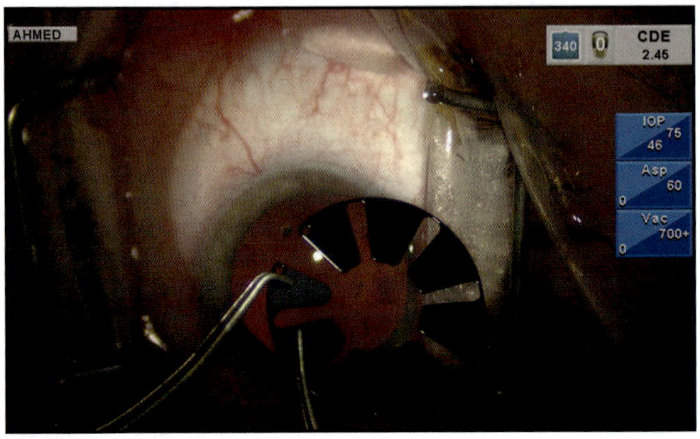

- After phacoemulsification and cortical cleanup, a cohesive OVD should be used to completely fill the capsular bag. Placing these devices in a bag that is not fully inflated may cause zonule and/or capsular trauma.
- The temporal wound is enlarged to at least 3.25 mm. Slightly larger wounds will make for easier entry, but excessively large wounds will promote anterior chamber shallowing. We recommend a 3.5- to 4-mm wound.
- Handle the device with nontoothed forceps because poly(methyl methacrylate) is susceptible to scratching by sharp instruments.

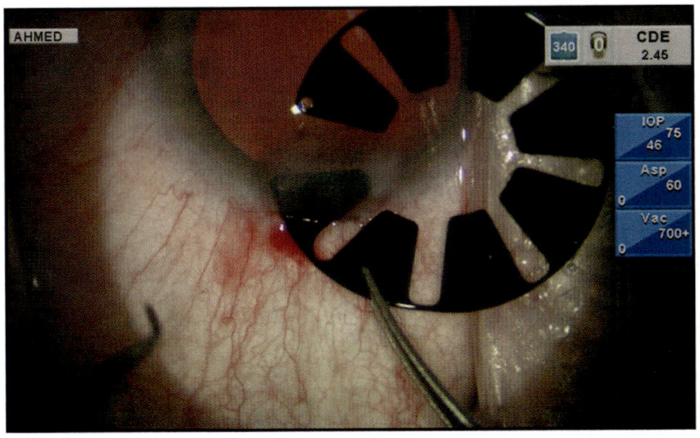

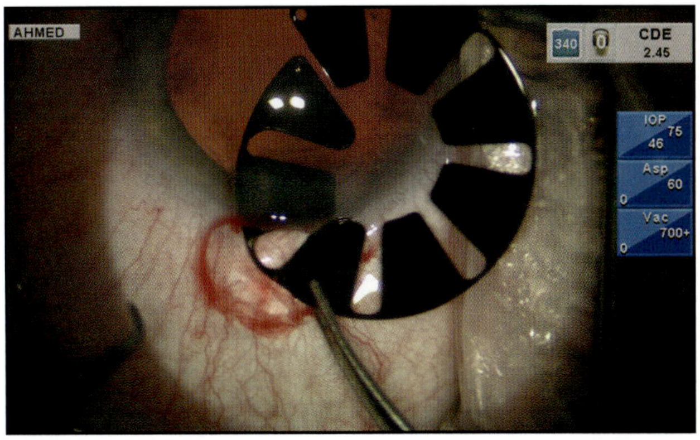

- Insert the device by placing the leading fin first (the leading fin is smaller and has a rounded out tip in both implants) using a nontoothed forceps.
- Continue to feed each fin through the temporal incision; the rings should be directed into the capsular bag. Before inserting more than 3 clock hours of the ring, ensure that the leading fin is inside the capsular bag and not in the ciliary sulcus.

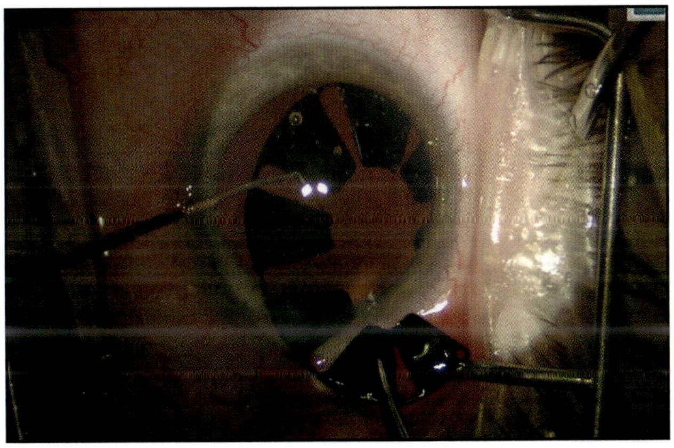

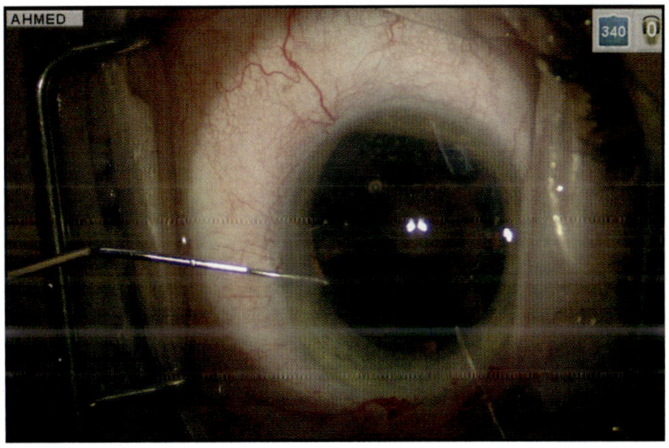

- Engaging a Sinskey hook in the perforation of the leading fin can help guide it into the capsular bag. Continue to feed the entire ring slowly until the final trailing fin (the hole is on the outside edge) is just at the wound. The Sinskey hook can then be engaged in the perforation of the last fin, guiding it posteriorly into the capsular bag.

The bag is filled with cohesive OVD, elevating the ring against the anterior capsule. The second ring goes behind this first ring. OVD is used again, refilling the entire capsular bag and ensuring that the first ring is displaced toward the anterior capsule.

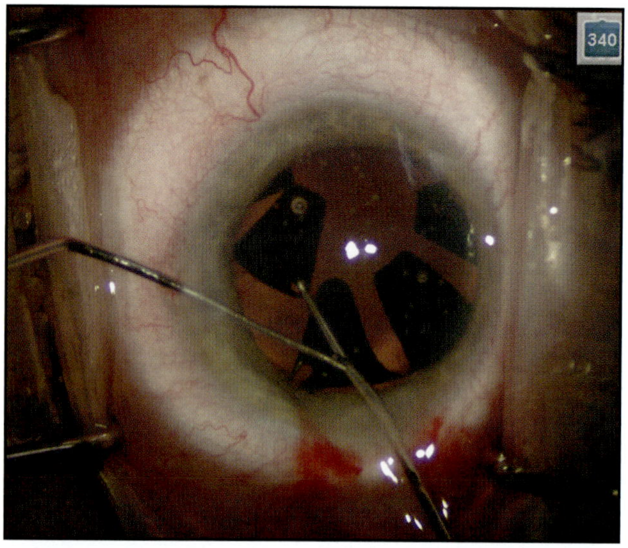

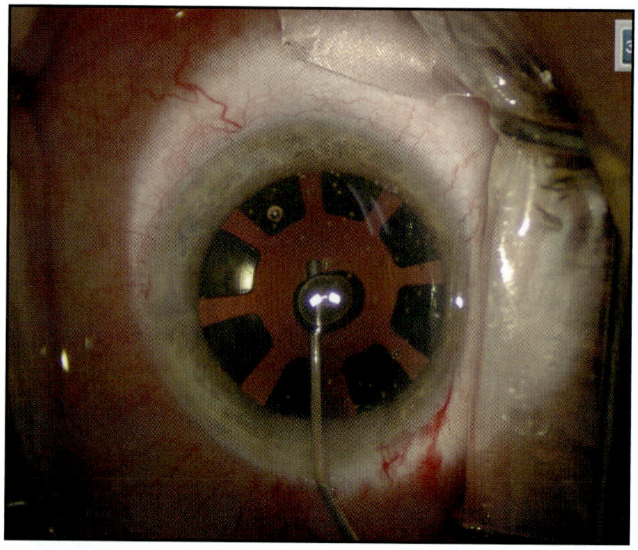

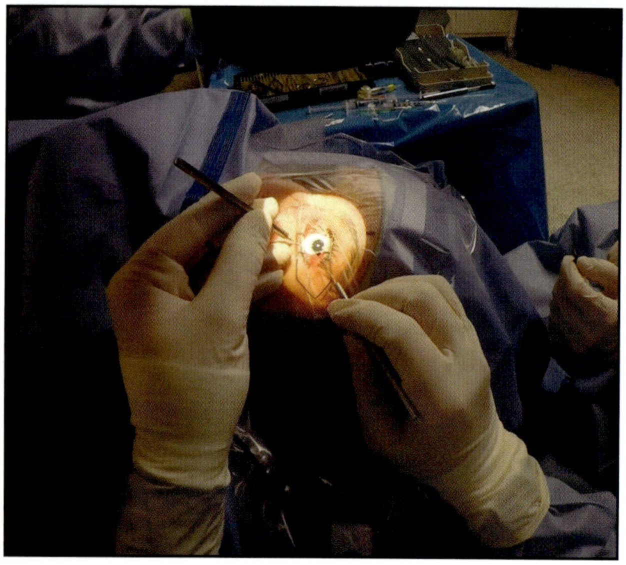

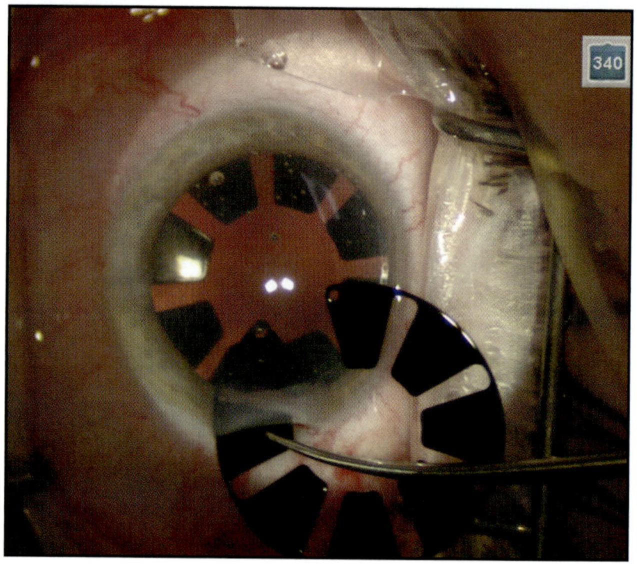

The first 2 fins of the second ring are inserted into the anterior chamber, through the center of the already implanted first ring. Through a paracentesis, a Kuglen hook is used to direct the ring downward behind the first ring while the rings are fed through the main incision with a blunt forceps.

- A Sinskey hook is used to engage the perforation on the final fin, guiding it through the main incision, while the Kuglen hook is used to ensure that the second ring remains below the first.
- Do not allow the fins to interdigitate as this could make rotation of the rings very difficult.

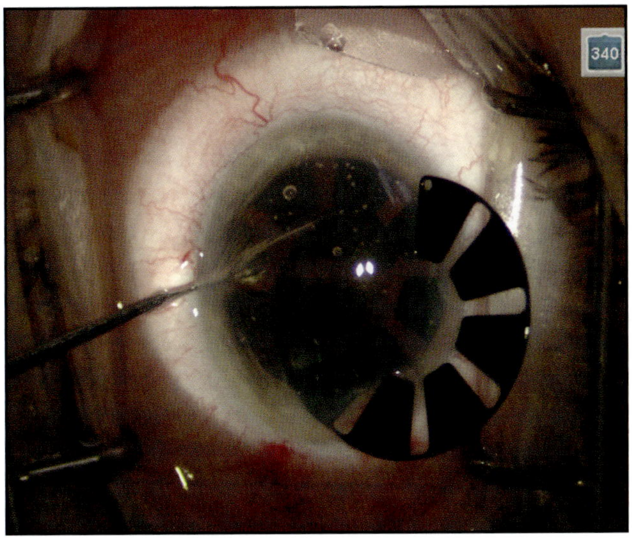

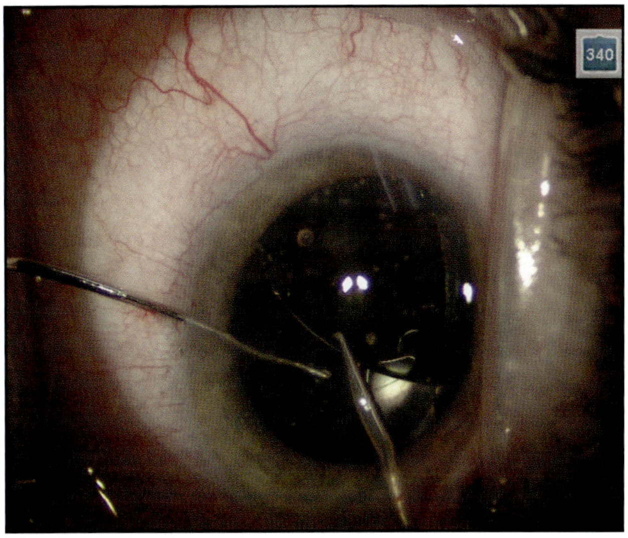

- Once the second ring is implanted, the Kuglen and Sinskey hooks are used to dial the superior ring until the fins overlap the empty spaces of the inferior ring. Using viscoelastic to separate these rings prior to rotation facilitates this process. Maintain a full capsular bag.
- Microforceps can be used to manually separate fins if they interdigitate. This is done by lifting the fin of the superior ring and with a Kuglen hook pushing back the fin of the inferior ring.

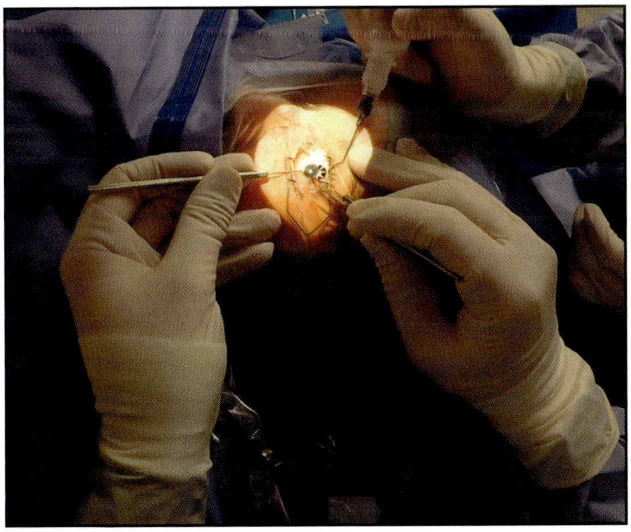

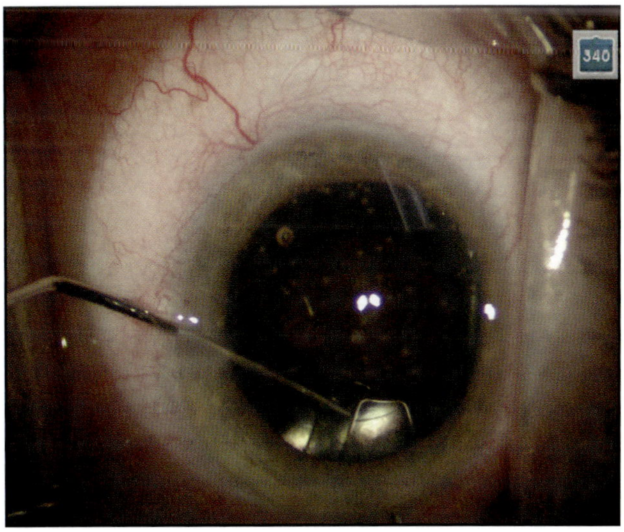

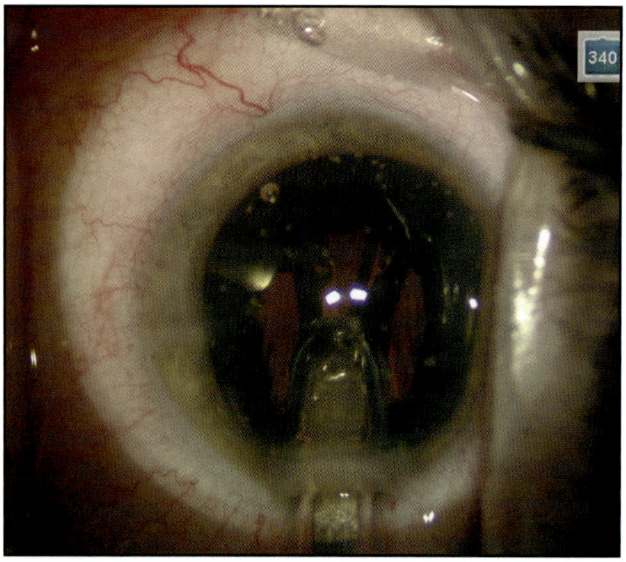

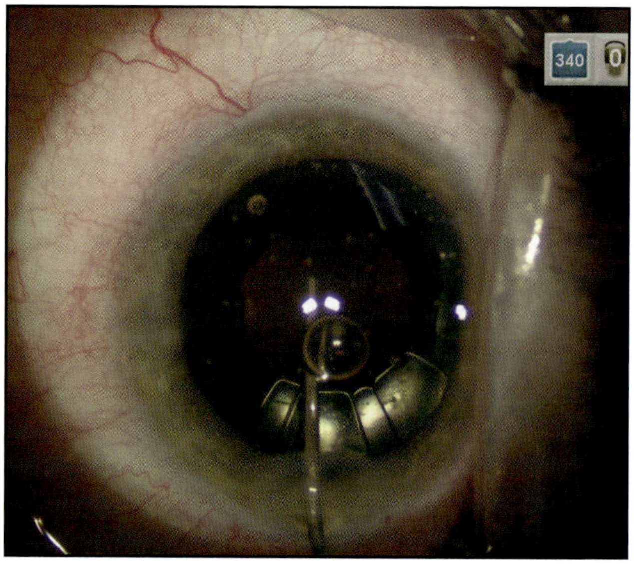

- Once all of the gaps in the rings are covered, there should be almost no red reflex viewed through the rings, except at the central pupil aperture.
- Cohesive OVD is used to elevate both rings anterior in the capsular bag. The IOL is delivered with the injector well within the capsular bag in order to ensure that the IOL is implanted posteriorly without catching the aniridia implants.
- Adjustments can be made to the aniridia rings to allow for complete occlusion of light penetration.

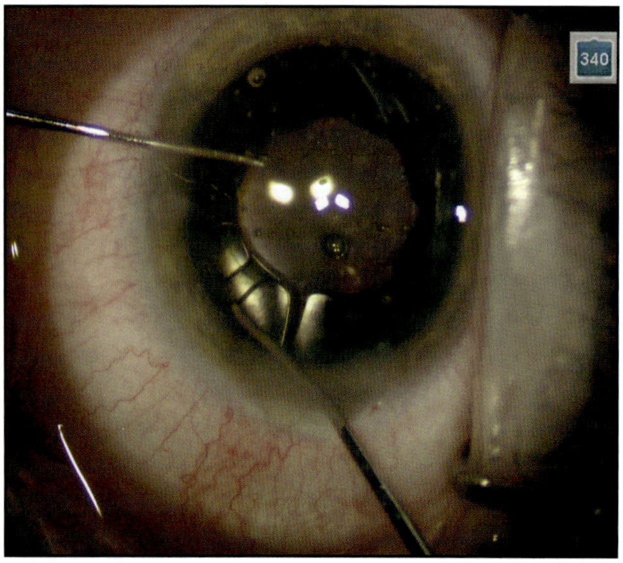

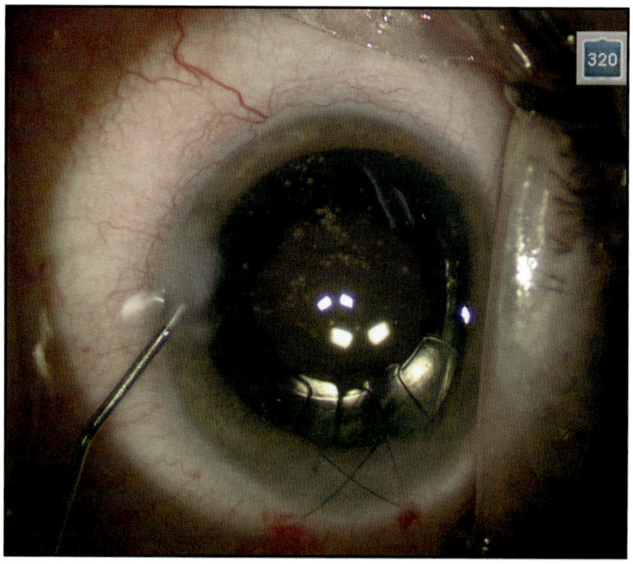

The main incision is sutured and OVD is removed manually to prevent movement of the implants that can occur with automated OVD removal.

HOW TO IMPLANT AN INTRACAPSULAR HUMANOPTICS ARTIFICIAL IRIS

This is a patient with congenital aniridia. Routine phacoemulsification and IOL implantation was performed. After insertion of a single-piece acrylic IOL in the capsular bag, the HumanOptics artificial, custom, hand-painted iris prosthesis (fiberless model) can be cut using a corneal trephine. Diameter of cut should be sized to 1 mm less than white-to-white distance.

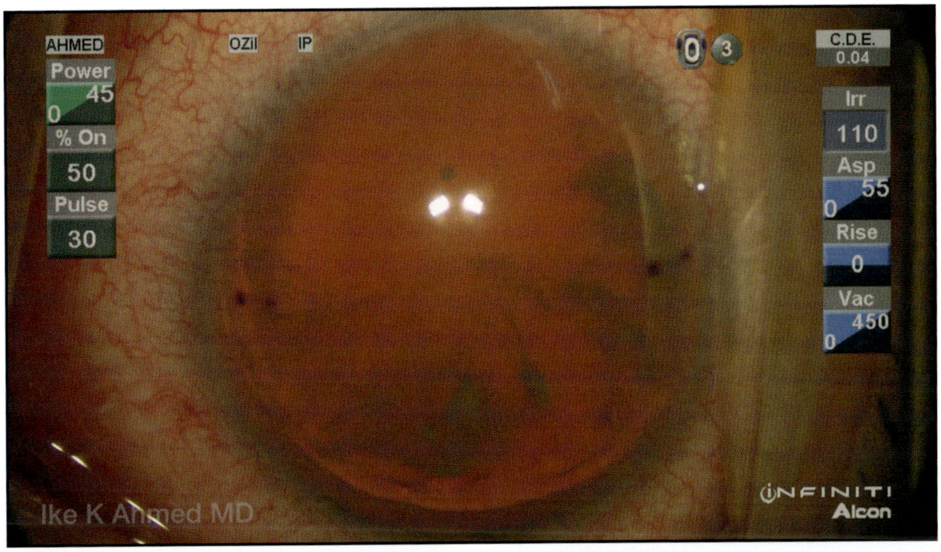

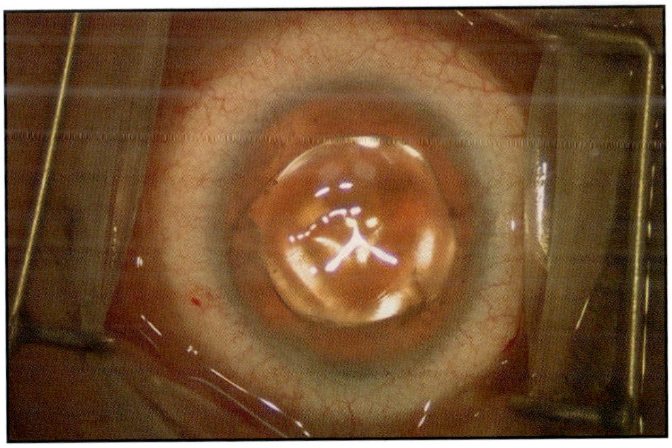

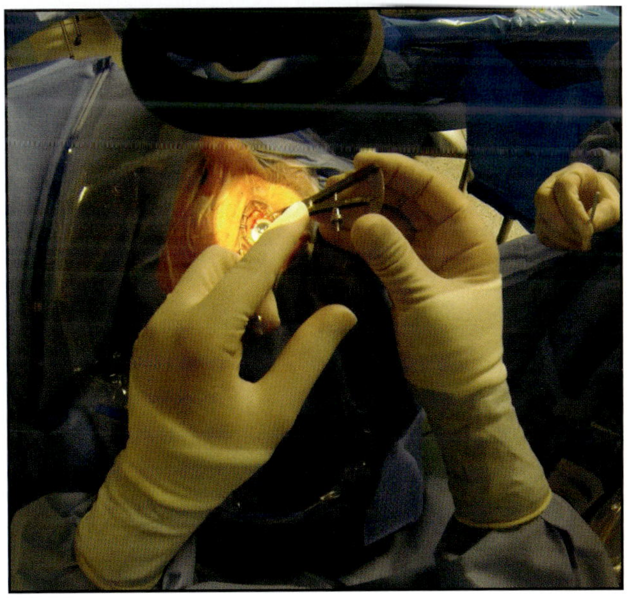

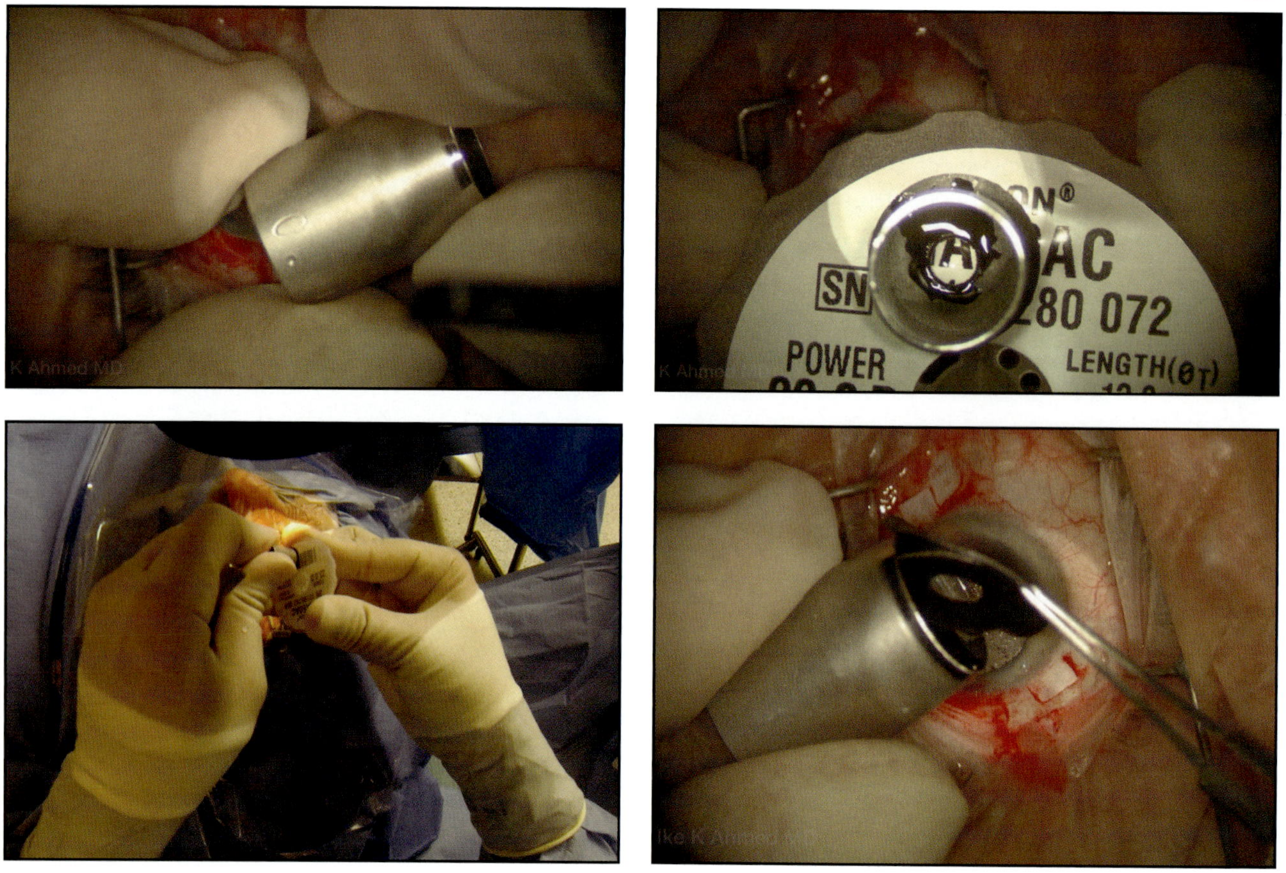

A corneal trephine can be used against an IOL case or any other small flat surface that can be held with one hand. Care must be taken to achieve a clean cut without leaving shards or pointed edges, which could cause uveal tissue chafing.

The HumanOptics implant must be tri-folded (rolled), color-side out, and inserted into an IOL injector cartridge with a toothless tyer to avoid damaging the customized color surface.

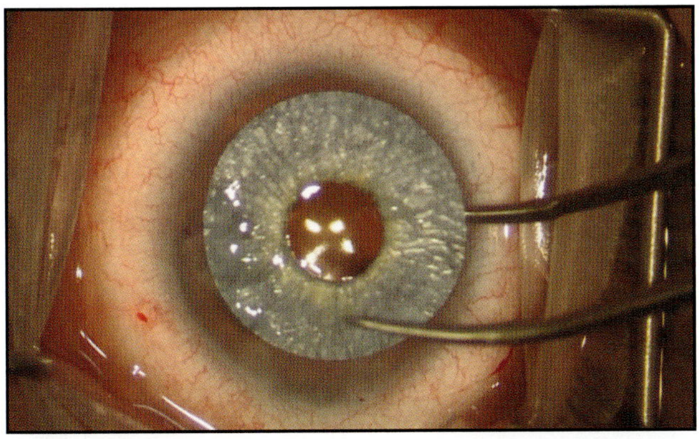

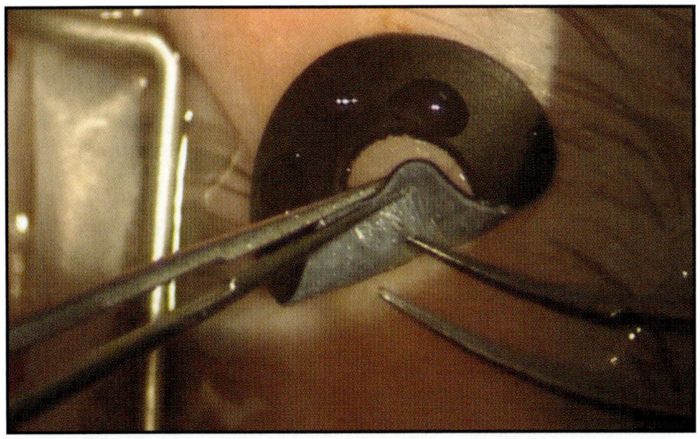

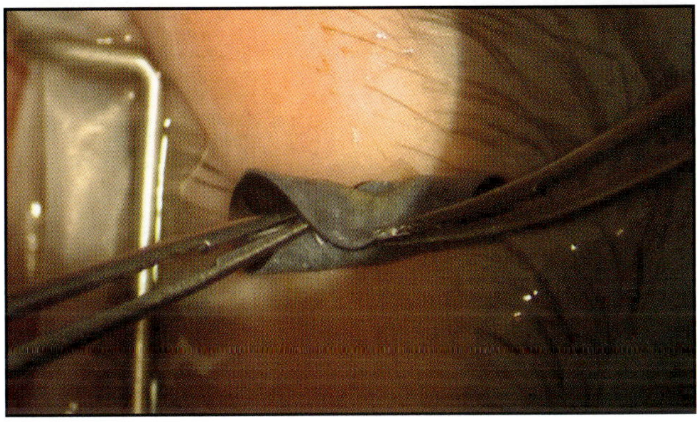

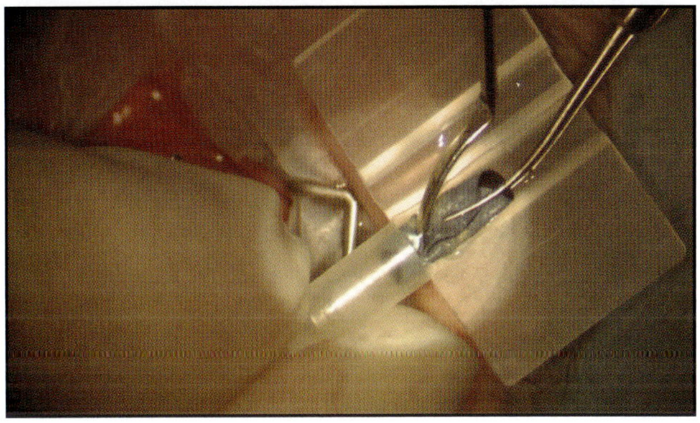

In this case, we used a hinge-style cartridge, but other nonhinged cartridges may also be used.

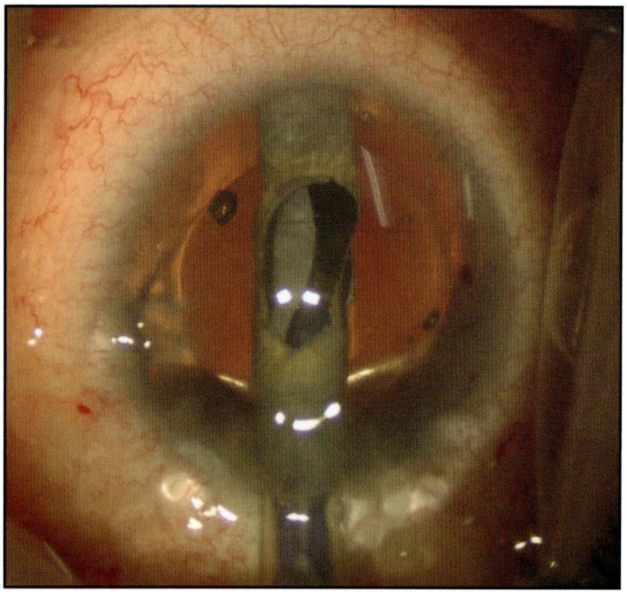

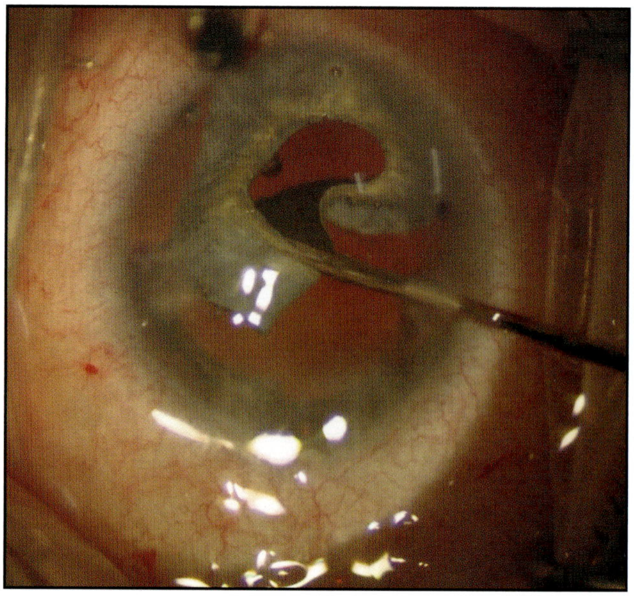

The cartridge bevel is inserted face down and the implant is injected directly inside or above the capsular bag. Do not use wound-assisted delivery. A second instrument keeps the implant in the eye as the injector is removed. Micrograspers and a Kuglen hook are used to position the implant completely inside the bag. Holding at the pupil border and pulling centrally allows the peripheral portion of the prosthesis to be placed beneath the bag with a Kuglen hook. OVD is removed manually using balanced salt solution on a blunt cannula. Take extra care to not allow anterior chamber shallowing. Postoperative intraocular pressure monitoring with glaucoma drops and sometimes oral medication is necessary after any manual OVD removal case.

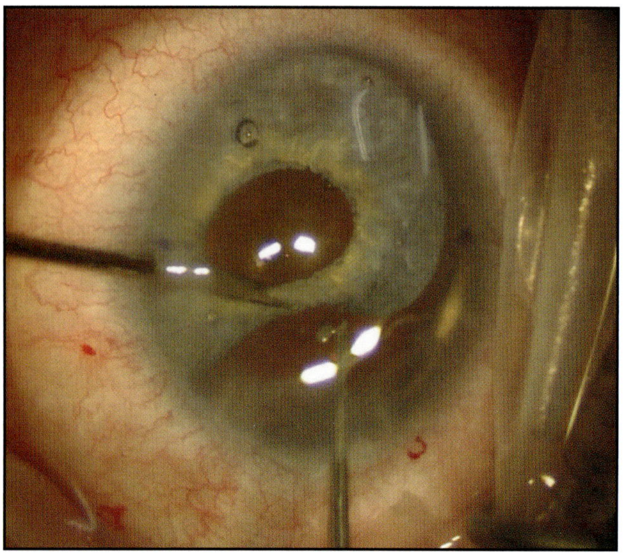

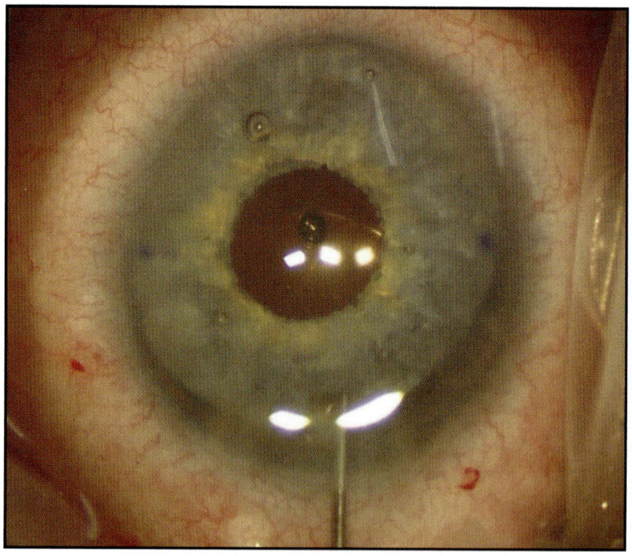

CHAPTER 31

HUMANOPTICS AND INTRASCLERAL HAPTIC FIXATION OF A THREE-PIECE IOL

INTRODUCTION

In the setting of aniridia and aphakia, the restorative options are limited to cosmetic contact lenses vs iris prosthetics that have intraocular lenses (IOLs) incorporated. Prefabricated surgical devices incorporating iris prosthetics with IOLs offer good outcomes in terms of visual recovery and resolution of photophobia, but are not cosmetically appealing.

The HumanOptics implant is cosmetically superior to current iris prostheses. However, it is not manufactured in combination with IOLs. This technique, although somewhat challenging surgically, provides excellent cosmetic outcomes as well as visual rehabilitation and improvement of photophobia.

KEY POINTS

- This technique is very similar to the intrascleral haptic fixation technique described in Chapter 20. An important difference is the need for a larger incision (7 mm) and the fixture of the 3-piece IOL onto the iris prosthesis by creating "belt loop" punctures on the prosthesis.
- IOL orientation must be correct when fixating the IOL through the "belt-loops" of the iris prosthesis. You must use HumanOptics artificial iris WITH FIBER for this technique.
- The wound should be at least 7 mm wide, otherwise too much force is needed to draw the iris prosthesis and IOL complex into the eye. This can decenter the IOL.
- Cut the iris prosthesis with a corneal trephine on a hard surface so that tags do not occur.
- If they exist, excise large stumps of residual iris tissue prior to placement of the iris prosthesis.

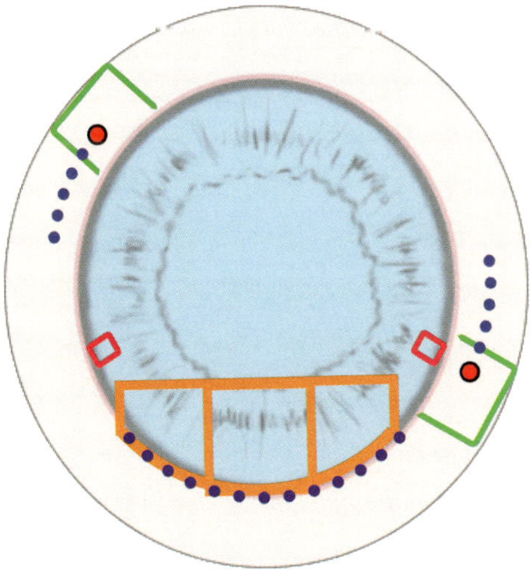

- Knife and fork
- 7-mm scleral groove, triplanar 3-step incision
- 23-g sclerotomies
- 30-g scleral tunnels 180 degrees apart beneath L-shaped conjunctival peritomies

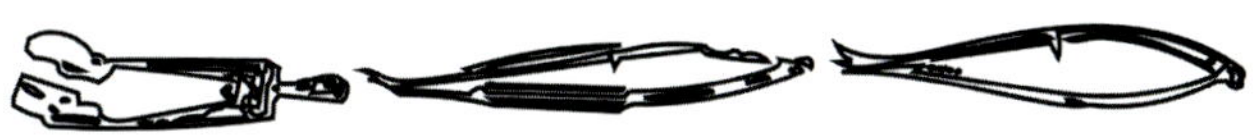

- Two Microsurgical Technology, Inc microtyers
- Anterior chamber maintainer or pars plana infusion
- 30-g needles (x2)
- 23-g trocar (microvitreoretinal [MVR] blade)
- HumanOptics artificial iris WITH FIBER
- Fibrin glue

Ahmed IK, Campos-Möller X, Shah M, Sheybani A. *Illustrated Advanced Anterior Segment Surgery: A Step-by-Step Guide for Challenging Cases* (pp 237-245).

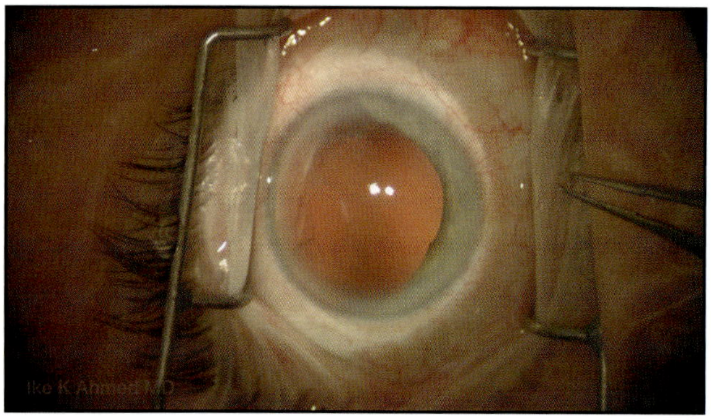

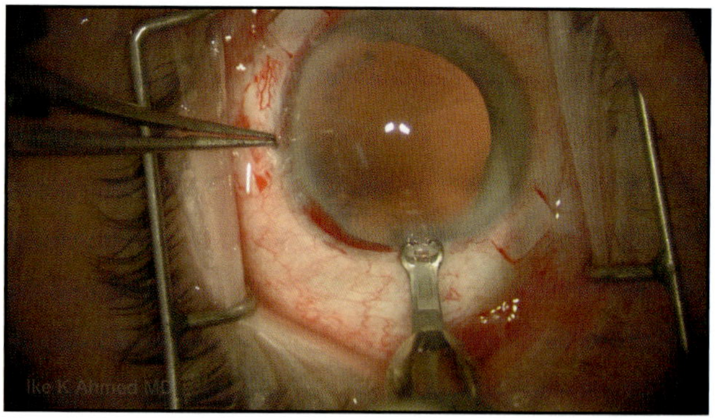

- This is a case of traumatic aphakia and partial aniridia with a history of pars plana vitrectomy and lensectomy.
- A 7-mm, 250-μm deep limbocorneal groove is created at the site of the main incision.
- Scleral flaps and tunnels for haptic tucking are created as for the intrascleral haptic fixated IOL technique described in Chapter 20.

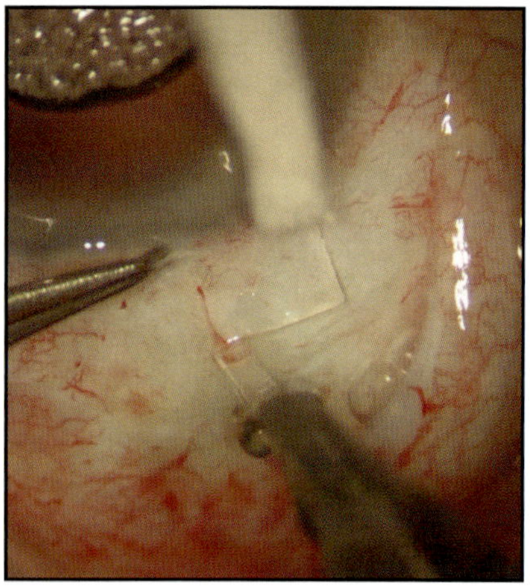

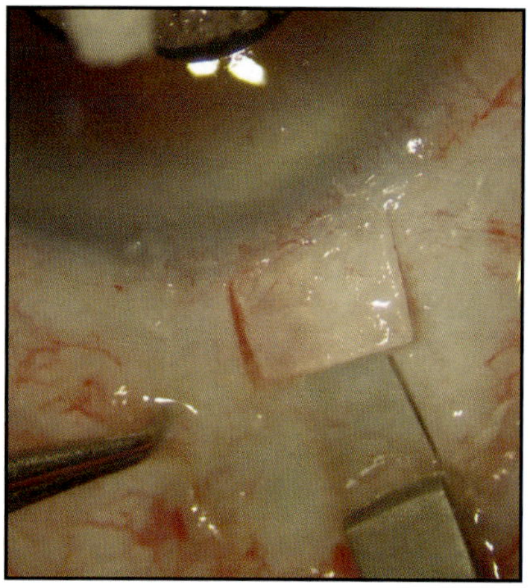

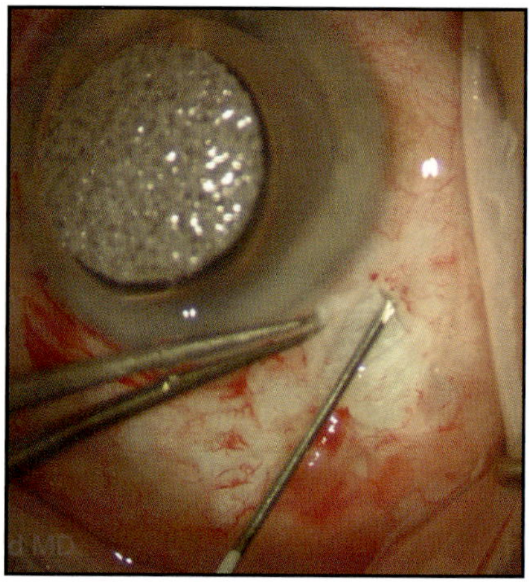

The HumanOptics implant comes standard in a 12.8-mm size. It must be cut to 10 mm for most eyes. This allows for sufficient clearance for the haptics of a 13-mm IOL to be tucked into the scleral tunnels. The implant has a colored side with tissue and a black side.

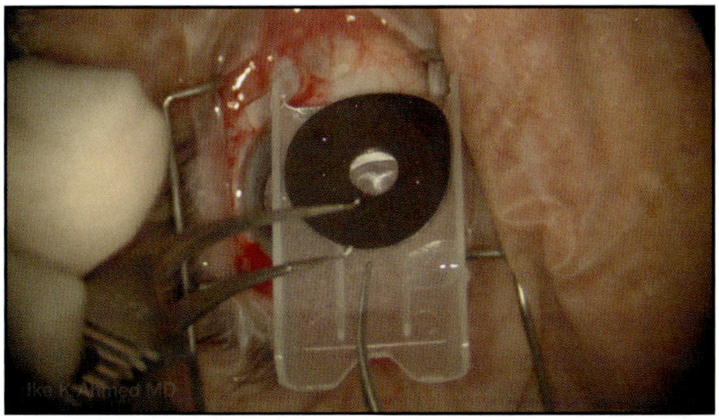

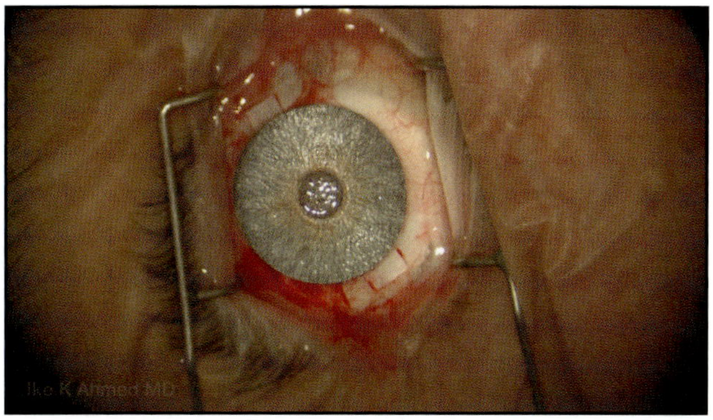

Cutting of the implant is best achieved using a 10-mm corneal trephine. Careful centration is important. The cutting motion requires a fair amount of pressure against the implant, as well as back-and-forth rotation of the trephine. Always place the implant colored face down to cut. It is important to cut all the way through the implant in one try and to avoid recentering to ensure the edges are smooth. Curved Westcott scissors can be used to free any remaining attachments between the 10-mm central implant and the surrounding ring.

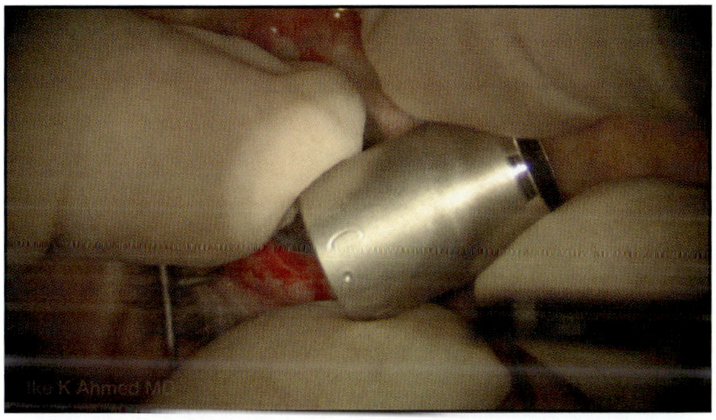

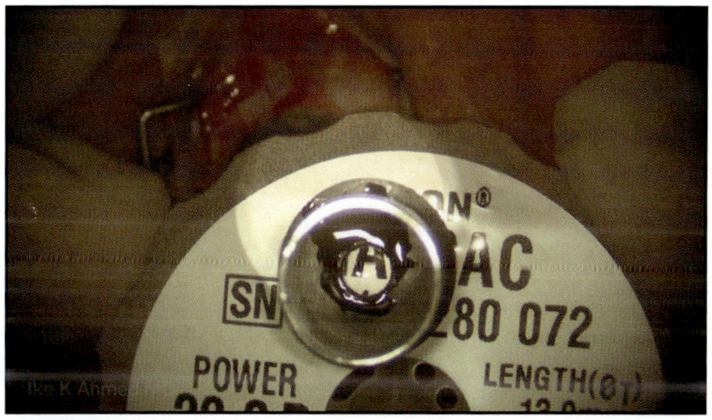

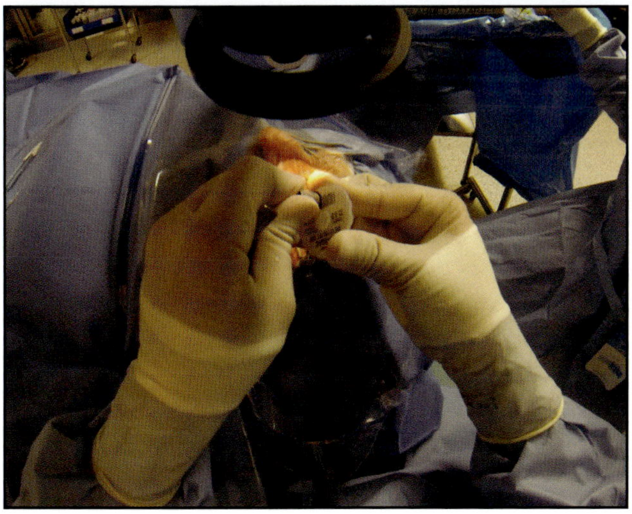

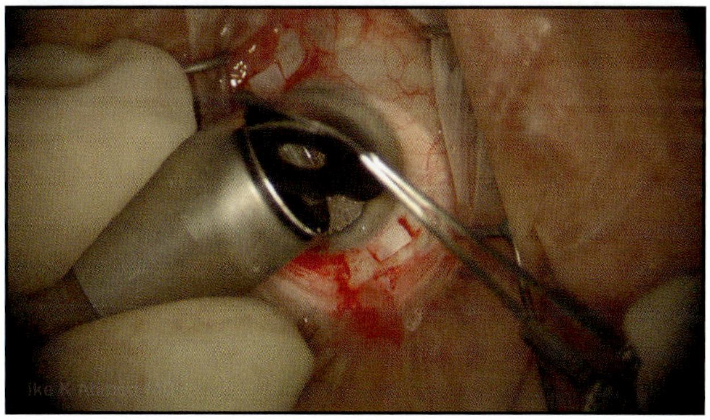

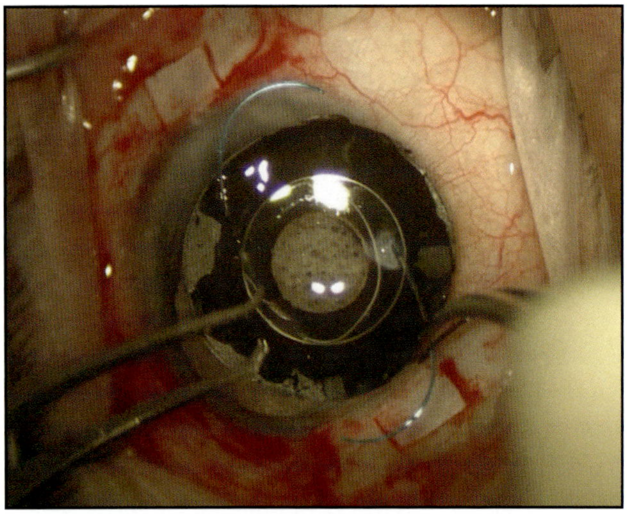

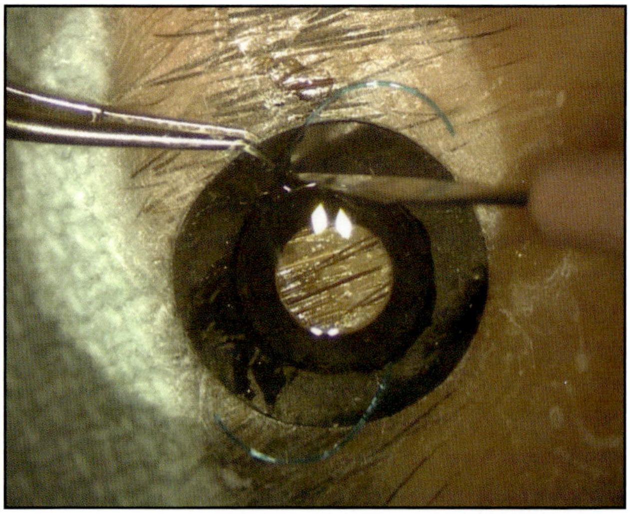

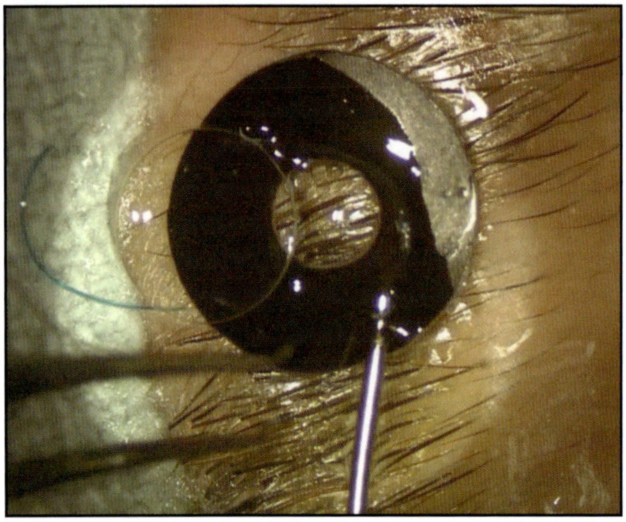

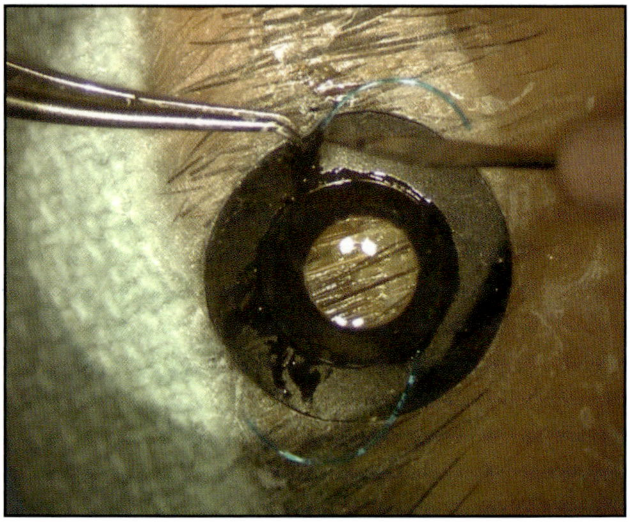

- Fixation of the IOL to the implant is achieved by creating 2 perforations that will act as belt loops for each haptic. The IOL and implant are flipped over for belt-loop creation. Center the inverted IOL over the artificial iris's aperture. This will serve as a template for the 2 punctures that are to be made in the artificial iris.
- Grasp the prosthesis with small toothed forceps and cut 2 full-thickness, 0.5-mm slits, 0.5 mm apart with a sharp-tipped blade running perpendicular to the haptic. This creates a belt loop through which the haptic will be placed in order to hold the IOL to the iris prosthesis implant.

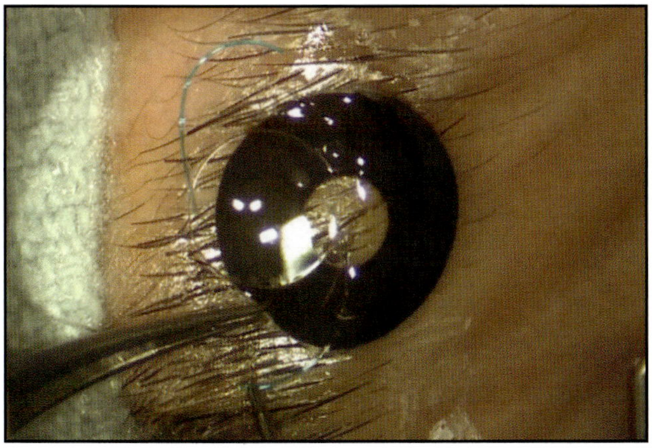

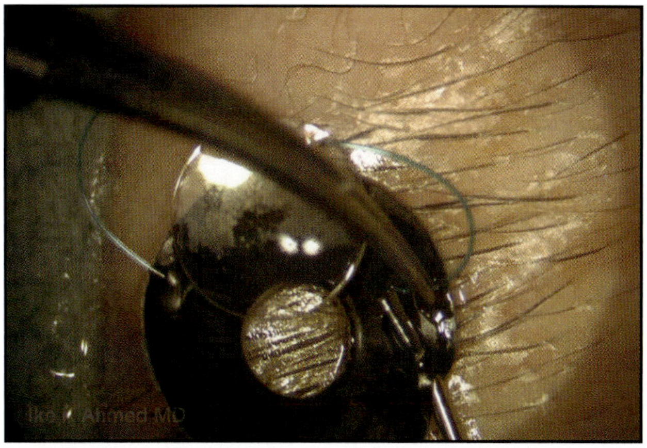

- Drawing of belt loops and attachment to IOL.

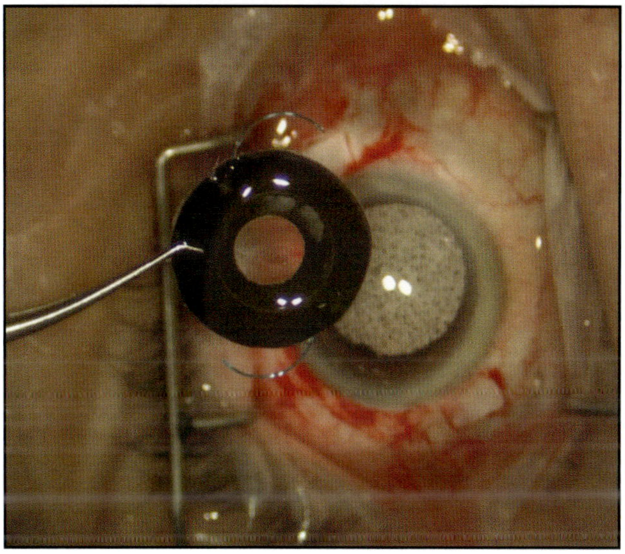

- Curved microforceps are placed through the slits. Proper placement of the microforceps results in a "bridge" of the iris prosthesis OVER the forceps.
- The proximal haptic is grasped at the distal tip of the haptic to prevent bending or breakage, and the micrograsper is retracted in reverse through the belt loop until the IOL is centered again in relation to the pupil.
- This is repeated for the distal haptic. In order to feed the second haptic through the belt loop while the first haptic has already been placed, shift the IOL as far through the first belt loop as possible to create more room so that the distal haptic is not kinked when it is fed through the loop.

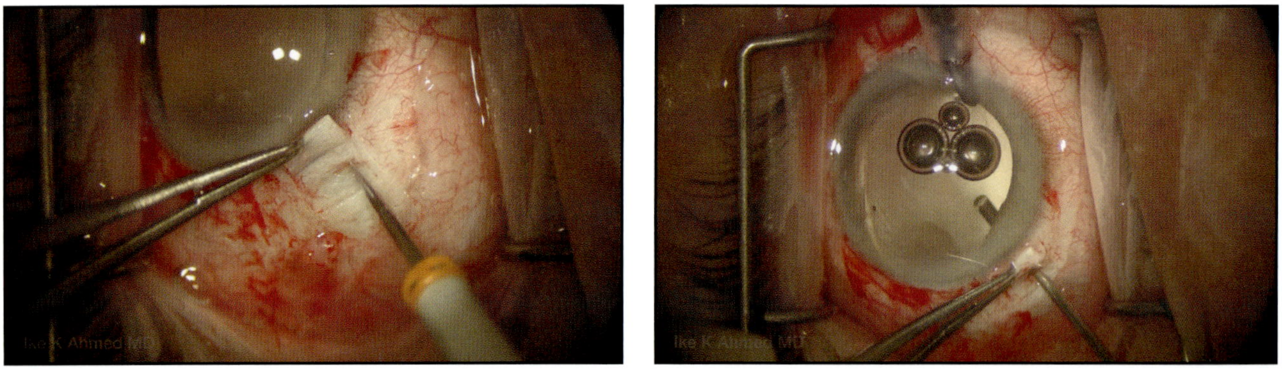

A 20-g MVR blade is used to make sclerotomies for haptic externalization. They are 0.5 mm back from the scleral spur (where the blue limbal fibers meet the white scleral fibers). They are not situated at the center of the square scleral bed—they should be shifted toward the site of haptic tunnel entry. This ensures that the externalized haptic travels through a long scleral tunnel. Here, we are using triamcinolone to stain the vitreous gel. Thorough vitrectomy should be performed from an anterior or posterior approach to remove vitreous from the anterior portion of the posterior segment, especially around the sclerotomies. An anterior chamber maintainer should be used from this point onward.

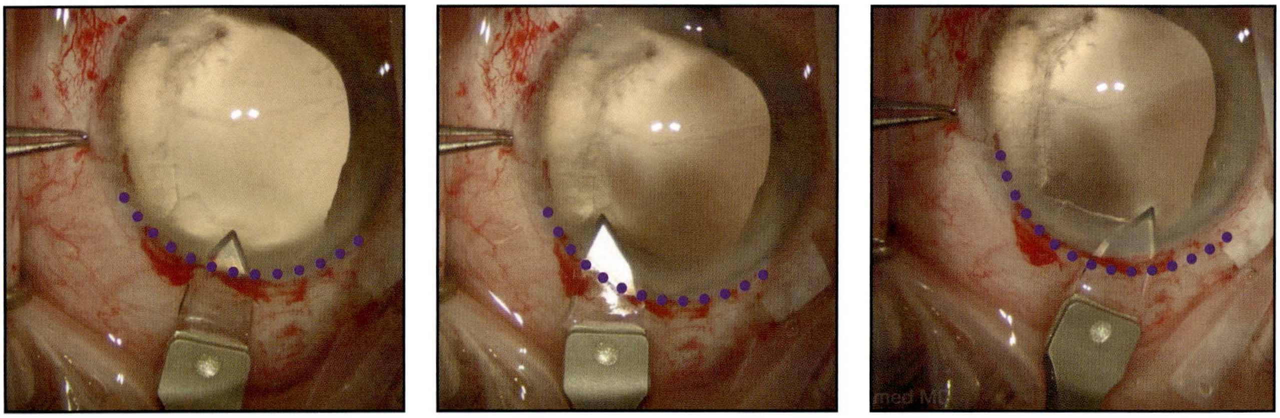

Creating an incision with a 3-plane architecture ensures adequate wound healing and minimizes astigmatism. Enter the anterior chamber with a 2.75- to 3-mm keratome at the center of the previously created limbal groove (purple dotted line) and then cut sideways to the left and right.

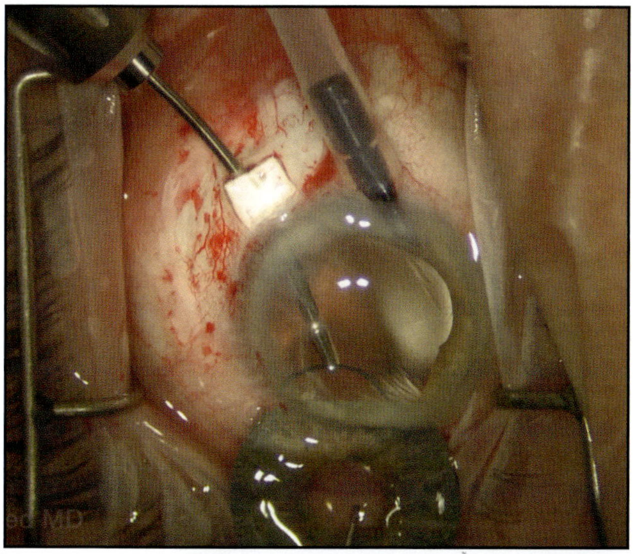

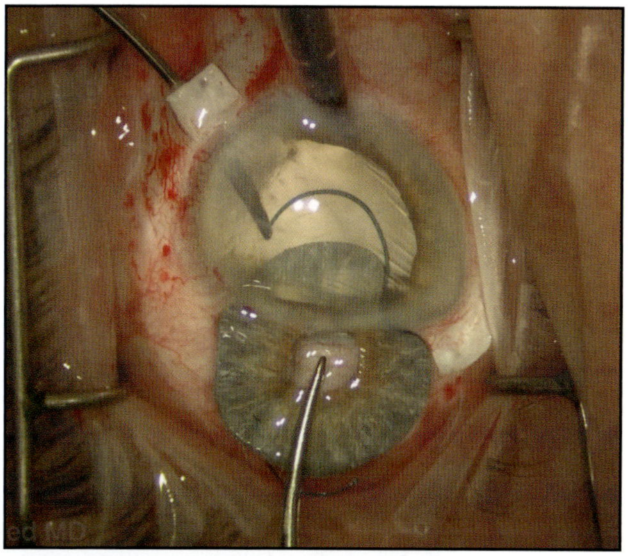

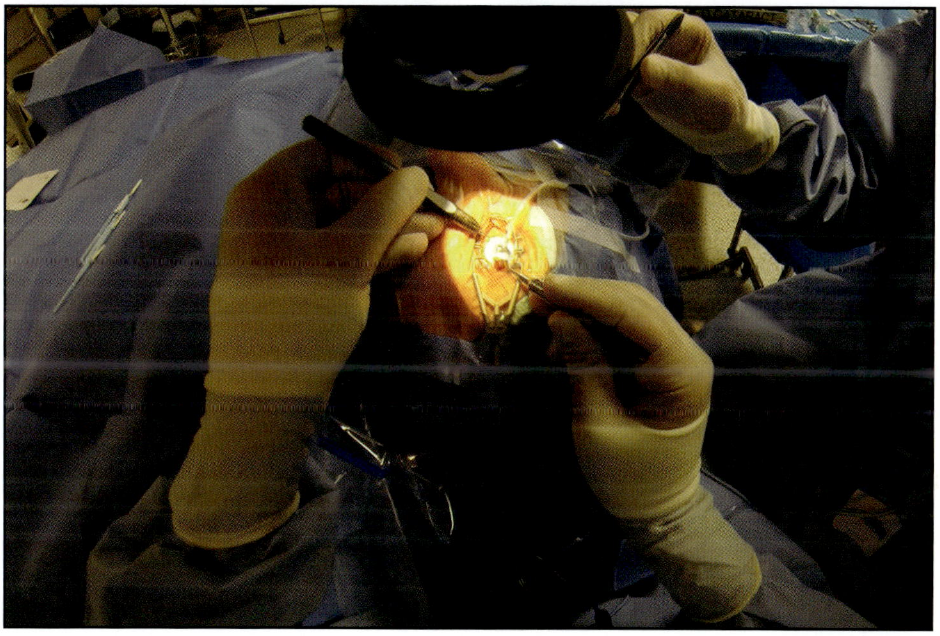

- Curved nontoothed forceps are used to grab the implant up to mid-pupil to prevent IOL slippage during insertion.
- The curved micrograsper is fed through the distal MVR incision (as in Chapter 20) and is used to grab the distal haptic as the IOL/prosthesis complex is inserted into the eye. DO NOT PULL, but push the implant into the eye. Remember to maintain chamber with posterior infusion or an anterior chamber maintainer.

The distal haptic is externalized and held with a nontoothed forceps by an assistant. The handshake maneuver is then performed by handing the trailing haptic with a micrograsper to another micrograsper that has been previously inserted through a sclerostomy 180 degrees apart to the site where the leading haptic was externalized (see Chapter 20). The implant can make visualization challenging, so performing the maneuver as peripherally as possible will provide the best visualization. Having made the scleral flap near the corneal incision will make this step more manageable.

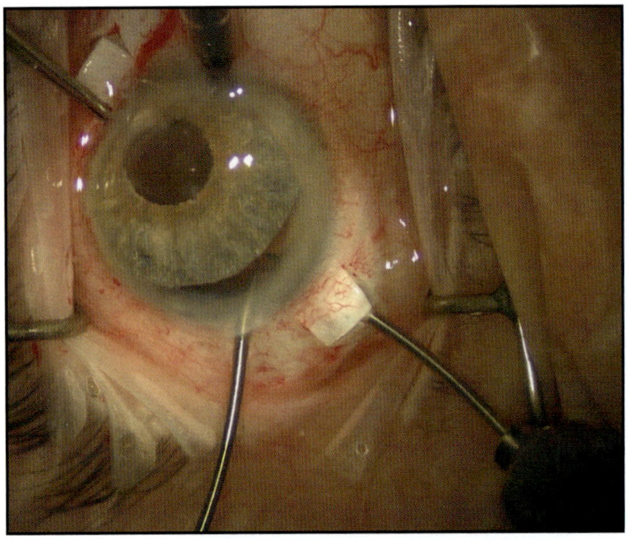

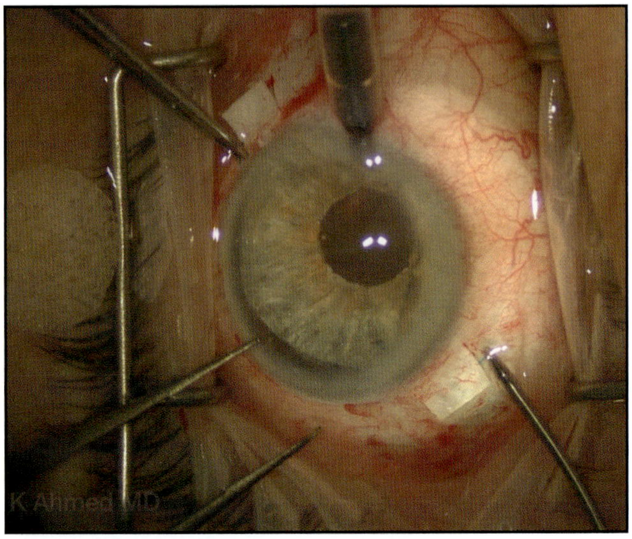

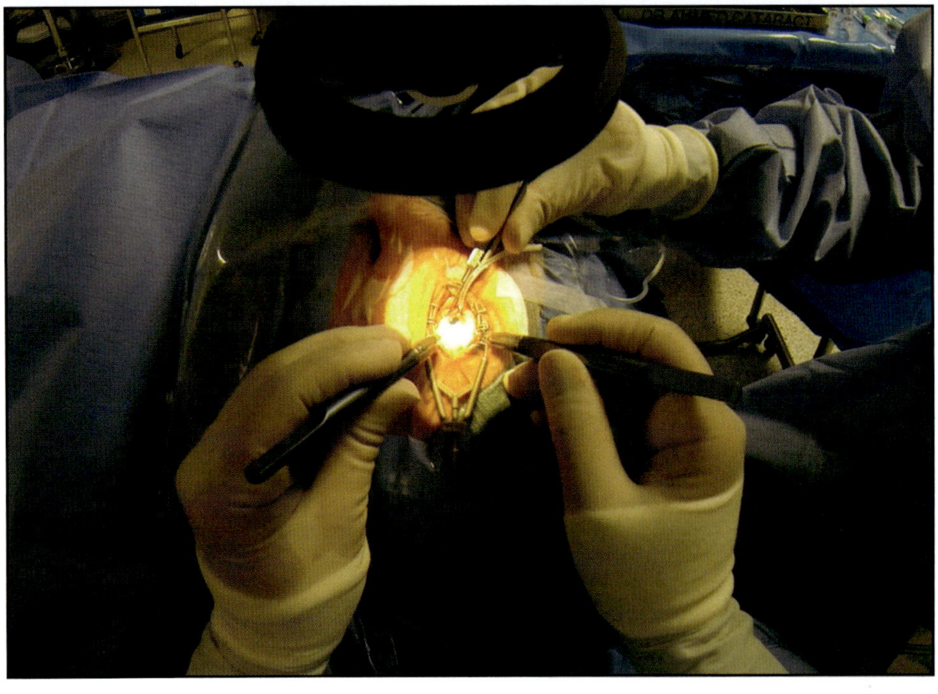

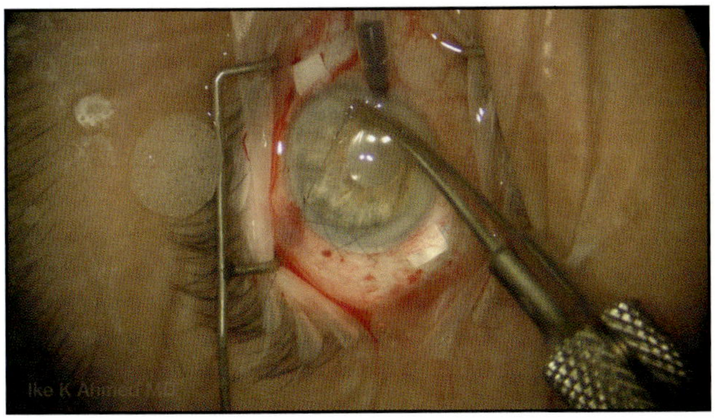

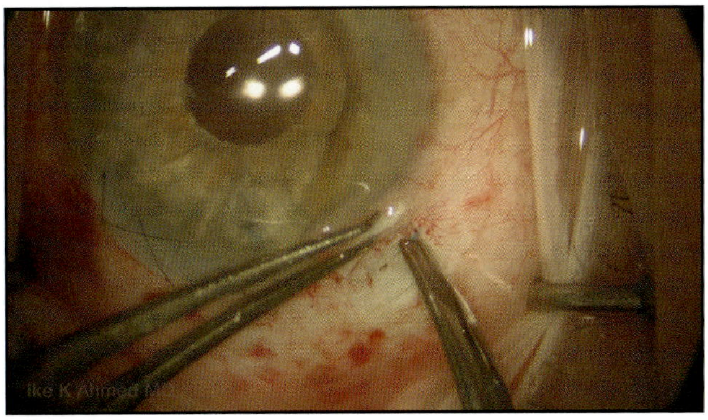

Wound closure should be prompt to avoid anterior chamber shallowing, vitreous prolapse, and especially choroidal expansion or detachment, which could lead to catastrophic complications. Our preferred suturing technique is a continuous "Z" technique. See Chapter 26 for a more detailed explanation of this suture.

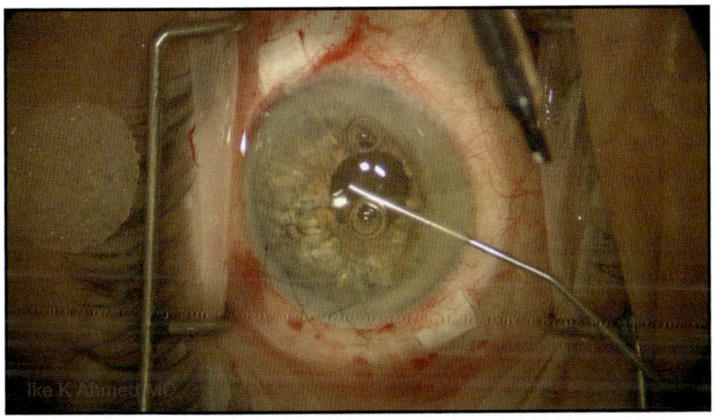

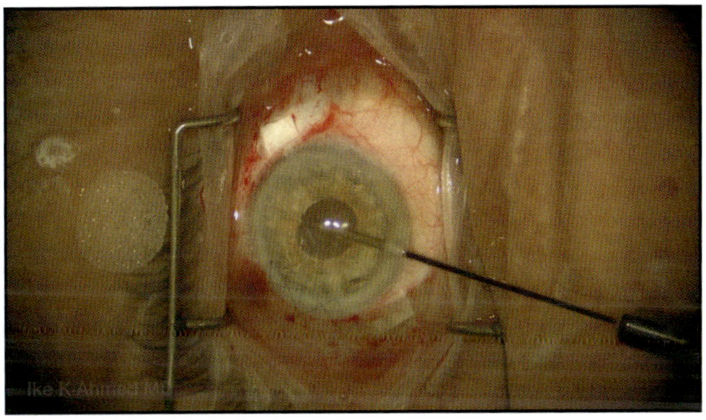

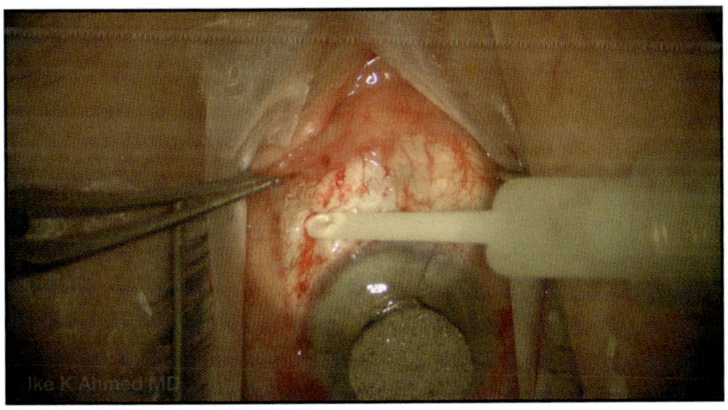

Centration of the implant can be achieved with a microforceps and by gently pulling on one haptic while holding onto the contralateral haptic to prevent dislocating it. Once centration is adequate, the haptics are tucked into their scleral tunnels and flap closure can be achieved with fibrin glue.

CHAPTER 32

HOW TO REPAIR AN IRIDODIALYSIS

INTRODUCTION

Iridodialysis repairs are performed when the patient has visual complaints that are attributed to the defect, including light sensitivity or monocular diplopia. This repair may need pupilloplasty in combination as drawing the iris to the iris root can sometimes result in mydriasis, especially when the iris sphincter is poor or nonfunctional.

KEY POINTS

- Identify the orientation of the iris; in iridodialysis, the iris can twist on itself and unless one is careful, the pupillary sphincter can be confused for peripheral iris root.
- Use a cohesive viscoelastic to flatten iris into position.
- Use a dispersive viscoelastic to tamponade vitreous.

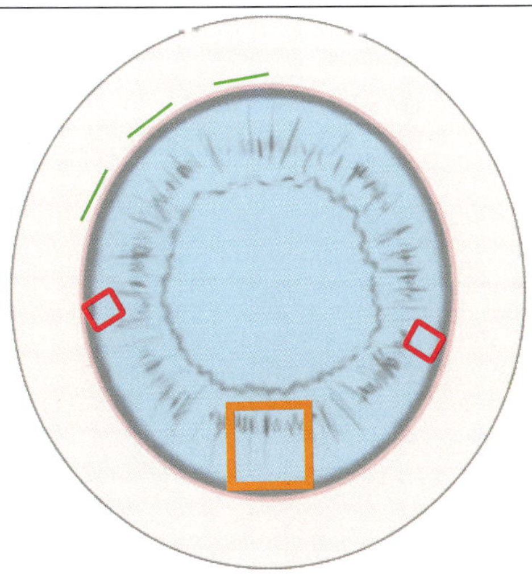

- Knife and fork, conjunctival peritomy, scratch grooves for suture burial (one groove per knot required)

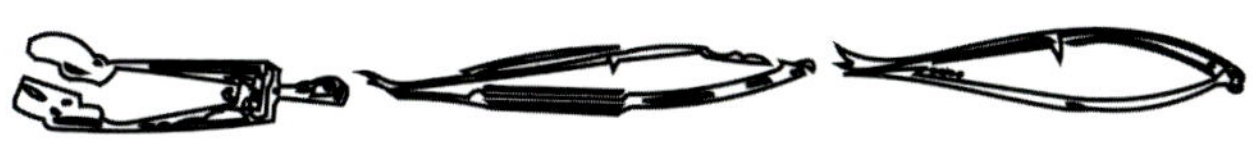

- Straight (STC-6) or curved (CIF-4 or PC-7) needle on a 10-0 polypropylene suture
- Micrograspers

Ahmed IK, Campos-Möller X, Shah M, Sheybani A. *Illustrated Advanced Anterior Segment Surgery: A Step-by-Step Guide for Challenging Cases* (pp 247-251).

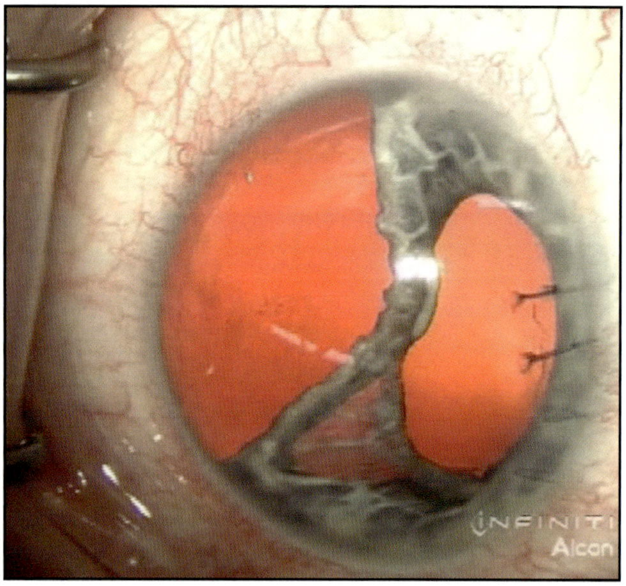

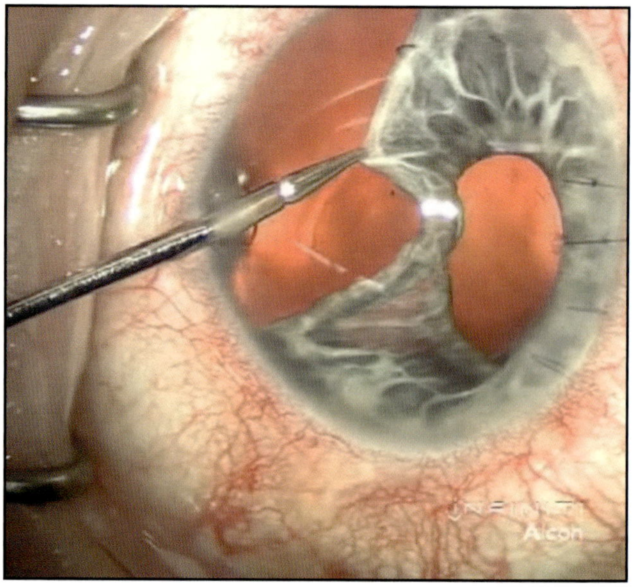

- Identify iris anatomy and position the iris with the pupil centered and the peripheral iris near the limbus. Micrograspers can be used to approximate the detached peripheral iris to the limbus, and cohesive ophthalmic viscosurgical device can be used to unroll any scrolls that may have curled up.
- Create a conjunctival peritomy along the length of the iridodialysis. Identify the scleral spur, looking for the blue-white junction. Create several 2-mm scleral "scratches" right at the scleral spur, parallel to the limbus, in the clock hours with iridodialysis.

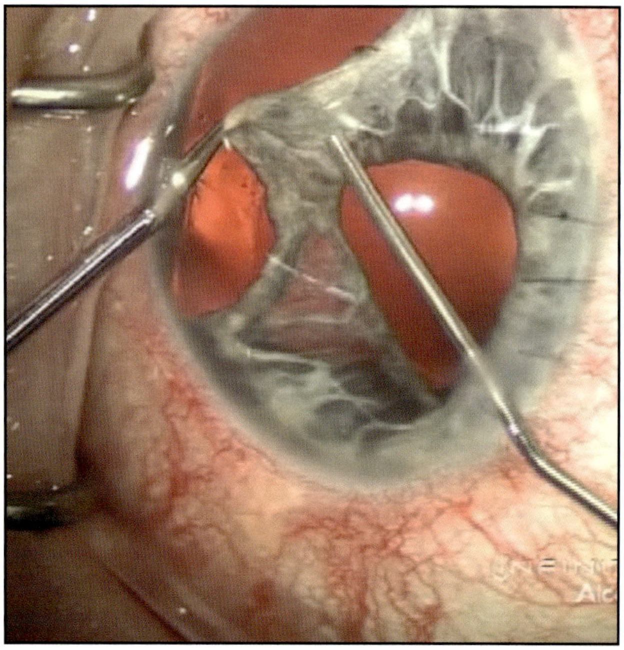

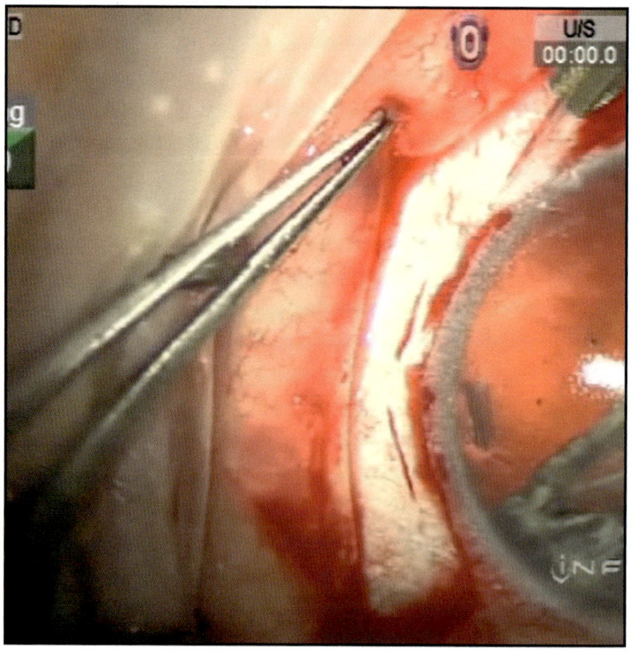

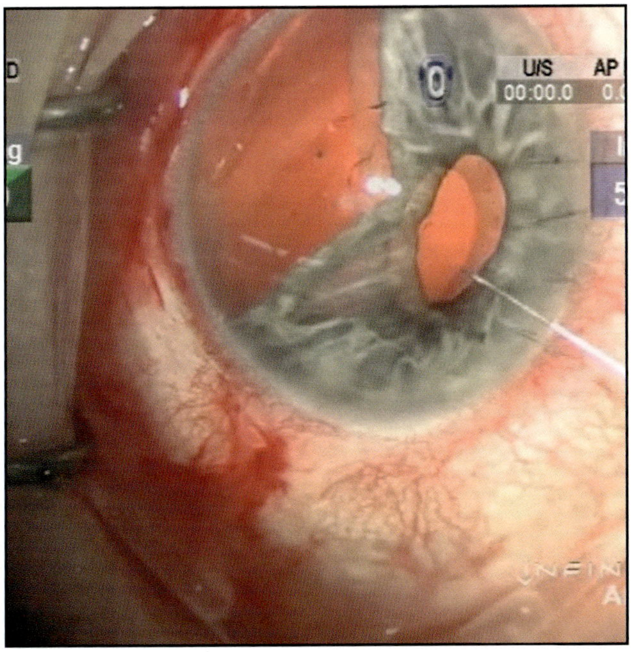

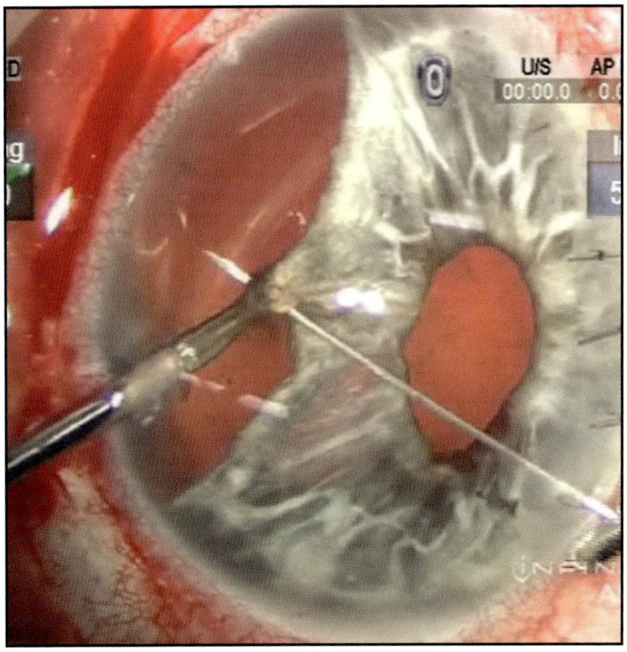

- The double-armed suture is passed through the peripheral iris and docked into a 27-g hypodermic needle that enters at the level of the scleral spur. A micrograsper can facilitate suture placement through iris.
- Withdraw the needle out of the eye.
- Alternatively, an ab interno approach can be performed, where there is no docking and the needle is passed through iris then through sclera.
- Repeat this step 1.5 clock hours apart with the second arm of the needle. The iris passes are closer together than the scleral passes so that the iris can stretch against the interior scleral wall.

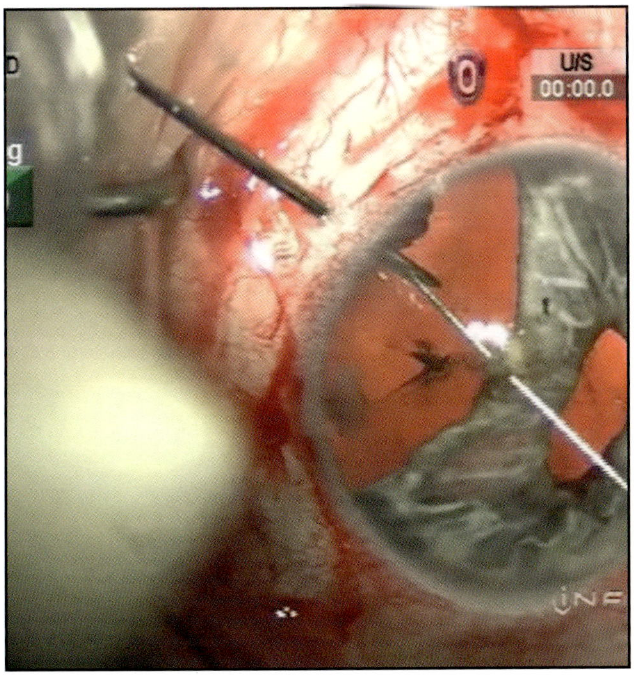

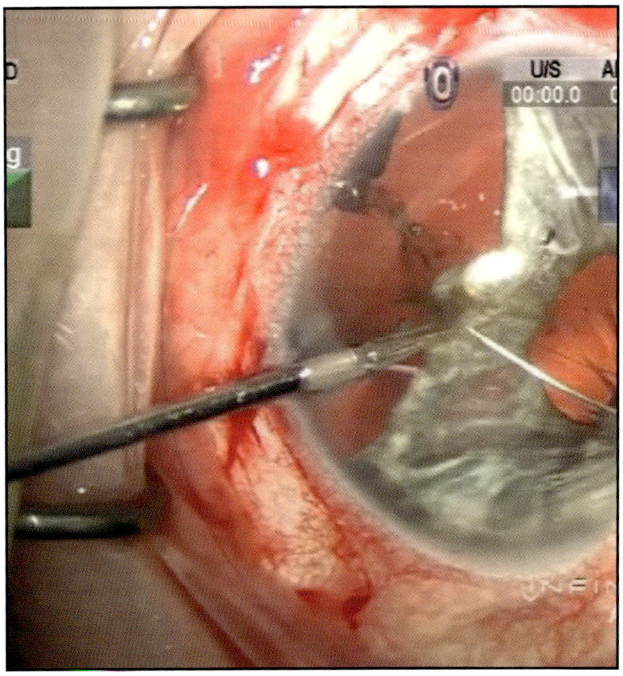

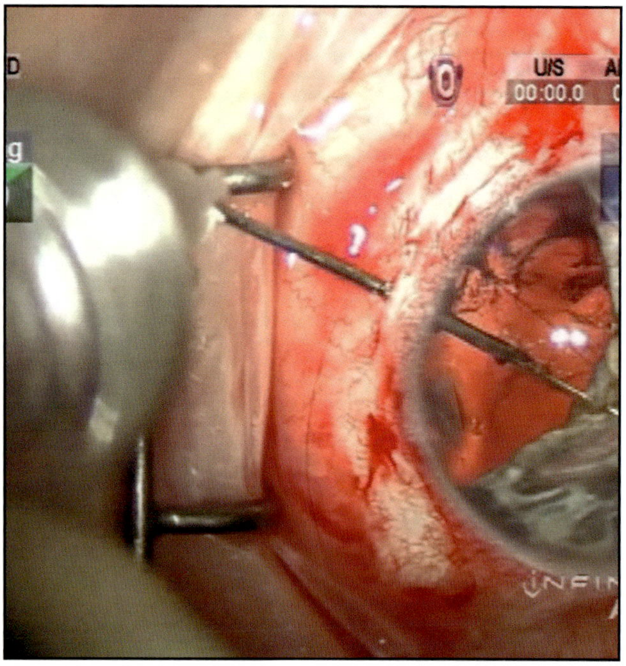

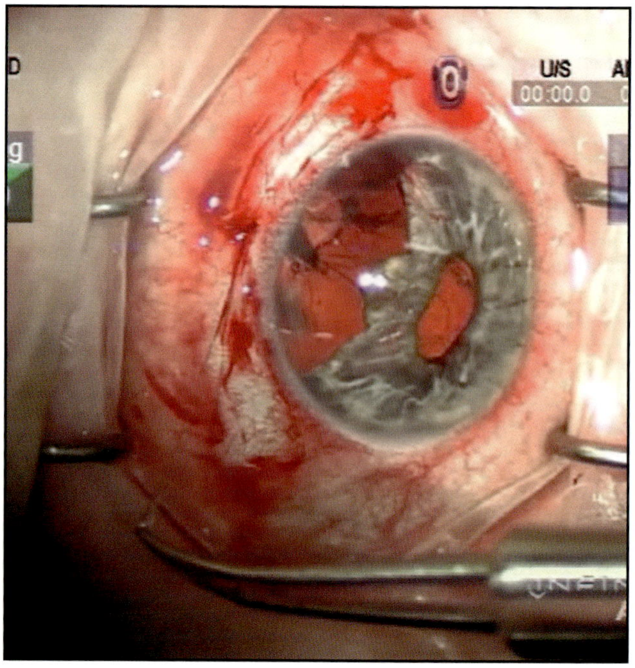

- The suture is tied externally, and this is repeated along the length of the defect. If multiple passes are required, DO NOT TIE the knots until all passes have been performed.
- Tie the sutures in a slip knot. Sometimes, the iris is allowed to hang back as to not overly draw the pupil toward the angle.
- The knots are rotated internally and buried with the help of a tyer.
- The conjunctiva is closed over the incision.

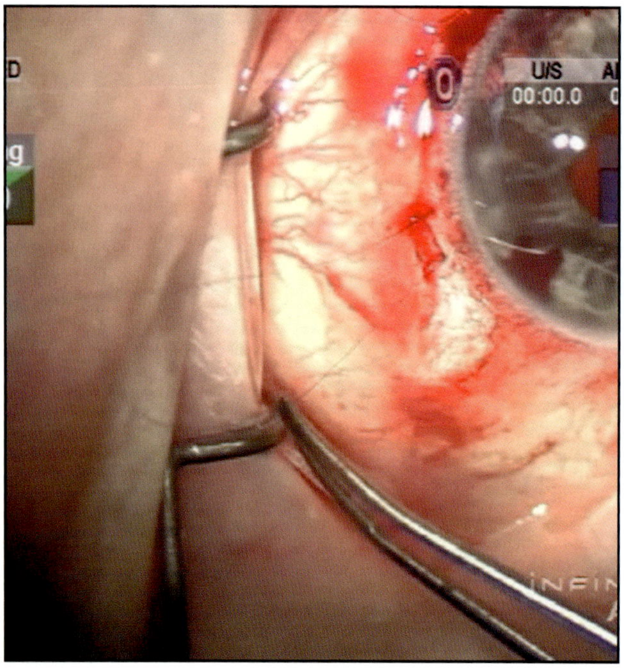

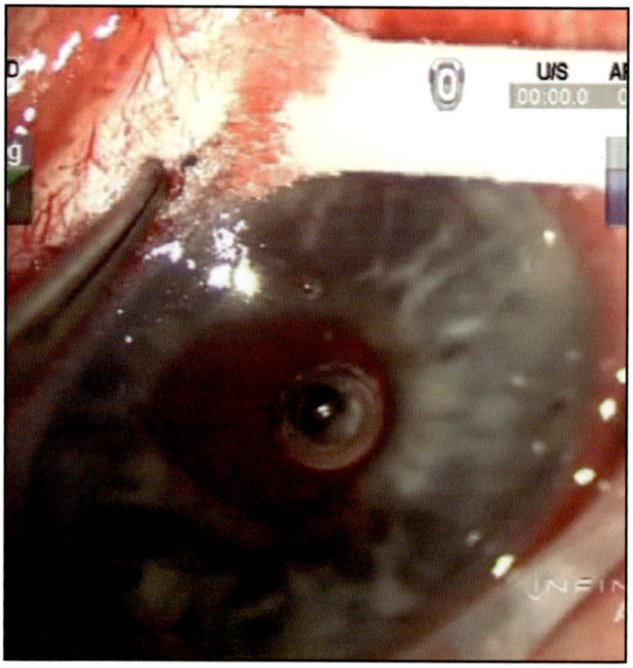

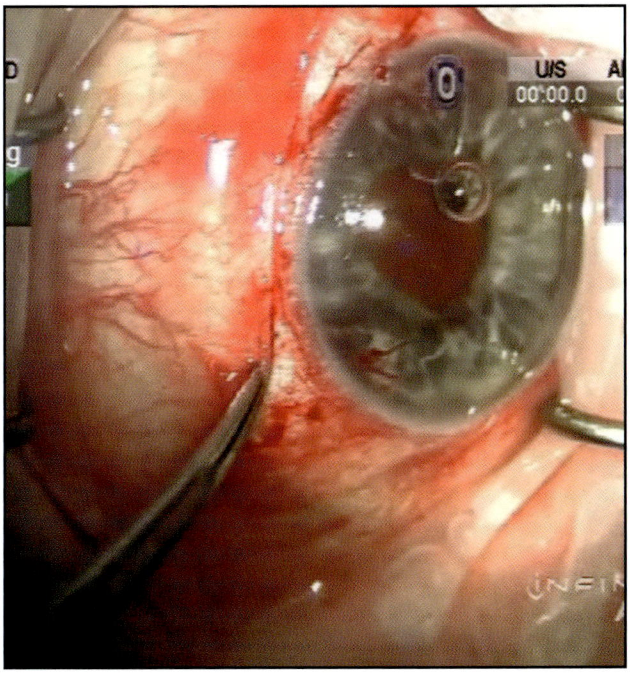
U/S
00:00.0

CHAPTER 33

HOW TO REPAIR A CYCLODIALYSIS CLEFT

INTRODUCTION

Cyclodialysis clefts can lead to hypotony as aqueous gains access to the suprachoroidal space. These clefts are a separation of the longitudinal fibers of the ciliary body from the scleral spur. Many can close spontaneously. Those that do not can lead to hypotony and its sequelae (hypotony maculopathy, choroidal effusions, disc edema, decreased vision). If conservative measures like atropine fail, laser therapy (argon or transscleral diode cyclophotocoagulation) can be attempted to close the cleft by inducing inflammation leading to scarring. If this fails, surgical therapy is performed to close the cleft.

KEY POINTS

- Closure requires proper intraoperative gonioscopy to delineate the borders of the cleft.
- Preoperative ultrasound biomicroscopy can potentially locate suprachoroidal fluid that extends beyond the clinically evident cleft.
- The choroid is highly vascular; care must be taken in patients on anticoagulation—direct surgical closure in patients who cannot stop anticoagulation can be high risk.
- Limit steroid use to induce scar tissue formation postoperatively.

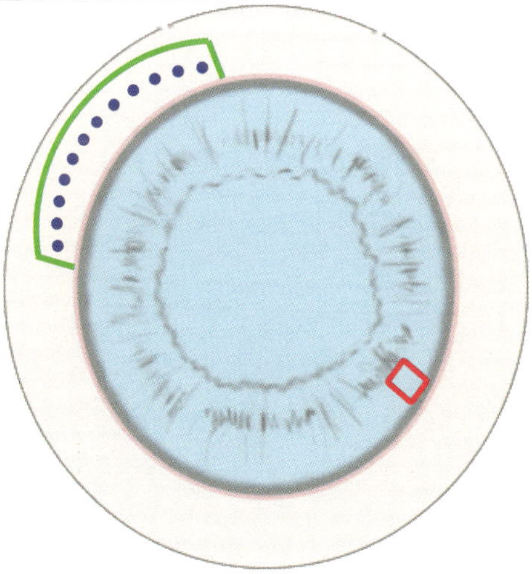

- Paracentesis
- Conjunctival peritomy and scleral flap over area of intended closure

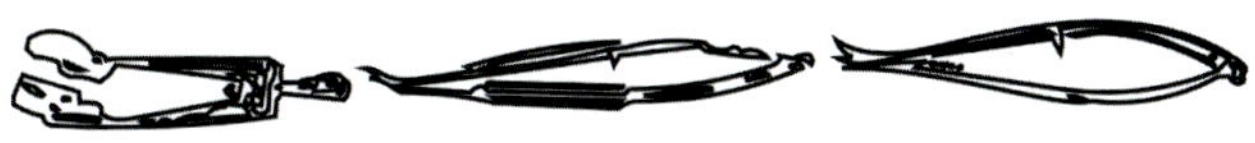

- 10-0 polypropylene on CIF-4 or PC-7 needle
- Single- or 4-mirror intraoperative gonioscopy lens
- Microsurgical Technology, Inc micrograspers
- Crescent blade

Ahmed IK, Campos-Möller X, Shah M, Sheybani A. *Illustrated Advanced Anterior Segment Surgery: A Step-by-Step Guide for Challenging Cases* (pp 253-257).

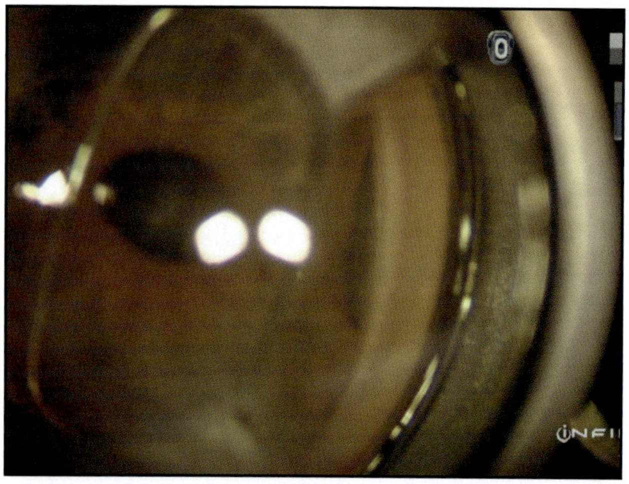

- In this case, we are repairing an iatrogenic cyclodialysis cleft (seen on gonioscopy to the left).
- After a paracentesis is made, the anterior chamber is filled with balanced salt solution to overpressurize the globe.
- Intraoperative gonioscopy can help delineate the borders of the cleft. These borders are marked on the corneal surface.

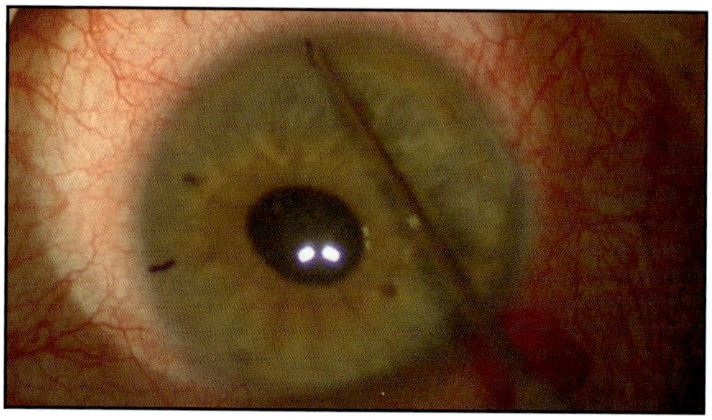

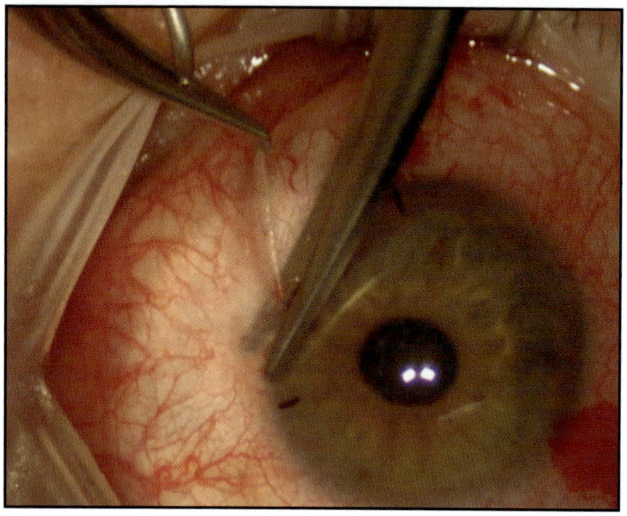

- A conjunctival peritomy extending 4 to 5 mm posterior to the limbus is performed about 1 mm beyond the borders of the cleft.
- A traction suture with a 7-0 Vicryl (polyglactin 910) or 6-0 silk can be placed to retract the globe.
- A scleral flap 50% to 75% thick is initiated 4.5 mm back from the limbus or 3.5 mm back from scleral spur.

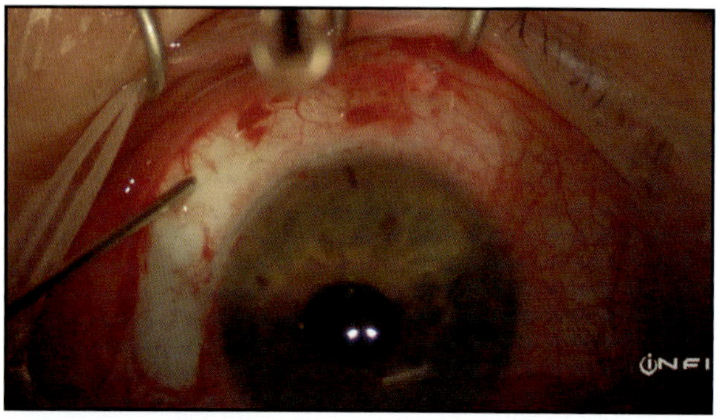

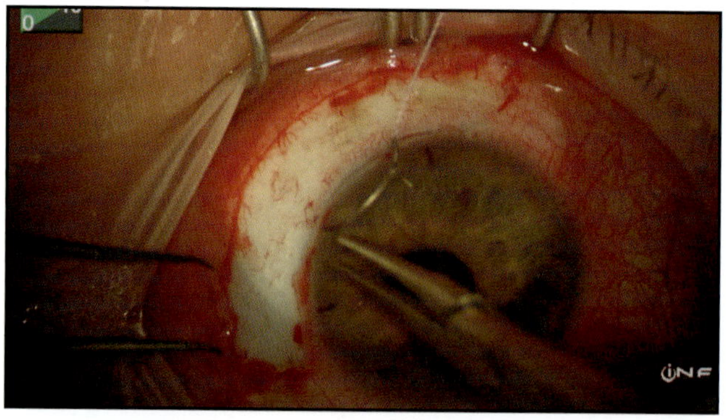

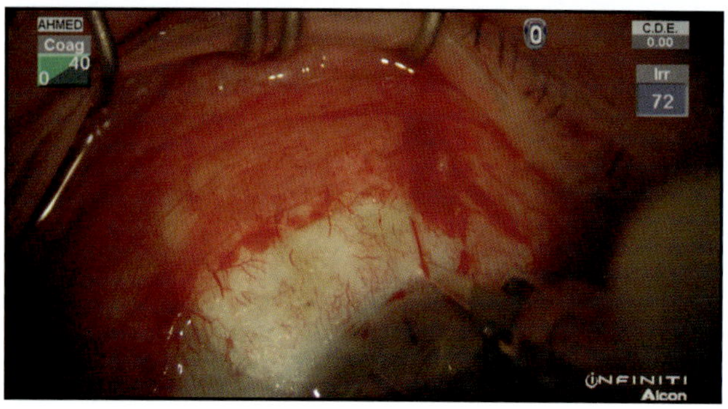

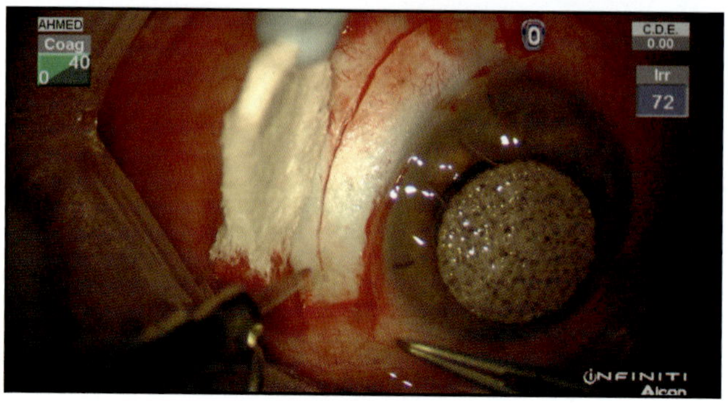

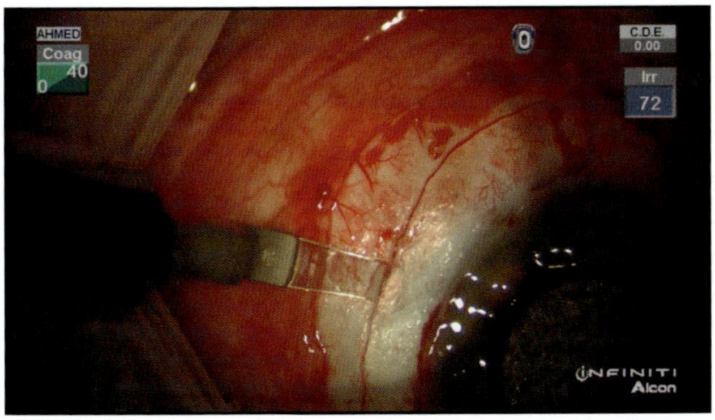

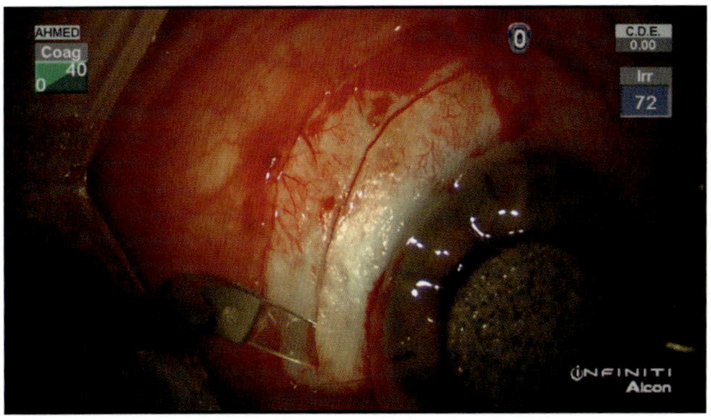

A crescent blade is used to dissect an approximately 250-μm thickness flap along the length of the dialysis and reflected over the limbus to expose the remaining sclera.

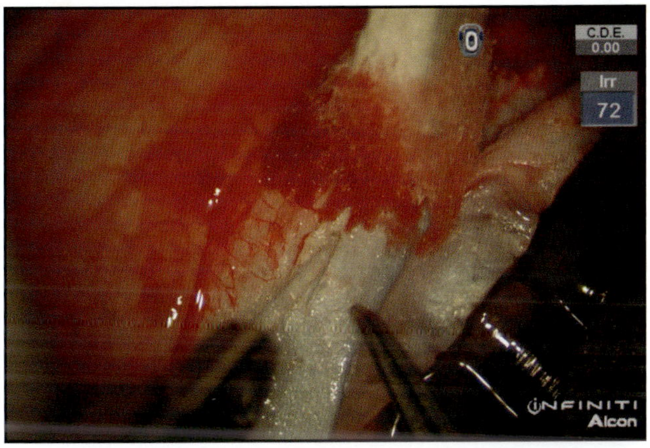

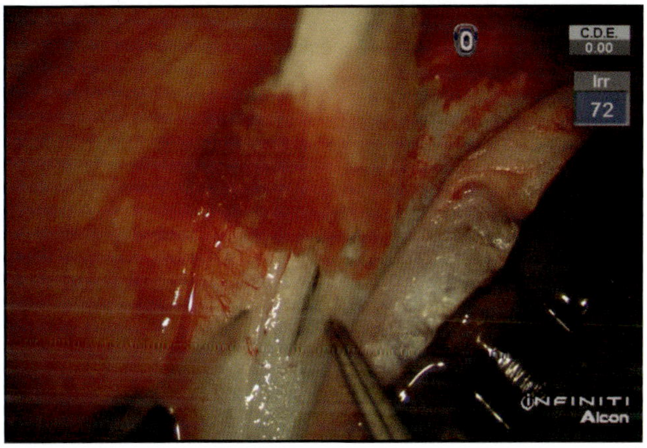

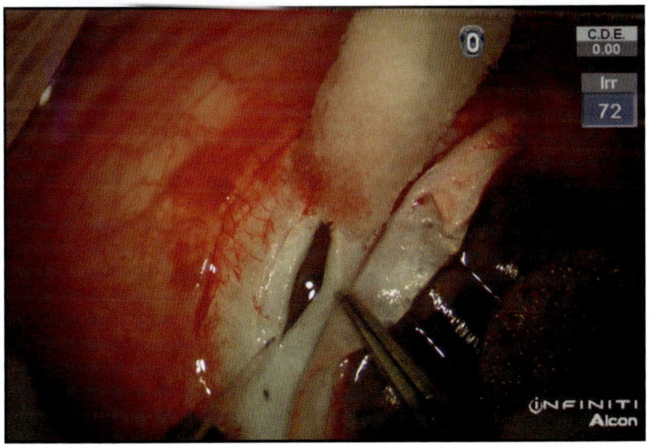

A groove is made along the length of the flap about 2.5 mm back from the scleral spur. If the eye is pressurized, fluid is seen as the dissection is carried out to expose bare uveal tissue (choroid).

- A polypropylene suture is passed through one side of the deep scleral groove, then incorporates a very thin and superficial bite of choroid before exiting through the other side of the scleral groove.
- Sutures can be placed in interrupted or mattress fashion.
- Sutures are tied to close the flap, incorporating choroid into the groove closure.

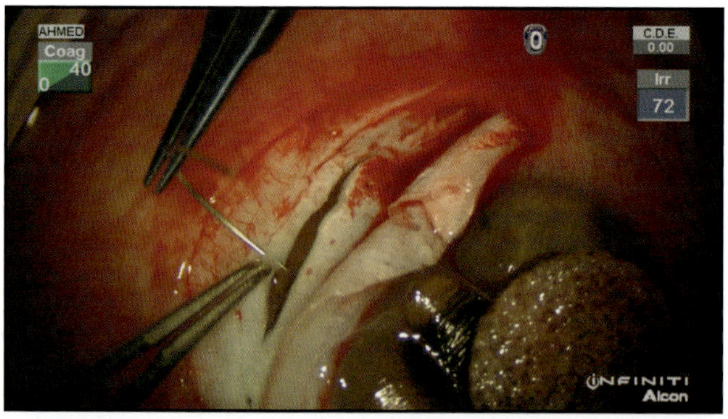

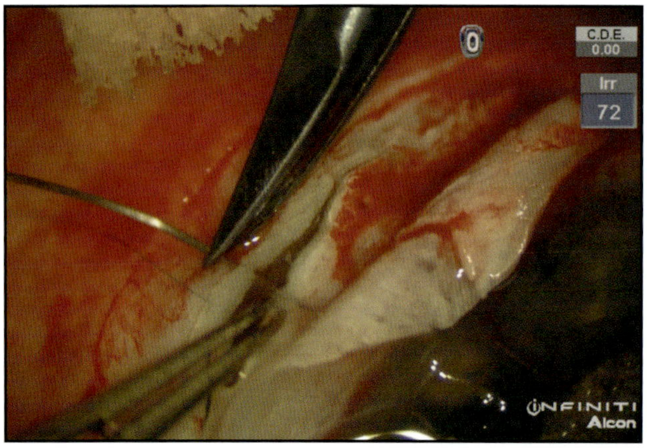

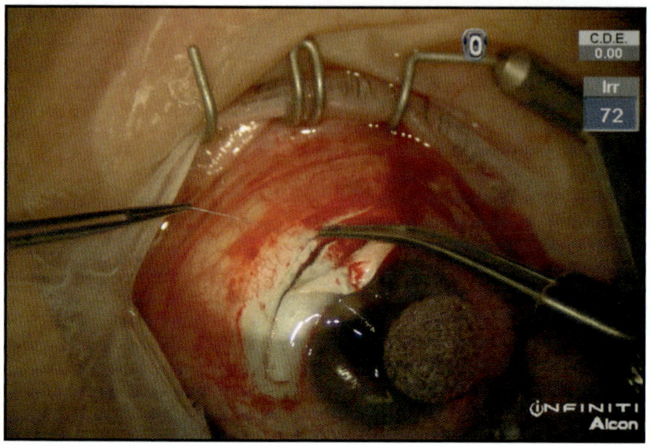

As this process is performed, if needed, the groove can be extended until the entire length of the cleft is exposed. Suturing in pieces then extending the groove can prevent a major hemorrhagic event that could expulse the contents of the eye through a very large scleral opening.

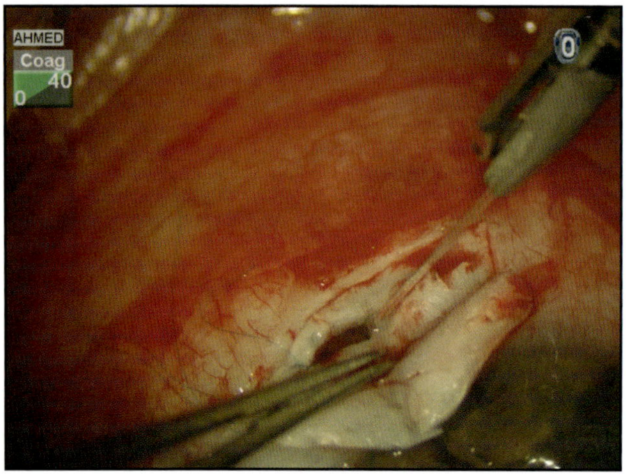

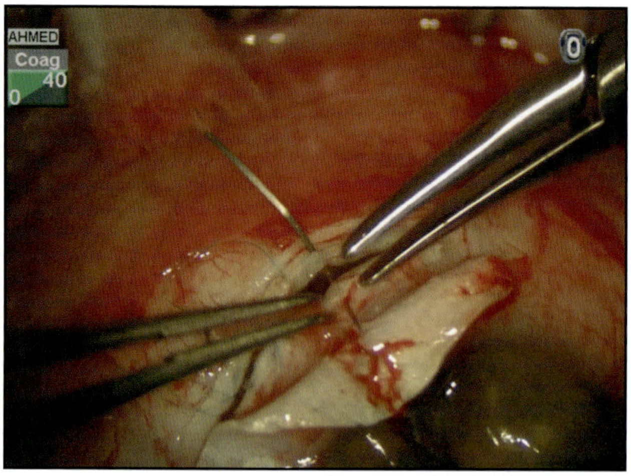

As choroid is sutured, iris may need to be drawn back into the eye using micrograsping forceps. Pulling too hard can, however, disinsert the choroidal bites. We would rather have the cleft closed than worry about the potential for mild mydriasis (which can certainly happen).

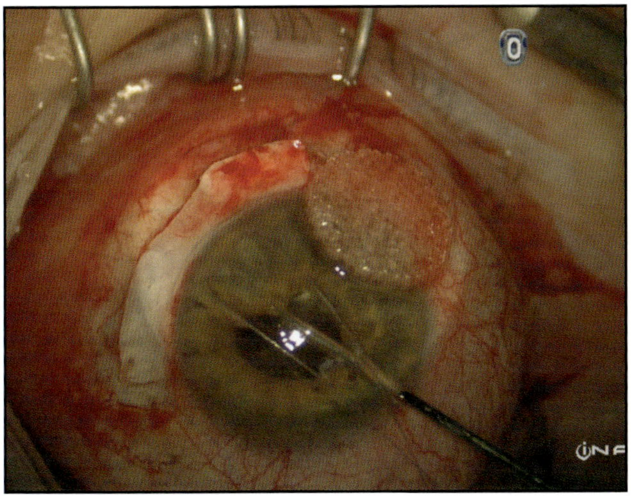

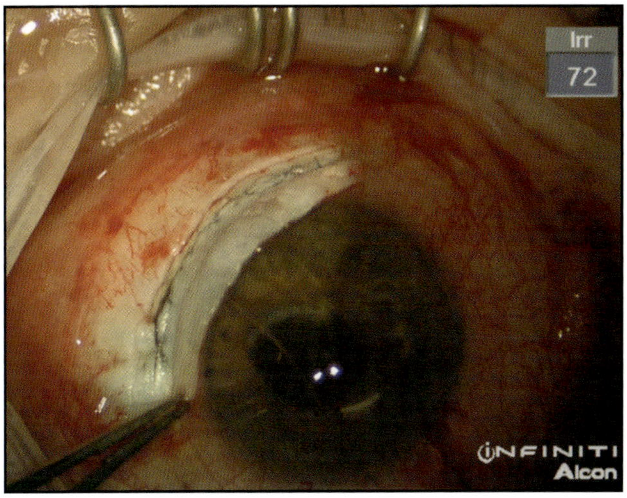

- After the cleft is closed, fibrin glue can be placed over the sclera to close the scleral flap; however, direct closure with suture (10-0 nylon or 7-0 Vicryl in this case) is usually required.
- Sometimes, intraoperative argon laser can be applied to the iris root to induce inflammation.
- The conjunctiva is then closed over the flap. In this case, we again use fibrin glue; however, direct closure with 7-0 Vicryl can be performed.
- The traction suture is removed, and sometimes viscoelastic can be left in the eye to elevated the intraocular pressure in the early postoperative period, especially in patients with pre-existing choroidal effusions.

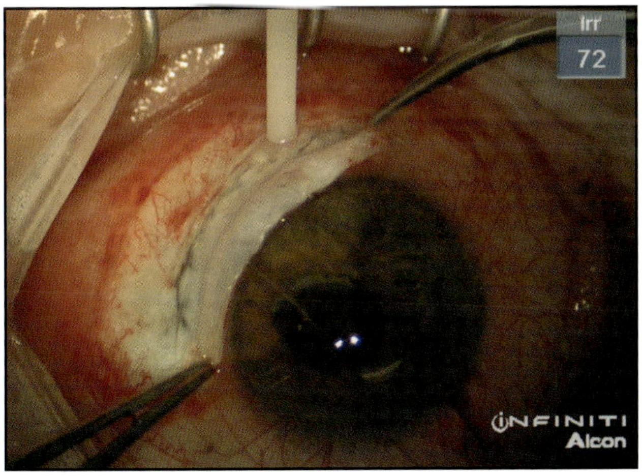

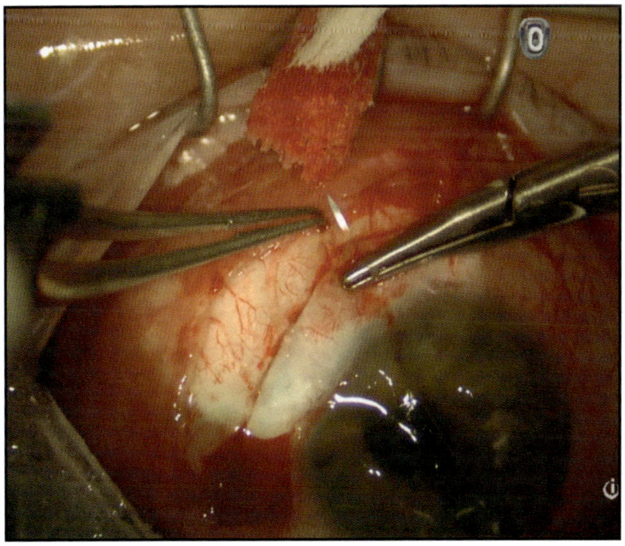

CHAPTER 34

HOW TO PREVENT AND TREAT MALIGNANT GLAUCOMA—IRIDO-ZONULO-HYALOIDO-VITRECTOMY

INTRODUCTION

Malignant glaucoma is a dreaded condition characterized by progressive axial shallowing of the anterior chamber. Although many theories exist regarding its pathogenesis, an emerging unifying explanation suggests the role of choroidal expansion in creating this cascade of events. Malignant glaucoma is more often encountered in eyes with small axial lengths and thicker sclera, so be wary of these risk factors whenever embarking on intraocular work.

KEY POINTS

- Prevention is key! Maintain anterior chamber pressurization to prevent transient hypotony and choroidal expansion.
- Use balanced salt solution (BSS) or ophthalmic viscosurgical device as needed to keep the chamber formed during all major instrument exchanges.
- Recognize the signs of intraoperative and postoperative malignant glaucoma. Remember that intraocular pressure does not always need to be elevated.
- Consider performing an irido-zonulo-hyaloido-vitrectomy (IZHV) in patients who are already suffering from malignant glaucoma or those who are at risk for developing it.
- Depending on the anterior chamber depth, one can perform IZHV from an anterior or posterior approach.
- Both approaches benefit from the absence of the crystalline lens, and both approaches can be combined with lens extraction or performed in pseudophakic eyes.
- Typically, an anterior approach is easier for the anterior segment surgeon given a potentially abnormal or short pars plana in at-risk eyes, but consider a posterior approach if concomitant deepening of the anterior chamber by removing vitreous is desired.
- The paracentesis for placement of the vitrector should be about 3 clock hours away from the site of planned IZHV. Otherwise, the eye will torque or one will not be able to dive the vitrector deep enough, especially if the paracentesis is further away requiring a long intraocular reach of the vitrector.

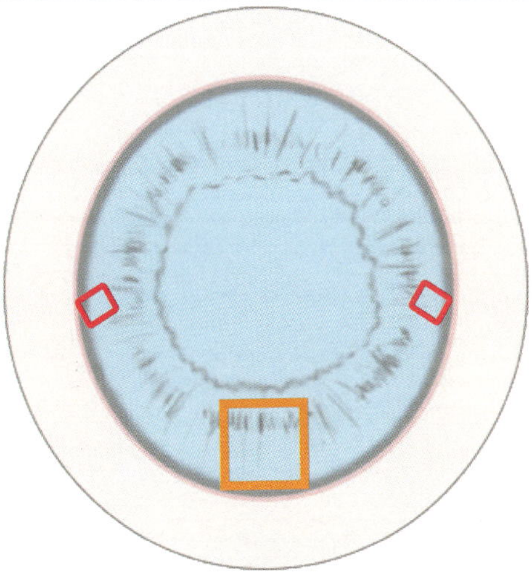

- Standard phaco with knife and fork

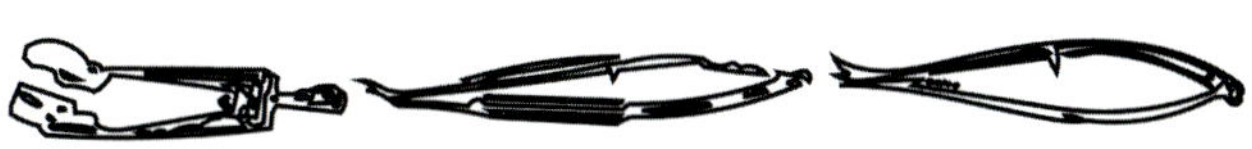

- 23-g anterior vitrectomy unit
- BSS 27-g cannula

Ahmed IK, Campos-Möller X, Shah M, Sheybani A. *Illustrated Advanced Anterior Segment Surgery: A Step-by-Step Guide for Challenging Cases* (pp 259-261).

Anterior Approach

Engage the peripheral iris with the vitrector with the cutting side pointed down. Arrow points to a pre-existing laser peripheral iridotomy. Using a high vacuum and a single cut, create a peripheral iridectomy. Given the large size of the iridectomy, ideally place this iridotomy superiorly.

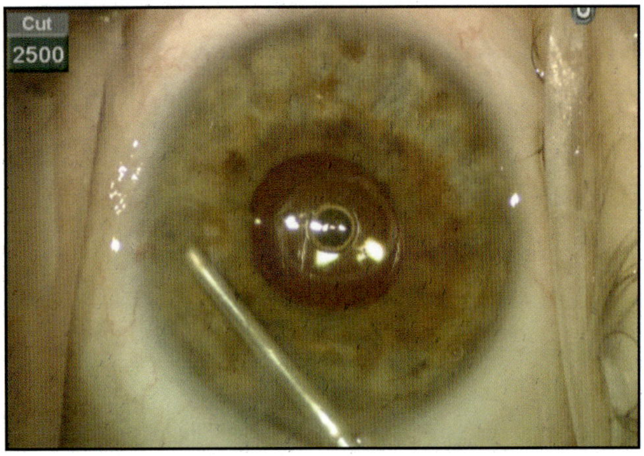

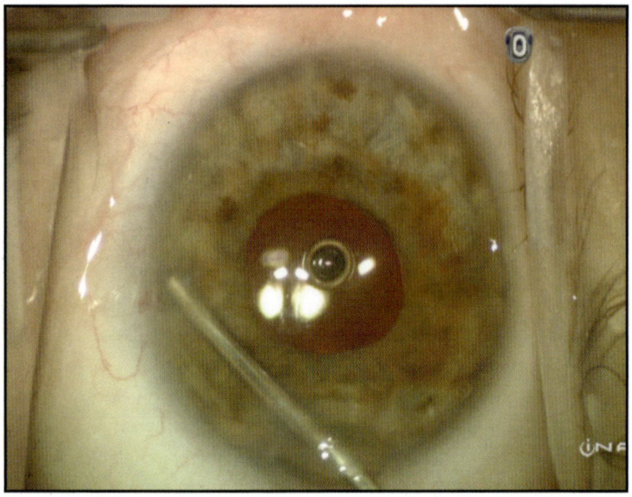

- Now that the iridotomy has been fashioned, turn the cutting port of the vitrector upward and enter the iridotomy without aspiration or cutting.
- Advance the vitrector through the iridotomy with cutter opening facing down and engage cut mode without aspiration (pedal step 2 on most machines).
- Advance the cutter approximately 2 to 3 mm, cutting the whole time. Aspirate some vitreous in the area of the anterior hyaloid.
- Withdraw the cutter toward the anterior chamber, taking care not to aspirate; doing so may bring vitreous forward.
- Pressurize the anterior chamber with viscoelastic to prevent vitreous prolapse.

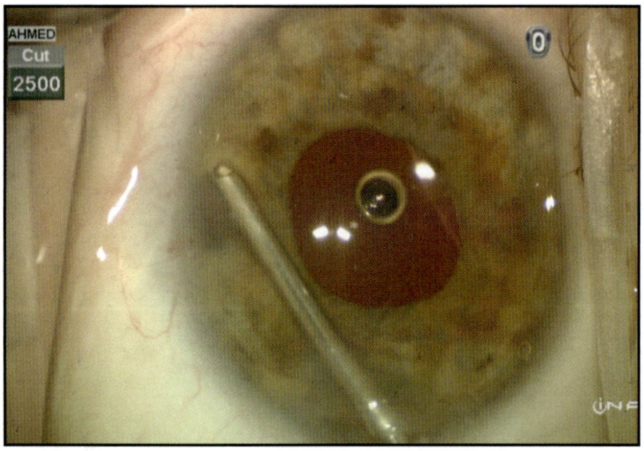

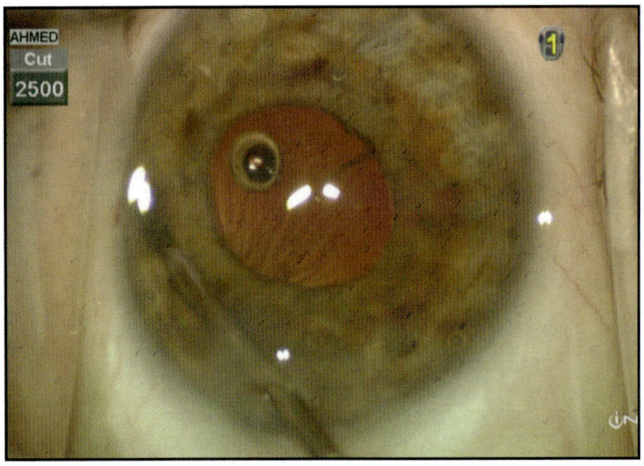

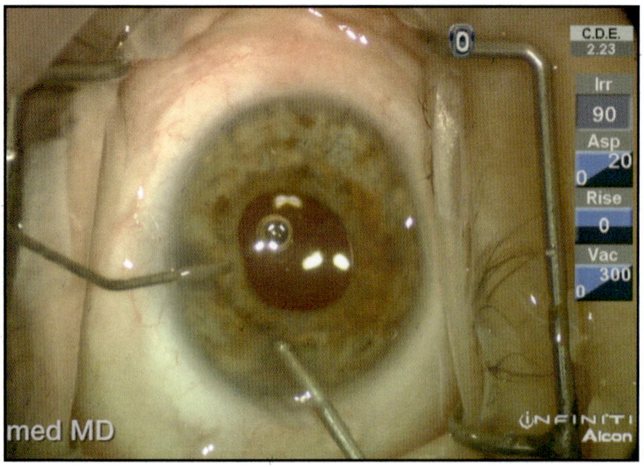

Posterior Approach

- In very small eyes that may require an IZHV, the pars plana can be incredibly small in size. Consider surgical comanagement with a vitreoretinal surgeon for placement and management of pars plana entry.
- Perform a limited anterior vitrectomy and bring the cutter peripherally with the port facing upward.
- Ideally, a peripheral iridotomy will already have been created for you to visualize your cutter through.
- Advance your cutter anteriorly through the peripheral zonules and enlarge the iridotomy.

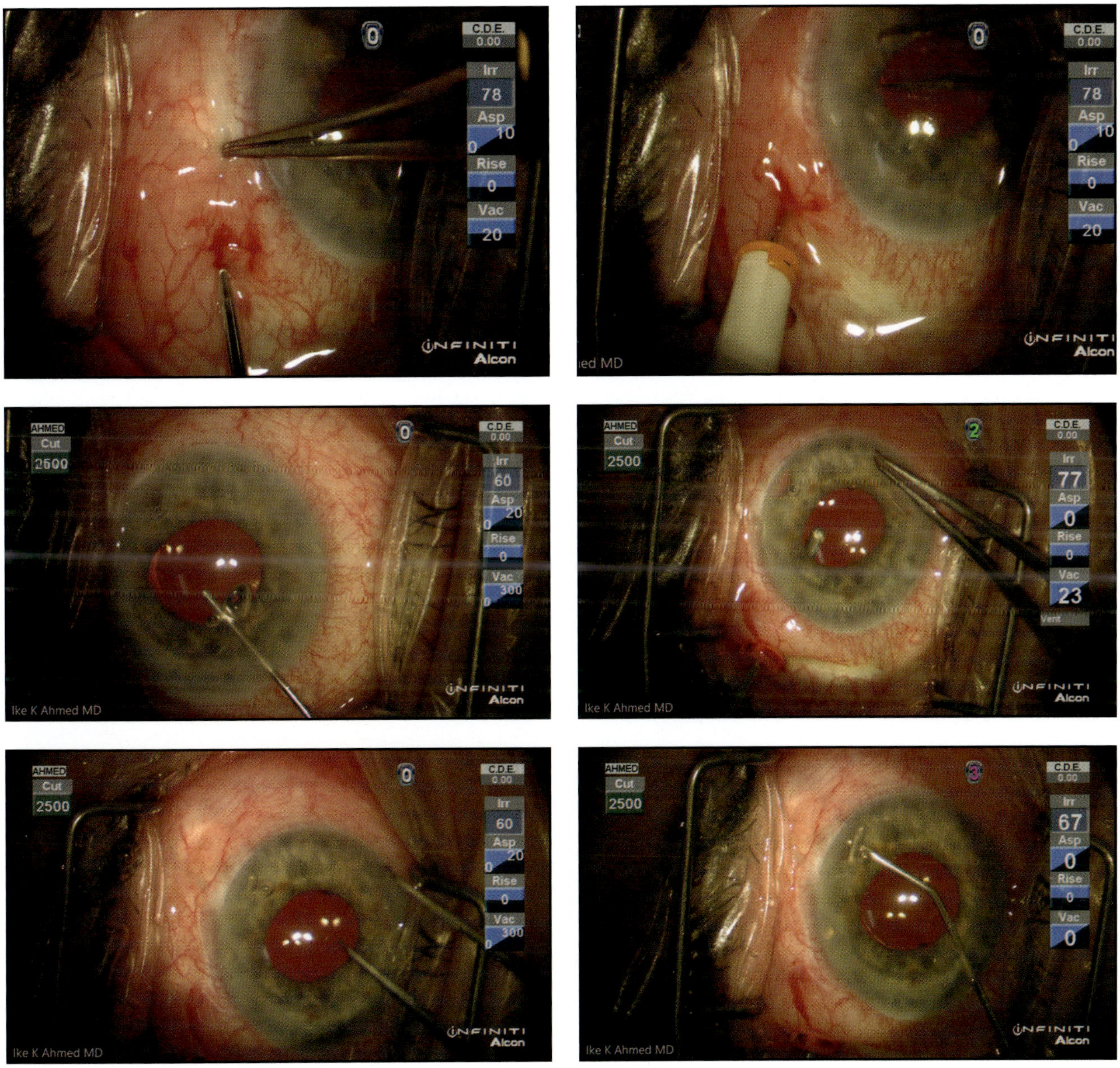

REFERENCES

Chapter 6

Malyugin B. Cataract surgery in small pupils. *Indian J Ophthalmol*. 2017;65(12):1323-1328. doi:10.4103/ijo.IJO_800_17.

Chapter 8

Little BC, Smith JH, Packer M. Little capsulorhexis tear-out rescue. *J Cataract Refract Surg*. 2006;32(9):1420-1422.

Marques FF, Marques DM, Osher RH, Osher JM. Fate of anterior capsule tears during cataract surgery. *J Cataract Refract Surg*. 2006;32(10):1638-1642.

Chapter 9

Blecher MH, Kirk MR. Surgical strategies for the management of zonular compromise. *Curr Opin Ophthalmol*. 2008;19(1):31-35.

Chapter 10

Hasanee K, Ahmed II. Capsular tension rings: update on endocapsular support devices. *Ophthalmol Clin North Am*. 2006;19(4):507-519.

Chapter 11

Hasanee K, Ahmed II. Capsular tension rings: update on endocapsular support devices. *Ophthalmol Clin North Am*. 2006;19(4):507-519.

Chapter 12

Li B, Wang Y, Malvankar-Mehta MS, Hutnik CM. Surgical indications, outcomes, and complications with the use of a modified capsular tension ring during cataract surgery. *J Cataract Refract Surg*. 2016;42(11):1642-1648. doi:10.1016/j.jcrs.2016.10.007. PubMed PMID: 27956292.

Chapter 14

Gimbel HV, DeBroff BM. Intraocular lens optic capture. *J Cataract Refract Surg*. 2004;30(1):200-206. Review. PubMed PMID: 14967291.

Chapter 15

Gimbel HV, DeBroff BM. Intraocular lens optic capture. *J Cataract Refract Surg*. 2004;30(1):200-206. Review. PubMed PMID: 14967291.

Chapter 16

Gimbel HV, DeBroff BM. Intraocular lens optic capture. *J Cataract Refract Surg*. 2004;30(1):200-206. Review. PubMed PMID: 14967291.

Ahmed IK, Campos-Möller X, Shah M, Sheybani A. *Illustrated Advanced Anterior Segment Surgery: A Step-by-Step Guide for Challenging Cases* (pp 263-265).

Chapter 17

Holt DG, Young J, Stagg B, Ambati BK. Anterior chamber intraocular lens, sutured posterior chamber intraocular lens, or glued intraocular lens: where do we stand? *Curr Opin Ophthalmol*. 2012;23(1):62-67. doi:10.1097/ICU.0b013e32834cd5e5. Review. PubMed PMID: 22081029; PubMed Central PMCID: PMC3306769.

Wagoner MD, Cox TA, Ariyasu RG, Jacobs DS, Karp CL; American Academy of Ophthalmology. Intraocular lens implantation in the absence of capsular support: a report by the American Academy of Ophthalmology. *Ophthalmology*. 2003;110(4):840-859. Review. PubMed PMID: 12689913.

Chapter 18

Holt DG, Young J, Stagg B, Ambati BK. Anterior chamber intraocular lens, sutured posterior chamber intraocular lens, or glued intraocular lens: where do we stand? *Curr Opin Ophthalmol*. 2012;23(1):62-67. doi:10.1097/ICU.0b013e32834cd5e5. Review. PubMed PMID: 22081029; PubMed Central PMCID: PMC3306769.

Wagoner MD, Cox TA, Ariyasu RG, Jacobs DS, Karp CL; American Academy of Ophthalmology. Intraocular lens implantation in the absence of capsular support: a report by the American Academy of Ophthalmology. *Ophthalmology*. 2003;110(4):840-859. Review. PubMed PMID: 12689913.

Chapter 19

Michaeli A, Assia EI. Scleral and iris fixation of posterior chamber lenses in the absence of capsular support. *Curr Opin Ophthalmol*. 2005;16(1):57-60. Review. PubMed PMID: 15650581.

Chapter 20

Agarwal A, Jacob S, Kumar DA, Agarwal A, Narasimhan S, Agarwal A. Handshake technique for glued intrascleral haptic fixation of a posterior chamber intraocular lens. *J Cataract Refract Surg*. 2013;39(3):317-322. doi:10.1016/j. jcrs.2013.01.019.

Agarwal A, Kumar DA, Jacob S, Baid C, Agarwal A, Srinivasan S. Fibrin glue-assisted sutureless posterior chamber intraocular lens implantation in eyes with deficient posterior capsules. *J Cataract Refract Surg*. 2008;34(9):1433-1438. doi:10.1016/j.jcrs.2008.04.040.

Gabor SGB, Pavlidis MM. Sutureless intrascleral posterior chamber intraocular lens fixation. *J Cataract Refract Surg*. 2007;33(11):1851-1854. doi:10.1016/j.jcrs.2007.07.013.

Kumar DA, Agarwal A. Glued intraocular lens: a major review on surgical technique and results. *Curr Opin Ophthalmol*. 2013;24(1):21-29. doi:10.1097/ICU.0b013e32835a939f. Review. PubMed PMID: 23080013.

Chapter 21

Güell JL, Barrera A, Manero F. A review of suturing techniques for posterior chamber lenses. *Curr Opin Ophthalmol*. 2004;15(1):44-50. Review. PubMed PMID: 14743019.

Yamane S, Sato S, Maruyama-Inoue M, Kadonosono K. Flanged intrascleral intraocular lens fixation with double-needle technique. *Ophthalmol*. 2017;124(8):1136-1142.

Chapter 23

Alio JL, Abdelghany AA, Fernández-Buenaga R. Management of residual refractive error after cataract surgery. *Curr Opin Ophthalmol*. 2014;25(4):291-297. doi:10.1097/ICU.0000000000000067. Review. PubMed PMID: 24865171.

Chapter 25

Dajee KP, Abbey AM, Williams GA. Management of dislocated intraocular lenses in eyes with insufficient capsular support. *Curr Opin Ophthalmol*. 2016;27(3):191-195. doi:10.1097/ICU.0000000000000260. Review. PubMed PMID: 26913739.

Chapter 26

Michaeli A, Assia EI. Scleral and iris fixation of posterior chamber lenses in the absence of capsular support. *Curr Opin Ophthalmol*. 2005;16(1):57-60. Review. PubMed PMID: 15650581.

Chapter 27

Campbell DG, Vela A. Modern goniosynechialysis for the treatment of synechial angle-closure glaucoma. *Ophthalmology*. 1984;91(9):1052-1060. PubMed PMID: 6493714.

Chapter 28

Ogawa GS. The iris cerclage suture for permanent mydriasis: a running suture technique. *Ophthalmic Surg Lasers*. 1998;29(12):1001-1009. Erratum in: *Ophthalmic Surg Lasers*. 1999;30(5):412. PubMed PMID: 9854714.

Tsao SW, Holz HA. Iris mattress suture: a technique for sectoral iris defect repair. *Br J Ophthalmol*. 2015;99(3):305-307. doi:10.1136/bjophthalmol-2014-305391. PubMed PMID: 24879808.

Chapter 29

Ogawa GS. The iris cerclage suture for permanent mydriasis: a running suture technique. *Ophthalmic Surg Lasers*. 1998;29(12):1001-1009.

Chapter 30

Farahi A, Hashemi H, Mehravaran S. Combined cataract surgery and aniridia ring implantation in oculocutaneous albinism. *J Cataract Refract Surg*. 2015;41(11):2438-2443. doi:10.1016/j.jcrs.2015.05.037. PubMed PMID: 26703494.

Weissbart SB, Ayres BD. Management of aniridia and iris defects: an update on iris prosthesis options. *Curr Opin Ophthalmol*. 2016;27(3):244-249. doi:10.1097/ICU.0000000000000253. Review. PubMed PMID: 26871656.

Chapter 31

Basarir B, Kaya V, Altan C, Karakus S, Pinarci EY, Demirok A. The use of a supplemental sulcus fixated IOL (HumanOptics Add-On IOL) to correct pseudophakic refractive errors. *Eur J Ophthalmol*. 2012;22(6):898-903. doi:10.5301/ejo.5000156. PubMed PMID: 22522392.

Chapter 32

Agarwal T, Singh D, Panda A. Guide needle-assisted iridodialysis repair. *J Cataract Refract Surg*. 2011;37(10):1918; author reply 1918-1919. doi:10.1016/j.jcrs.2011.08.009. PubMed PMID: 21930063.

Chapter 33

Ioannidis AS, Barton K. Cyclodialysis cleft: causes and repair. *Curr Opin Ophthalmol*. 2010;21(2):150-154. doi:10.1097/ICU.0b013e3283366a4d. Review. PubMed PMID: 20051856.

Chapter 34

Varma DK, Belovay GW, Tam DY, Ahmed II. Malignant glaucoma after cataract surgery. *J Cataract Refract Surg*. 2014;40(11):1843-1849. doi:10.1016/j.jcrs.2014.02.045.

FINANCIAL DISCLOSURES

Dr. Iqbal K. Ahmed is a consultant or receives consulting fees from Aequus, Aerie Pharmaceuticals, Akorn, Alcon, Allergan, Aquea Health, Inc, ArcScan, Bausch Health, Beaver Visitec, Beyeonics, Carl Zeiss Meditec, Centricity Vision, Inc, CorNeat Vision, ELT Sight, ElutiMed, Equinox, Genentech, Glaukos, Gore, Iantrek, InjectSense, Iridex, iStar, Ivantis, Johnson & Johnson Vision, LayerBio, Leica Microsystems, Long Bridge Medical, Inc, MicroOptx, MST Surgical, New World Medical, Ocular Instruments, Ocular Therapeutix, Oculo, Omega Ophthalmics, PolyActiva, Radiance Therapeutics, Inc, Ripple Therapeutics, Sanoculis, Santen, Shifamed, LLC, Sight Sciences, Smartlens, Inc, Stroma, Thea Pharma, ViaLase, and Vizzario.

He receives speakers honoraria from Alcon, Allergan, Carl Zeiss Meditec, Johnson & Johnson Vision, MST Surgical, and Mundipharma. He also receives research grant/support from Aerie Pharmaceuticals, Alcon, Allergan, Glaukos, Ivantis, Johnson & Johnson Vision, New World Medical, and Santen.

Dr. Xavier Campos-Möller has no financial or proprietary interest in the materials presented herein

Dr. Manjool Shah is a consultant for Allergan/Abbvie, Katena, Ivantis, ONL Therapeutics, and Glaukos.

Dr. Arsham Sheybani is a consultant for Allergan and Alcon.

INDEX